Equine Ophthalmology

Editor

MARY LASSALINE

VETERINARY CLINICS OF NORTH AMERICA: EQUINE PRACTICE

www.vetequine.theclinics.com

Consulting Editor
THOMAS J. DIVERS

December 2017 • Volume 33 • Number 3

ELSEVIER

1600 John F. Kennedy Boulevard • Suite 1800 • Philadelphia, Pennsylvania, 19103-2899

http://www.vetequine.theclinics.com

VETERINARY CLINICS OF NORTH AMERICA: EQUINE PRACTICE Volume 33, Number 3
December 2017 ISSN 0749-0739, ISBN-13: 978-0-323-55304-9

Editor: Colleen Dietzler
Developmental Editor: Donald Mumford

Veterinary Clinics of North America: Equine Practice (ISSN 0749-0739) is published in April, August, and December by Elsevier Inc., 360 Park Avenue South, New York, NY 10010-1710. Business and Editorial Offices: 1600 John F. Kennedy Blvd., Suite 1800, Philadelphia, PA 19103-2899. Subscription prices are $270.00 per year (domestic individuals), $506.00 per year (domestic institutions), $100.00 per year (domestic students/residents), $315.00 per year (Canadian individuals), $637.00 per year (Canadian institutions), $365.00 per year (international individuals), $637.00 per year (international institutions), and $180.00 per year (international and Canadian students/residents). To receive student/resident rate, orders must be accompanied by name of affiliated institution, date of term, and the signature of program/residency coordinator on institution letterhead. Orders will be billed at individual rate until proof of status is received. Foreign air speed delivery is included in all *Clinics* subscription prices. All prices are subject to change without notice. **POSTMASTER:** Send address changes to *Veterinary Clinics of North America: Equine Practice*, 3251 Riverport Lane, Maryland Heights, MO 63043. Customer Service (orders, claims, online, change of address): Elsevier Health Sciences Division, Subscription **Customer Service, 3251 Riverport Lane, Maryland Heights, MO 63043. Tel: 1-800-654-2452 (U.S. and Canada); 314-447-8871 (outside U.S. and Canada). Fax: 314-447-8029. E-mail: journalscustomerservice-usa@elsevier.com (for print support);** E-mail: **journalsonlinesupport-usa@elsevier.com (for online support).**

Reprints. For copies of 100 or more of articles in this publication, please contact the Commercial Reprints Department, Elsevier Inc., 360 Park Avenue South, New York, NY 10010-1710. Tel.: 212-633-3874; Fax: 212-633-3820; E-mail: reprints@elsevier.com.

Veterinary Clinics of North America: Equine Practice is covered in *MEDLINE/PubMed (Index Medicus), Excerpta Medica, Current Contents/Agriculture, Biology and Environmental Sciences, and ISI.*

Contributors

CONSULTING EDITOR

THOMAS J. DIVERS, DVM
Diplomate, American College of Veterinary Internal Medicine; Diplomate, American College of Veterinary Emergency and Critical Care; Steffen Professor of Veterinary Medicine, Section of Large Animal Medicine, College of Veterinary Medicine, Cornell University, Ithaca, New York

EDITOR

MARY LASSALINE, DVM, PhD
Diplomate, American College of Veterinary Ophthalmologists; Associate Professor of Clinical Equine Ophthalmology, Department of Surgical and Radiological Sciences, University of California, Davis, Davis, California

AUTHORS

REBECCA R. BELLONE, PhD
Associate Adjunct Professor, Department of Population Health and Reproduction, Veterinary Genetics Laboratory, UC Davis School of Veterinary Medicine, Davis, California

GIL BEN-SHLOMO, DVM, PhD
Diplomate, American College of Veterinary Ophthalmologists; Diplomate, European College of Veterinary Ophthalmologists; Associate Professor, Department of Veterinary Clinical Sciences, College of Veterinary Medicine, Iowa State University, Ames, Iowa

KRISTA ESTELL, DVM
Diplomate, American College of Veterinary Internal Medicine; Clinical Assistant Professor, Department of Equine Internal Medicine, Marion DuPont Scott Equine Medical Center, Virginia-Maryland College of Veterinary Medicine, Leesburg, Virginia

BRITTA MARIA FISCHER, DVM
Large Animal Internal Medicine, Auburn University, Auburn University College of Veterinary Medicine, JT Vaughan Large Animal Teaching Hospital, Auburn, Alabama

BRIAN C. GILGER, DVM, MS
Diplomate, American College of Veterinary Ophthalmologists; Professor of Ophthalmology, Department of Clinical Sciences, NC State University College of Veterinary Medicine, Raleigh, North Carolina

AMY L. JOHNSON, DVM
Diplomate, American College of Veterinary Internal Medicine (Large Animal Internal Medicine & Neurology); Assistant Professor of Large Animal Medicine and Neurology, Department of Clinical Sciences, Clinical Studies–New Bolton Center, University of Pennsylvania School of Veterinary Medicine, Kennett Square, Pennsylvania

ERIC C. LEDBETTER, DVM
Diplomate, American College of Veterinary Ophthalmologists; Associate Professor of Ophthalmology, Department of Clinical Sciences, Cornell University College of Veterinary Medicine, Cornell University Hospital for Animals, Ithaca, New York

RICHARD JOSEPH McMULLEN Jr, Dr med vet
Diplomate, American College of Veterinary Ophthalmologists; Diplomate, European College of Veterinary Ophthalmologists; Associate Professor of Ophthalmology, Department of Clinical Sciences, Auburn University, Auburn University College of Veterinary Medicine, JT Vaughan Large Animal Teaching Hospital, Auburn, Alabama

TAMMY MILLER MICHAU, DVM, MS, MSpVM
Diplomate, American College of Veterinary Ophthalmologists; BluePearl Veterinary Partners, Tampa, Florida; Brandon Equine Medical Center, Brandon, Florida

KATHERN E. MYRNA, DVM, MS
Diplomate, American College of Veterinary Ophthalmologists; Associate Professor of Ophthalmology, Department of Small Animal Medicine and Surgery, Veterinary Medical Center, University of Georgia, Athens, Georgia

CARYN E. PLUMMER, DVM
Diplomate, American College of Veterinary Ophthalmologists; Associate Professor, Comparative Ophthalmology, Departments of Small Animal Clinical Sciences and Large Animal Clinical Sciences, College of Veterinary Medicine, University of Florida, Gainesville, Florida

WENDY M. TOWNSEND, DVM, MS
Diplomate, American College of Veterinary Ophthalmologists; Associate Professor of Ophthalmology, Department of Veterinary Clinical Sciences, Purdue University, West Lafayette, Indiana

KATHRYN L. WOTMAN, DVM
Diplomate, American College of Veterinary Internal Medicine (Large Animal Internal Medicine); Diplomate, American College of Veterinary Ophthalmologists; Assistant Professor, Comparative Ophthalmology, Department of Clinical Sciences, College of Veterinary Medicine and Biomedical Sciences, Colorado State University, Fort Collins, Colorado

Contents

Preface: The Science and Practice of Equine Ophthalmology: A Quarter Century Later

ix

Mary Lassaline

Corneal Response to Injury and Infection in the Horse

439

Caryn E. Plummer

This article describes the natural responses of the immune system and the cornea to injury and infection. The process of reepithelialization and reformation of stromal collagen is discussed, as are the clinical signs and manifestations of the effects of the healing response when it is routine and when it is pathologic. Excessive inflammatory or immune responses by host tissues can cause further damage that may be present from the antecedent injury or the effect of a pathogen. The clinical signs and manifestations of wound healing as well as potential therapeutic interventions are described.

Medical and Surgical Management of Equine Recurrent Uveitis

465

Richard Joseph McMullen Jr and Britta Maria Fischer

Equine recurrent uveitis (ERU) is characterized by recurrent bouts of inflammation interrupted by periods of quiescence that vary in duration. There is little consensus on the clinical manifestations, the underlying causes, or the management. The 3 commonly recognized syndromes of ERU (classic, insidious, and posterior) do not accurately separate the clinical manifestations of disease into distinct categories. An accurate diagnosis and early intervention are essential to minimizing the effects of disease and preserving vision. There are multiple medical and surgical options for controlling ERU as long as the disease is recognized early and targeted treatment is initiated immediately.

Disease and Surgery of the Equine Lens

483

Wendy M. Townsend

Examination of the lens is critical, particularly when evaluating horses with visual impairment or performing prepurchase examinations. To adequately evaluate the lens, the pupil must be pharmacologically dilated. A cataract is any lens opacity. The size, density, and position of a cataract determine the impact on vision. Cataracts may be congenital or inherited or occur secondary to trauma or equine recurrent uveitis. Surgical removal is the only treatment option for vision-impairing cataracts, but careful selection of surgical candidates is critical for successful outcomes.

The Equine Fundus

499

Gil Ben-Shlomo

Fundus is an anatomic term referring to the portion of an organ opposite from its opening, and the fundus of the eye is the back portion of the posterior segment of the globe, including the optic nerve, retina, and choroid. Clinically, the fundus can be visualized by direct or indirect ophthalmoscopy. Understanding the normal anatomy and appearance of the equine fundus is crucial for differentiating normal variations from abnormalities. This article reviews the normal anatomy and appearance of the equine fundus and discusses basic and advanced examination techniques. It also discusses common findings in the equine fundus and their interpretation.

Equine Glaucoma   519

Tammy Miller Michau

Glaucoma is a multifactorial neurodegenerative ocular disease leading to progressive loss of retinal ganglion cells and their axons that form the optic nerve, causing blindness. Knowledge of the pathogenesis and development of equine glaucoma is in its infancy compared with human glaucoma. Glaucoma occurs most commonly secondary to uveitis and may be underdiagnosed or misdiagnosed in horses suffering from uveitis. Recognition and clinical diagnosis of glaucoma in the horse is improved with clinician awareness and the availability of handheld tonometers. Therapy for glaucoma is aimed at decreasing aqueous humor production through medical and surgical means. Even with therapy, long-term prognosis for vision is poor.

Neuro-ophthalmology in the Horse   541

Kathern E. Myrna

This article provides a brief, clinically relevant review of neurologic disorders of the eye. A description of the neuro-ophthalmic examination is provided. Stepwise descriptions of the most common neuro-ophthalmic abnormalities are provided along with common rule outs.

Periocular Neoplasia in the Horse   551

Krista Estell

Periocular neoplasia is common in horses. Treatment of the periocular skin and ocular adnexal structures can be technically challenging. Common neoplastic conditions, a treatment algorithm, surgical principles, and therapeutic modalities are reviewed. Regardless of the type of neoplasia found or the treatment that is applied, success is most likely when the neoplastic tumor is small.

Ocular Manifestations of Systemic Disease in the Horse   563

Kathryn L. Wotman and Amy L. Johnson

Many systemic diseases have ocular manifestations. In some cases, ocular abnormalities are the most obvious or first recognized sign of disease that prompts veterinary evaluation. In other cases, the systemic disease leads to secondary ocular changes that might lead to loss of vision or globe if not addressed. Therefore, recognition of ocular abnormalities that might result from systemic diseases is an essential skill for the equine practitioner. This article provides practitioners with information regarding the most common systemic diseases of horses in North America that have ocular manifestations, organized by ocular signs.

Antifungal Therapy in Equine Ocular Mycotic Infections   583

Eric C. Ledbetter

Fungi are clinically important causes of ocular infections in the horse. Keratomycosis is the most common; however, a diverse range of mycotic infections, affecting numerous ocular tissues, may be encountered. Many equine mycoses are diagnostic and therapeutic challenges. Prompt and appropriate treatment is essential to minimize morbidity and reduce the likelihood of vision loss. Knowledge of the characteristics and properties of equine ophthalmology antifungal medications is essential to selecting an optimal treatment strategy, including selection of appropriate medication and effective administration route. Newer delivery methods and devices are available and can contribute to an improved outcome in select situations.

Advanced Imaging of the Equine Eye   607

Brian C. Gilger

This article reviews the literature for studies describing advanced imaging of the equine eye as a reference for practitioners to help in the selection of image modalities, describe how to use the instruments, and help interpret the image findings. Indications for, technique of, and image interpretation of advanced imaging modalities, such as ultrasound imaging, computed tomography, MRI, optical coherence tomography, confocal microscopy, and angiography, are reviewed. The article is organized anatomically, not by instrument, so that the reader will be able to quickly research ways to image specific disease entities or anatomic locations that are affecting their equine patients.

Genetic Testing as a Tool to Identify Horses with or at Risk for Ocular Disorders   627

Rebecca R. Bellone

Advances in equine genetics and genomics resources have enabled the understanding of some inherited ocular disorders and ocular manifestations. These ocular disorders include congenital stationary night blindness, equine recurrent uveitis, multiple congenital ocular anomalies, and squamous cell carcinoma. Genetic testing can identify horses with or at risk for disease and thus can assist in clinical management. In addition, genetic testing can identify horses that are carriers and thus can inform breeding decisions. Use of genetic tests in management and breeding decisions should aid in reducing the incidence of these disorders and improving the outcomes for horses at highest risk.

VETERINARY CLINICS OF
NORTH AMERICA: EQUINE PRACTICE

FORTHCOMING ISSUES

April 2018
**Advances in the Diagnosis and Management
of Equine Gastrointestinal Disease**
Henry Stämpfli and Angelika Schoster,
Editors

August 2018
Equine Sports Medicine
Jose Garcia-Lopez, *Editor*

December 2018
Wound Management
Earl Michael Gaughan, *Editor*

RECENT ISSUES

August 2017
Orthopedic Disorders of the Foal
Ashlee. E. Watts, *Editor*

April 2017
Equine Pharmacology
K. Gary Magdesian, *Editor*

December 2016
**Advances in Diagnostic and Therapeutic
Techniques in Equine Reproduction**
Marco A. Coutinho da Silva, *Editor*

RELATED ISSUE

Veterinary Clinics of North America: Equine Practice
August 2016 (Vol. 32, Issue 2)
Geriatric Medicine
Catherine M. McGowan, *Editor*

THE CLINICS ARE NOW AVAILABLE ONLINE!
Access your subscription at:
www.theclinics.com

Preface

The Science and Practice of Equine Ophthalmology: A Quarter Century Later

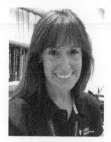

Mary Lassaline, DVM, PhD
Editor

It has been 25 years since Steven Roberts edited an issue of *Veterinary Clinics of North America: Equine Practice* with a focus on ophthalmology. Throughout those 25 years, the science and practice of equine ophthalmology have been challenged by some of the same diseases, including complicated corneal ulcers, fungal keratitis, uveitis, cataracts, glaucoma, and squamous cell carcinoma; however, progress has been made. There have been advances in pharmacology, genetics, diagnostics, imaging, and surgery, some of which are discussed within this issue, that have changed how ocular disease in the horse can be approached. The formation of the International Equine Ophthalmology Consortium, which first met in 2009, has provided a forum for collaboration and the exchange of ideas that previously was not as easily available. The volume of material in the literature, both as peer-reviewed articles and as reviews, has increased exponentially. Opportunities for continuing education are more available than previously. Finally, the sheer number of people engaged in the science and practice of equine ophthalmology has grown to better support the need and includes general equine practitioners, basic scientists, internists, and surgeons as well as ophthalmologists in this field that is truly interdisciplinary. It is hoped the momentum will continue.

The goal of this issue is to summarize current knowledge across an array of topics within equine ophthalmology in a format in which each article can stand alone as a valuable source of information, yet together provide a state-of-the-art summary. It has been a privilege to shepherd the current issue from concept to the articles contained within it. These articles represent some of the advances that have been made in the past 25 years as well as the current thinking of some of the individuals who have been deeply engaged in the science and practice of equine ophthalmology

Vet Clin Equine 33 (2017) ix–x
https://doi.org/10.1016/j.cveq.2017.09.001
0749-0739/17/© 2017 Published by Elsevier Inc.

throughout their careers. Without them, a collaborative effort such as this would not be possible.

This issue is dedicated to Tim Cutler, who thirteen years ago served as guest editor of the second *Veterinary Clinics of North America: Equine Practice* issue devoted to ophthalmology. His wisdom and wit are missed; would that he were here to witness where we've come and help move us forward.

Mary Lassaline, DVM, PhD
Department of Surgical and Radiological Sciences
University of California, Davis
One Shields Avenue
Davis, CA 95616, USA

E-mail address:
lasutter@ucdavis.edu

Corneal Response to Injury and Infection in the Horse

Caryn E. Plummer, DVM[a,b],*

KEYWORDS

- Cornea • Wound healing • Protease • Inflammation • Keratomalacia
- Infectious keratitis • Fibrosis

KEY POINTS

- The cornea is the transparent anterior aspect of the fibrous tunic of the eye that is responsible for refraction and protection of the interior ocular structures.
- Corneal wound healing is a complex process that occurs in a series of interconnected and concurrent steps to reform the integrity of the protective tunic.
- Corneal wound healing may be associated with the formation of fibrosis, haze, or other opacities that decrease corneal clarity and its refractive function.
- Clinical signs associated with corneal disease are the direct consequence of the effects of a pathogen (if present) and corneal response to injury or infection.
- Medical and surgical therapy should be aimed at modulating the natural healing response to decrease the effects of pathogens and host cells on tissue destruction.

CORNEAL ANATOMY

Corneal disease is, unfortunately, a common complaint in our equine patients. Injuries and infections of the cornea are often due to a combination of factors, including the lateral position of the globes, the prominence of the corneas, the environment in which patients reside, the opportunistic nature of the ocular flora, and the quick-to-react behavior of this prey species. A good understanding of the normal anatomy and responses to injury of the horse cornea is critical to the development of treatment plans and the ability to make accurate and reasonable prognostic predictions.

The cornea is the transparent, anterior-most part of the fibrous tunic of the globe. It is protected mechanically by the palpebrae and nictitating membrane, and is

Disclosure Statement: The author has nothing to disclose.
[a] Comparative Ophthalmology, Department of Small Animal Clinical Sciences, College of Veterinary Medicine, University of Florida, PO Box 100101, 2015 Southwest 16th Avenue, Gainesville, FL 32610, USA; [b] Comparative Ophthalmology, Department of Large Animal Clinical Sciences, College of Veterinary Medicine, University of Florida, PO Box 100101, 2015 Southwest 16th Avenue, Gainesville, FL 32610, USA
* PO Box 100101, 2015 Southwest 16th Avenue, Gainesville, FL 32610, USA.
E-mail address: PlummerC@ufl.edu

nourished anteriorly by the tear film and posteriorly by the aqueous humor. In healthy animals, the cornea is avascular and is the major contributor to light refraction or focusing capacity.[1,2] The horse cornea ranges in thickness from 0.770 to 0.893 mm, with the peripheral cornea being relatively thicker than the central regions.[3,4] When a defect is present in the cornea, there is not that much tissue separating the inside of the eye from the outside world! This underscores the critical need for prompt and aggressive therapy for ulcers that are deep or infected, because perforation can occur rapidly in the unstable cornea.

The cornea is composed of 3 main layers, an outer epithelium, a middle stroma, and an internal endothelium. The epithelium consists of stratified squamous epithelium in 8 to 12 cell layers and is anchored to its basement membrane by hemidesmosomes.[1,2,5] The epithelium provides the outermost protective barrier for the eye and, when intact, is very effective at preventing invasion of the deeper corneal structures by pathogens. The corneal epithelium itself can be divided into several regions. Two to 3 layers of nonkeratinized squamous cells make up the outermost part of the epithelium, which is in contact with the environment. Deep to this lies a transitional zone consisting of 2 to 3 layers of polyhedral wing cells that rest on a single layer of columnar basal cells. The basal cell layer is attached to a basement membrane, which represents the caudal boundary of the corneal epithelium. Analogous to the epithelia of other organs, the corneal epithelium undergoes continuous desquamation as the outermost cells are replaced by those beneath them, which are continuously produced at the level of the basal cell layer.[1,2,5]

The stroma makes up 90% of the corneal thickness and is poorly cellular. It consists of very regularly arranged collagen fibers and a matrix of proteoglycans.[1,2,6] The stroma is made up of thick bands of parallel collagen lamellae that are uniformly 25 nm in diameter, and extend across the entire cornea.[6] The lamellae are formed from parallel bundles of collagen fibrils and are arranged in repeating orthogonal layers, with each layer extending at right angles to the bundles positioned above and below. Each fibril's small, uniform diameter, combined with the overall organized lamellar arrangement and carefully controlled fibril volume fraction, provide an optimal structure for light transmission in the healthy cornea.[1,2,6–9] Taken together, these attributes make the stroma an extremely important layer for maintaining corneal transparency, allowing up to 99% of light to pass through unimpeded.[9] The stroma is composed mainly of type I collagen with trace amounts of type III collagen and proteoglycans, mainly keratin sulfate and chondroitin/dermatin sulfate.[1,2,8–10] Collagen types IV, V, VI, and VII also play a role in corneal structure and repair. Throughout the stroma, specialized cells known as keratocytes are fixed between the lamellae. These cells have characteristically narrow nuclei, thin cell membranes, and contain crystallins, which are thought to aid in light transmission.[11] Keratocytes produce the majority of the extracellular matrix (ECM), both the collagen and the proteoglycans. In the normal cornea, keratocytes contribute to the maintenance of the stromal lamellae and, in the wounded cornea, keratocytes undergo apoptosis or transformation into myofibroblasts, which are integral to the healing process.[1,2,5,9–11] Also present in the stroma are migratory leukocytes, which are responsible for immune surveillance and response.

Deep to the stroma is the basement membrane of the innermost endothelium, known as Descemet's membrane. This structure is much more easily appreciable than the epithelial basement membrane and thickens with age owing to continued secretion. Descemet's membrane is composed of many types of collagen. Collagen types III and IV comprise the posterior banded zone, types IV and VIII comprise the anterior banded zone, and types V and VI comprise the anterior unbanded zone.[1,5]

Type VIII is interesting in that it is found in the iridocorneal angle only, and is not present anywhere else in the cornea.[1,2,5]

The endothelium is the innermost monolayer of interdigitating hexagonal cells, which function via a Na^+/K^+-ATPase to keep water and solutes out of the cornea.[1–3] They constantly pump fluid out of the stroma to maintain that tissue in a relative state of deturgescence, which is necessary for stromal collagen fibril organization and optical clarity. After experimental removal of the endothelium in otherwise normal eyes, cornea edema results in a 500% increase in corneal thickness.[3,5] These cells exhibit much less regenerative potential than other corneal cells throughout life, as evidenced by decreased cell density over time.[3]

The regular arrangement of fibers and relatively dehydrated status of the cornea allow for its clarity. To maintain the degree of sensation necessary for avoidance behavior and protection, it is innervated diffusely by the long ciliary nerves, which arise from the ophthalmic division of the trigeminal nerve (cranial nerve V) and terminate in naked nerve endings in the anterior stroma and among the wing cells of the corneal epithelium.[12,13]

IMMUNE RESPONSES OF THE OCULAR SURFACE

The immune system of the ocular surface can be divided into 2 types, similar to the generalized immune system for the rest of the body, innate immunity and active immunity. The first line of defense is innate immunity, which is nonspecific and consists of a concert of anatomic, cellular, and biochemical adaptations.[14] The orbit and adnexal tissues and the blink reflex limit access of foreign material and agents to the ocular surface. The eyelids, the aqueous portion of the tear film, and the phenomenon of reflex tearing flush debris and organisms from the ocular surface. Mucin and lipid in the tear film prevent microbial adhesion.[15] The corneal epithelium provides a mechanical barrier to microbial penetration. Numerous antiinflammatory and antimicrobial proteins also exist in the tear film, including lysozyme, lactoferrin, lipocalins, secretory immunoglobulin A, and complement, which function to either prevent adhesion, enhance clearance, inactivate proteases elaborated by microbes, or degrade the cell walls of microbes.[16] Phagocytic cells, such as macrophages and polymorphic mononuclear cells (PMNs), reside in the conjunctiva and eyelid skin ingest microbes and digest them with potent proteases. Additionally, the presence of commensal bacteria that coat the eyelids, conjunctiva, and corneal epithelium limit the growth and attachment of pathogenic microbes by depleting the tear film of nutrients, occupying binding sites, and secreting bacteriocidins.[15]

Active immunity responds to specific pathogens and establishes memory for a particular antigen after initial exposure. Active immunity requires that the foreign antigen be recognized (by the innate immune system) and presented to T lymphocytes by antigen-presenting cells.[14] The antigen is then processed, and expressed on the surface of the antigen-presenting cells in association with major histocompatibility complex class antigens, and B and T lymphocytes are activated.[14–16] The activated lymphocytes then destroy the offending agent. The humoral response involves the production of antigen-specific immunoglobulin that is capable of killing and clearing microbes.[14] The cell-mediated response involves the activation of cytotoxic T cells.[14] The cell-mediated immune response is particularly important for combating viral infections of the ocular surface. The major antigen-presenting cells in the ocular surface is the Langerhans cell, a dendritic cell related to the macrophage, which is found in eyelid skin, conjunctival mucosa, and the limbal and peripheral corneal epithelium.[15]

An important facet of the immune response of the ocular surface is the mucosal immune defense system associated with the conjunctiva, termed the conjunctival-associated lymphoid tissue.[15] Resident immunocompetent cell populations in the conjunctiva, including lymphocytes, mast cells, plasma cells, dendritic cells, epithelial cells, fibroblasts, and vascular endothelial cells, actively participate in the ocular immune response to foreign antigens, and are complemented by cellular functions of the lacrimal gland, tear film, and cornea.[15,16]

Fibroblasts, vascular endothelium, conjunctival epithelium, and keratocytes may be induced to express major histocompatibility complex class II antigens, which allows them to participate in antigen presentation.[15] This function may facilitate or hasten an immune response during an active infection, but may possibly be a contributing factor in instances of noninfectious, chronic, and immune-mediated keratitis (IMMK).

CORNEAL REACTION TO INJURY

When the cornea sustains an injury, the subsequent steps necessary for wound healing depend on the extent, location, and type of the injury. A complex orchestration of cytokine and growth factor activity, cellular migration, transformation, and tissue remodeling is triggered, much of which is still only partially understood. The sequence of events begins with stabilization of the wound, followed by tissue reaction to produce cells and ECM and finally tissue remodeling.[2] Cell death is necessary for the initiation of a response from uninjured surrounding cells.[17,18] This death may be accomplished by either necrosis, in which there is damage to the cell's membrane, accompanied by cell swelling, rupture, and release of cytoplasmic contents, which can be damaging to adjacent cells and induce inflammation, or by apoptosis. Apoptosis is induced either by the loss of trophic factors (survival signals) or by the action of killing factors. Apoptosis results in cell shrinkage with maintenance of the cell membrane until late in the process and allows removal of the cell without inducing injury to surrounding tissues.[17]

The basic response to injury occurs with little variation, regardless of whether the stromal wound was created by trauma, infectious disease, surgical intervention, or other etiologies.[1,2] Epithelial defects will generally heal rapidly (as much as 0.6 mm/d in the uncomplicated wound) via migration of basal epithelial cells surrounding the wound into the defect and mitotic replication of limbal stem cells to reform the normal epithelial structure (**Fig. 1**).[2] When a stromal defect is present, the edges of the wound are initially debrided by PMNs and then keratocytes adjacent to the wound transform into fibroblasts and begin to synthesize collagen and proteoglycans to replace that missing from injury or infectious destruction (**Fig. 2**).[5,19,20] Because the

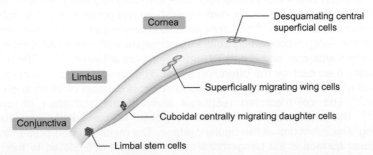

Fig. 1. Migration of corneal epithelial cells during steady-state homeostasis. The process is accelerated and enhanced after injury.

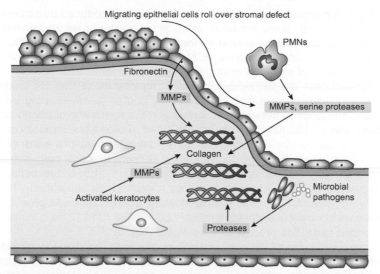

Fig. 2. Proteases play critical roles in normal wound healing to permit the migration of epithelial cells and stromal fibroblasts and in removing damaged cells and extracellular matrix (ECM). However, if levels of proteases are either elevated or chronically persistent, they may impair corneal wound healing. Delayed reepithelialization may occur as well as increased degradation of stromal ECM (delayed production of replacement ECM or keratomalacia, both of which can compromise the integrity of the globe). Levels are often elevated in the face of infection or persistent inflammation. MMPs, matrix metalloproteinases.

process of stromal regeneration is more complex than that of reepithelialization, it can be considerably more time consuming. An epithelial defect might heal in a matter of days, whereas a stromal wound might take weeks or longer. The stroma that is initially laid down is disorganized and results in a scar. Over time, this hastily produced collagen will be reorganized, which is how scars fade and become less dense.[2,5] However, the injured cornea does not return to normal and never achieves the tensile strength and transparency of native cornea.

When the endothelium is damaged, its ability to regenerate is quite limited. Cells that die are not replaced by new cells; instead, the adjacent cells spread out and hypertrophy. Once the endothelial cell density or function declines below a certain threshold (generally regarded to be 400–700 cells/mm^2), persistent corneal edema results.[1,3–5]

Epithelial Wound Healing

Replacement of damaged and destroyed epithelial cells is nearly immediate. The first priority is to bridge the wounded area and reestablish a continuous cellular barrier across the defect. Signals generated by the damaged cells or from exposure of the epithelial basement membrane to tear fluid or the circulation are sent to surrounding intact epithelial cells. There is a short latent phase of approximately 1 hour during which the cell cytoskeleton and intracellular junctions are modified. Flattening, retraction, and release of hemidesmosomal attachments to the epithelial basement membrane by the basal epithelial cells nearest the wound edge occurs.[21] These cells begin to extend actin-rich pseudopodia via their microfilament structure over the denuded wound surface. Cell membrane receptors, such as those for integrin, bind to extracellular proteins, such as fibronectin, collagen, and laminin, which initiates migration of the basal cells onto the wound surface at a rate of 0.75 μm/min.[22–24]

Fibronectin, which appears immediately after injury and is produced by adjacent cells or is delivered through tears, aqueous, or plasma, creates a temporary matrix for epithelial cell migration on the wound surface.[22–24] A variety of endogenous growth factors and their receptors, cytokines, ECM proteins, and proteases are also important in the regulation of epithelial wound healing.

New epithelial cells are formed by mitosis to replace those that are leading the march forward. The healing epithelium draws on a pool of rapidly dividing stem cells at the limbus, the junction between the cornea and the sclera and overlying conjunctiva. Limbal stem cells have an almost unlimited proliferative capacity and lifespan.[25,26] Their division by mitosis gives rise to daughter cells that either replenish the stem cell pool or give rise to transiently amplifying cells that in turn give rise to terminally differentiated epithelial cells. The cells in the basal layer of the epithelium have some mitotic capability, but as they migrate more superficially, they lose their ability to multiply.[25,26] The normal corneal epithelium undergoes constant self-renewal with complete epithelial turnover occurring in 10 to 12 days in the horse.[2] In the wounded state, this process is accelerated (**Fig. 3**).

Depending on the size of the epithelial defect, the cells may have to migrate over several millimeters, which requires the simultaneous formation and destruction of attachments between the cells and the underlying ECM.[25] The destruction of those attachments is accomplished by the action of proteases, such as the serine proteases (tissue plasminogen activator, urokinase-plasminogen activator, plasmin, neutrophil elastase) and matrix metalloproteinases (MMPs).[27–30] Migrating epithelial cells move forward in a sheetlike formation until contact inhibition occurs by physical contact with adjacent cells. Once the epithelial defect is closed, the basal epithelial cells reform their adhesion complexes, the epithelium thickens with basal cells moving

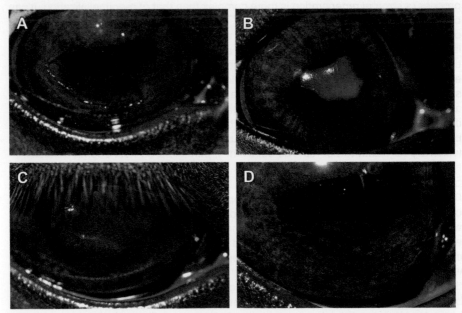

Fig. 3. (*A*) Superficial, noninfected ulcer in a horse. (*B*) Same eye 3 days later. The epithelium is migrating over the exposed stroma. The exposed stroma is retaining fluorescein. (*C*) Same eye 4 days after presentation. The epithelium continues to migrate over the defect. (*D*) Same eye 6 days after presentation.

superficially when they are replaced by new basal cells incoming from the limbus, and the superficial epithelial cells terminally differentiate.[25,26]

A healthy epithelium is critical to maintenance of the health of the rest of the cornea. An intact corneal epithelium prevents stromal degradation and loss, and is a prerequisite for stromal wound healing.

Stromal Wound Healing

Even as the epithelium begins to proliferate and migrate in earnest, there are important changes taking place within the wounded corneal stroma.[1,2] The stimulus that initiates corneal stroma reaction is keratocyte death. The degree of the response depends on the number of keratocytes that expire as a result of apoptosis or necrosis. Apoptosis of keratocytes plays a central role in initiating corneal wound healing cascades. If only a small number of keratocytes undergo apoptosis, the stromal response may be negligible or minimal.[17,18] Even when the original insult is only to the overlying epithelium, but the basement membrane or some denuded stroma is exposed, keratocytes in the superficial stroma undergo apoptosis as a secondary effect. With more significant or stromal wounds, a larger number of keratocytes die, resulting in a more profound stromal reaction. Keratocytes within a few hundred microns of the wound undergo apoptosis and die, and those beyond that zone become "activated," enlarge in size, and alter their biochemical apparatus. They become migratory and transform into a fibroblast-like phenotype to be capable of replacing damaged stromal collagen fibrils, synthesizing ECM material, and restoring natural curvature to the cornea.[21,31,32]

Once the site of the injury has been cleared of damaged tissue and debris by the action of inflammatory cells, the activated keratocytes start to produce replacement collagen. These new collagen fibers, although made of type I collagen, are generally larger and more variable in caliber than native corneal collagen and the new proteoglycans differ in character and proportion as well.[25] These differences contribute to corneal opacity.

Some of the activated keratocytes and other recruited keratocyte-like fibroblasts, derived from circulating monocytes and cells of bone marrow origin or from epithelial to mesenchymal cell transformation of corneal epithelial or endothelial cells, differentiate into myofibroblasts that have large amounts of α-smooth muscle actin, which enables the cells to contract the surrounding matrix in the wound bed. Myofibroblasts are crucial to the survival and repair of the wounded cornea owing to their unique ability to secrete ECM, produce adhesions in the surrounding stroma by crosslinking the ECM, and contract wound edges.[31-37] In addition, myofibroblasts produce MMPs, which are very active in collagen remodeling.[37,38] However, with prolonged myofibroblast activity, there is an increase in corneal haze.[39-46] Myofibroblasts express greater quantities of vimentin, α-smooth muscle actin, and desmin as they mature, which has been associated with the formation of corneal haze.[35,36] In addition, activated keratocytes and myofibroblasts decrease production of their internal crystalline proteins, which are responsible for helping the cells to maintain transparency. Crystallins are water-soluble proteins that control optical clarity in the lens and cornea, and are normally abundantly expressed in corneal cells.[11,37] In the face of this change, there is an increased reflectance of the cells and a corresponding increase in corneal haze.

Inflammation

The most obvious evidence of inflammation in most tissues is the appearance, proliferation, and dilation of blood vessels. Blood vessels dramatically facilitate delivery of immune and inflammatory cells to the site of injury and may prevent perforation. Because the cornea is normally devoid of blood vessels, the delivery of cells and protein factors (coagulation factors, growth-stimulating factors, and oxygen ion–regulating factors) necessary for initial clearing of debris and subsequent restoration of structure in a corneal ulcer is accomplished through the tear fluid externally and the aqueous humor internally. Within the first 12 to 24 hours of injury, inflammatory cells such as neutrophils, lymphocytes, macrophages, and monocytes enter the stroma via the precorneal tear film and conjunctival blood vessels at the limbus.[1,2,15,25,47] Limbal blood vessels dilate and their endothelial cell walls become increasingly permeable and adhesive for intraluminal inflammatory cells. Adherent leukocytes migrate through the vessel walls via diapedesis and are drawn toward the wound between the corneal lamellae by variable gradients of cytokines.[25] Once present, the inflammatory cells work to scavenge the remnants of necrotic and apoptotic cells and remove any invasive microorganisms in the vicinity. They do so by liberating proteolytic enzymes and phagocytizing cellular and noncellular debris. If upregulated or produced in excessive amounts, these proteolytic enzymes, which include the serine proteases and MMPs, can contribute to progression of the original injury.[27–30,37,38]

If the stimulus for inflammation persists, episcleral vascular endothelial cells at the limbus will proliferate and migrate forming capillary tufts that sprout into the cornea between the stromal lamellae toward the injury or stimulus.[25,40,46] The cells then form a lumen for an incipient vessel. The ECM surrounding the new blood vessel is degraded by enzymes such as MMPs and a basal lamina forms around the vessel as it matures. Significant vascular invasion and the transitional tissues surrounding it lead to the development of granulation tissue (**Fig. 4**). Neovascularization is an expected healing response and can provide a range of cells and growth factors that encourage healing and structural integrity; however, blood vessels have the unwanted consequence of increasing corneal opacity.

Although inflammation is an essential response to injury and infection, it can be a significant source of additional injury to host tissues and can initiate or exacerbate

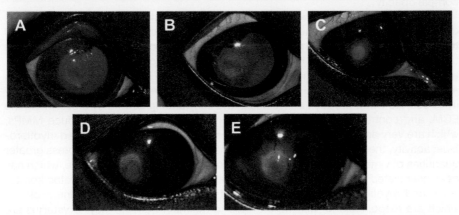

Fig. 4. (*A*) Stromal ulcer in a young Quarter Horse. Note the mild diffuse corneal edema, dense edema, and early keratomalacia in the central defect and the absence of corneal vascularization. (*B*) Same eye 12 days after presentation and the initiation of medical support. There is vascularization approaching the wound from the dorsotemporal limbus. The keratomalacia has resolved and the secondary anterior uveitis is well-controlled. (*C*) Same eye on same day as (*B*). Fluorescein is only retained in the central portion of the defect, indicating that the wound is reepithelializing. (*D*) Same eye 4 weeks after initial presentation. The wound has reepithelialized and missing stroma is being reformed. Note the further migration of vascularization along the dorsal aspect of the wound. (*E*) Same eye 6 weeks after initial presentation. The wound bed has filled in with granulation tissue.

tissue scarring. Judicious modulation of corneal inflammation is a therapeutic goal in many instances of corneal disease.

Endothelial Wound Healing

Because of the limited capacity of endothelial cells to undergo mitosis, defects of the endothelium are covered by spreading and hypertrophy of adjacent cells, followed by the formation of a new Descemet's membrane.[1,3] If the total number and density of cells decreases below a critical threshold, the capacity of those cells to remove ions from the stroma decreases precipitously and corneal hydration results.[3] The highly ordered orthogonal arrangement of the corneal lamellae is distorted and corneal opacity results. Persistent and severe corneal edema may result in focal accumulations of fluid or microbullae in the superficial stroma that are subject to rupture, which may result in corneal ulceration.

The reason for the limited mitotic ability of corneal endothelial cells is not well-established, but it is possible that the environment of the anterior chamber does not support extensive mitosis either because of the lack of factors necessary to stimulate it or the presence of factors that block it.[25]

When prolonged inflammation or mechanical damage affect the corneal endothelium, a retrocorneal membrane composed of fibroblast-like cells, collagen and basement membrane-like material will form posterior to Descemet's membrane and influence conversion of the endothelial cells into fibroblast-like cells which cease to perform their solute-pumping function.[3,25]

Perforating Injury

If a wound results in a full-thickness rent in the cornea, the exposed hydrophilic stroma swells when exposed to tears and aqueous humor (**Fig. 5**).[25] This swelling may seal the wound if there is not a large gap or a large degree of tissue loss. Alternatively, acute phase

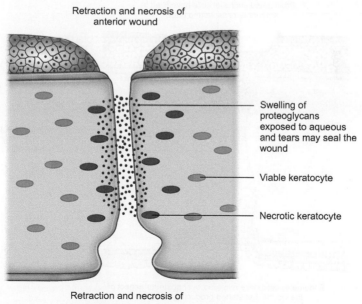

Retraction and necrosis of
anterior wound

Swelling of
proteoglycans
exposed to aqueous
and tears may seal the
wound

Viable keratocyte

Necrotic keratocyte

Retraction and necrosis of
posterior wound

Fig. 5. Characteristics of an acute perforating corneal wound.

inflammatory proteins, particularly fibrin, which are generated from the aqueous humor and from transudation of factors from surrounding blood vessels, will arrive to form a temporary plug.[25] If the wound is too expansive to be supported by this fibrin plug, surgical stabilization is indicated to replace missing tissue. The anterior and posterior aspects of the wound gape and retract with subsequent curling of the epithelial basement membrane and Descemet's membrane. Biochemical signals then recruit distant cells toward the wound center with the epithelial cells being first to act. Epithelial cells at the leading edge of the wound loosen their attachments and migrate along a layer of newly accumulated fibronectin across the surface of the wound.[22–25] Activated keratocytes react much more slowly and in some instances may not begin their migration until the epithelial cells have covered the wound surface. Once they migrate to the wound edges, these fibroblasts and fibroblast-like cells will begin producing collagen and proteoglycans to replace the tissue missing as a result of the injury and clean up processes (**Fig. 6**).[25,31–35] The endothelial cell response occurs between those of the epithelium and the stroma. These cells thin and flatten and migrate over a provisional matrix of fibronectin toward the center of the wound.[22–24] The epithelium and endothelium reform their respective basement membranes much later in the course of healing. Basement membrane and cellular adhesion sites may take up to 6 weeks after the insult to become well-established.[2,19,25] The formation of a stromal scar is a dynamic process and may continue for months or years after the initiating event (**Fig. 7**). The wounded site will never regain the degree of tensile strength it originally had. Estimates range from 25% to 70% of normal, depending on the extent and orientation of the wound.[25]

CORNEAL INFECTION

Infection of the cornea requires 4 steps: access of the microbe to the ocular surface, attachment of the microbe to the ocular surface, penetration of the microbe through the

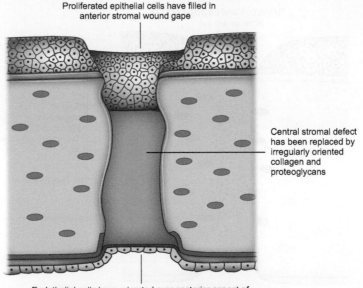

Proliferated epithelial cells have filled in
anterior stromal wound gape

Central stromal defect
has been replaced by
irregularly oriented
collagen and
proteoglycans

Endothelial cells have migrated over posterior aspect of
the wound and started producing new DM

Fig. 6. Intermediate stage of healing of a perforating wound demonstrating replacement epithelium and randomly arranged stromal extracellular matrix. DM, Descemet's membrane.

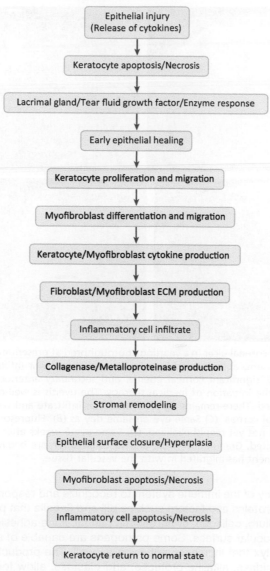

Fig. 7. The steps of the corneal wound healing cascade. ECM, extracellular matrix.

epithelium, and subsequent growth and expansion of the organism.[48] In instances when the physical, innate, and active immune responses of the ocular surface do not prevent infection of the cornea, a robust inflammatory and immune reaction will be triggered in the attempt to maintain ocular integrity (**Figs. 8** and **9**).[14,19,47]

Fortunately, the corneal immune system is robust and corneal infections are rare. In fact, most cases of corneal infection with bacteria or fungi require some sort of antecedent trauma or preexisting disease process. However, opportunistic pathogens are very adept at evolving ways around host defenses. Bacteria and fungi have several important virulence factors that can improve their ability to cause disease in immunocompetent hosts. Many bacteria express a thick capsule to

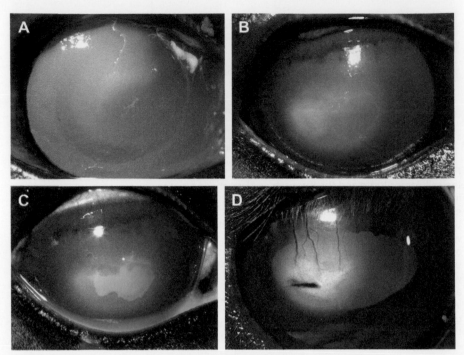

Fig. 8. (*A*) Infected corneal ulcer in a yearling Thoroughbred at presentation. A large super-ficial wound is present, accompanied by a creamy yellow cellular infiltrate (polymorphic mononuclear cells), significant corneal edema, and secondary anterior uveitis. (*B*) Same eye 1 week after the initiation of medical therapy. The uveitis is well-controlled and the edema has improved. There remains significant cellular infiltrate and vessel migration has begun in the dorsal cornea. (*C*) Same eye on same day as (*B*). Fluorescein delineates area of cornea that has not yet reepithelialized. (*D*) Same eye 6 weeks after presentation. The wound has contracted. Granulation tissue and vascularization are beginning to recede. A small focus of pigment has migrated in with the vascular tissue.

minimize the ability of the immune system to recognize and respond to them. A va-riety of surface proteins and factors such as pili and flagella that permit pathogens to bind to epithelium, collagen, or fibronectin can facilitate adhesion to and migra-tion through the ocular surface. Some pathogens are capable of secreting a slime layer, or glycocalyx that increases adhesion as well. The production of enzymes, such as hyaluronidase, alkaline protease, and elastase, allow for the destruction of the ECM, which creates space for migration and invasion.[27–30,37] Some patho-gens secrete proteins, such as coagulase, catalase, and leucocidin, which in-crease resistance to phagocytosis. Others produce exotoxins that directly damage host tissue.[48]

Once a pathogen has eluded the passive adaptations of the innate immune system, the corneal response to infection is a combination of innate and active immune re-sponses and inflammation. The nonspecific responses include the production and upregulation of antimicrobial proteins that either prevent adhesion, inactivate bacterial proteases, impair microbial growth, or physically degrade the cell walls of pathogens and the recruitment of phagocytic cells that kill and remove microbes.[14,15] Infla-mmation results in increased blood flow and leukocyte delivery and recruitment from the conjunctiva, tear film, and areas of corneal vascularization.[25] Although the

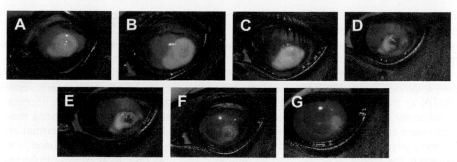

Fig. 9. (A) Stromal infected corneal ulcer in a middle-aged Tennessee Walking Horse. Note the cellular infiltrate and the intense vascular response. (B) Same eye as (A) 2 days after the initiation of medical therapy. Note that the blood vessels seem less perfused and have not migrated significantly. This is due to the effects of the systemic nonsteroidal antiinflammatory flunixin. A balance must be struck between allowing the healing cascade to progress while minimizing inflammation that might lead to further damage to host tissues (corneal and intraocular structures). (C) Same eye 6 days after initial presentation. The cellular infiltrate has begun to dissipate and the epithelium is migrating in from the periphery of the wound. Although blood vessels continue to move centrally, they are not well-perfused and changes in the peripheral stroma peripheral to the vasculature are occurring, resulting in fibrosis. (D) Same eye 12 days after initial presentation. Vessels have taken a more targeted path. (E) Same eye 12 days after initial presentation. The wound continues to reepithelialize. (F) Same eye 3 weeks after initial presentation. The wound bed has granulated and is beginning to contract. Note the peripheral fibrosis. (G) Same eye 6 weeks after initial presentation.

profound response to infection is necessary for elimination of the offending organism, it may contribute to further damage of host tissue and the formation of fibrosis and corneal opacity.

MODULATION OF CORNEAL WOUND HEALING

Although a concert of epithelial cells, keratocytes, myofibroblasts, and bone marrow–derived cells is crucial for repairing a corneal wound and preventing rupture of the globe, it often results in significant haze within the previously clear corneal stroma. The terms corneal fibrosis or haze are used to describe any changes in cellular characteristics, ECM arrangement, or cell infiltrates that contribute to an overall decrease in light transmission through the corneal stroma.[31,32,34–36,41–44] Taken together, these changes to the stromal cell morphology and the organization of its surrounding ECM contribute significantly to haze formation after a corneal wound. Because the degree of haze is directly proportional to a decrease in vision, and the cornea is responsible for approximately 70% of ocular light transmission, its effect on functional vision and quality of life cannot be overstated.

The goals of medical and surgical therapy of corneal disease include sterilizing the infected wound, arresting and reversing tissue destruction, enhancing and encouraging reepithelialization and reformation of stromal tissue, and, ideally, minimizing the formation of secondary corneal haze. A variety of approaches to enhance epithelial wound healing have been explored including the addition or upregulation of certain growth factors such as fibroblast growth factors, epidermal growth factors, or by ECM components like soluble fibronectin derived from plasma.[1,24,25,40] Proteases inhibitors, many derived from or present in plasma or serum, such as aprotinin, may improve epithelial healing, hence, the recommendation to use plasma or serum topically on corneal ulcers.[49]

Despite our best intentions, any exogenous interventions that we apply or promote may modulate the process of corneal wound healing in a negative fashion. Epithelial wound healing may be impaired by the application of topical medications that contain preservatives such as benzalkonium chloride, ethylenediaminetetraacetic acid (EDTA), or thimerosal.[49] Superficial ulcers that are refractory to healing, may improve significantly with the use of preservative-free medications. Topical antibiotics may also retard epithelial regeneration to varying degrees. Although critical to combat infections, which will also delay corneal healing, topical antibiotics should be used judiciously in the sterile ulcer. Aggressive antibiotic use until an infection is controlled is indicated, but once the wound is sterilized, their use should be minimized. Aminoglycoside and fluoroquinolone antibiotics tend to have the most harsh effects on healing epithelial cells.[49]

Enhancement of stromal wound healing aims to decrease the destruction of the corneal ECM, increase the production of new ECM, or minimize the development of fibrosis leading to haze. Of course, stromal wound healing is complex. Factors that have been shown to increase the rate of stromal regeneration and tensile wound strength very often result in increased scar formation and opacity. The transforming growth factor-beta system regulates key aspects of corneal wound healing, but has been shown to promote scar deposition. The growth factor connective tissue growth factor is chemotactic and mitogenic for fibroblasts and stimulates the production of ECM material.[19,24,25,40,49] Both of these factors, although they hasten the formation of new stroma, promote the development of haze and are therefore targets for the modulation of scar formation.

Protease inhibitors such as those agents that inhibit MMPs by chelating the essential zinc cation in the active site of the enzyme, including EDTA and acetylcysteine, or by competitive inhibition, such as tetracyclines and ilomastat, have been repeatedly demonstrated to decrease collagenolysis. Structural and biochemical support may be enhanced with the application of amniotic membrane to a stromal wound.[27–30,49] Amnion has a variety of properties that enhance wound healing, including growth factors and protease inhibitors, as well as antiinflammatory factors and antiangiogenic factors.[49,50] Additionally, it suppresses the transforming growth factor-beta system and myofibroblast differentiation. In both acute and chronic inflammatory conditions of the cornea, amnion successfully reduces scarring, vascularization, and loss of corneal stem cells, and may restore stromal tissue in instances of its loss.

When considering methods of intervention, it is advisable to consider both potential positive and negative outcomes and interactions of potential therapies. Future advances should strive to achieve or maintain a balanced approach to therapy.

IMPLICATIONS OF THE WOUND HEALING CASCADE ON INJURY AND DISEASE IN THE EQUINE CORNEA
Keratomalacia

Corneal inflammation, regardless of the etiology, causes release of cytokines (interleukins, tumor necrosis factor alpha, and interferons) from host cells, which results in the upregulation of a variety of intracellular adhesion molecules that recruit and facilitate migration and infiltration of the cornea by leukocytes. These PMNs, once activated, release MMPs and other lysosomal enzymes that are capable of corneal destruction and ulceration. Keratomalacia, or corneal melting, results when there is an overabundance of these enzymatic proteins elaborated by these recruited inflammatory cells, activated resident host cells, and any pathogens present.[27–30] The destructive forces overwhelm the restorative responses and result in dissolution of corneal collagen and necrosis of cells. The production of elastase and alkaline phosphatase by *Pseudomonas*, hyaluronidase by *Staphylococcus* and other extracellular proteases by fungal organisms can greatly augment this melting process.[48] Even when an infection is eradicated by the frequent use of an effective antimicrobial, residual proteases may continue to destroy the corneal matrix, even after microbial replication has ceased (**Fig. 10**).

Infectious Keratitis

Most instances of infectious keratitis in the horse are ulcerative in nature. Corneal ulcers infected with a bacterial or fungal agent can be very serious and may manifest with extensive cellular infiltrate and extensive destruction of corneal tissue. The most important route of therapy is antimicrobial medication directly aimed at the causative or complicating microbe. Culture and susceptibility testing are imperative, because so many pathogens are increasingly demonstrating resistance to available antimicrobial medications. Initial empiric antimicrobial therapy should be chosen after samples from a corneal scraping have been examined for cytologic evidence of infection and the morphologic appearance of the infectious agents. The healing cascade of an infected corneal wound generally proceeds as described, but with increased levels of corneal and tear film proteases and

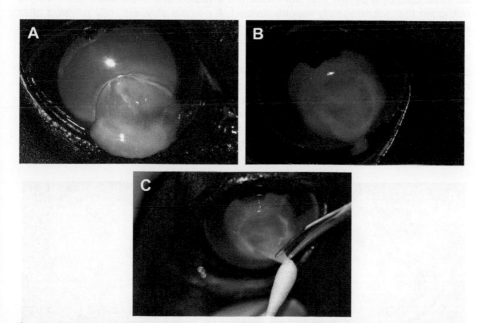

Fig. 10. (*A*) Severe keratomalacia in a weanling Thoroughbred. Note the soft, drooping cornea running over the eyelid margin. (*B*) Keratomalacia in an infected corneal ulcer (*Streptococcus* spp.) in a yearling Thoroughbred. Note the anterior uveitis indicated by relative miosis and hypopyon. (*C*) Same eye as (*B*). A keratectomy is being performed with Wescott scissors to remove necrotic tissue and decrease the load of inflammatory products, pathogens and antigens.

a more robust inflammatory response.[27–30,48] This results in the greater likelihood of stromal destruction (loss of ECM, keratomalacia) than in a sterile wound and subsequently a greater risk for perforation, intraocular damage from secondary uveitis, and scar tissue formation. Often, especially in corneas infected with fungi, a groove or furrow will develop at the periphery of the lesion owing to increased concentrations and activity of proteases elaborated both by host tissues and the pathogens (**Fig. 11**).[28,29,51,52] It can almost seem as if the lesion is attempting to be sloughed. Unfortunately, corneal thickness is finite. Infections that travel to the deeper layers of the cornea, especially fungal organisms that are chemoattracted to Descemet's membrane, are more likely to result in a full-thickness rupture.[48,51] Antiprotease agents are critical to successful treatment of these infected wounds. Autologous serum or plasma, EDTA, acetylcysteine, doxycycline, and ilomostat are the current favorites.[27–29,52–54] Surgical debridement of infected wounds with structural stabilization (corneal grafts, conjunctival grafts, or amniotic membrane transplantation) are often necessary to prevent or treat full-thickness corneal compromise.[50,55] Surgical procedures that hasten the advance of vascular invasion of the host or donor tissues will expedite healing, but generally result in greater degrees of scarring (**Fig. 12**). Amniotic membrane transplantation for superficial wounds may provide excellent cosmetic results and minimize corneal opacity; however, it is not recommended for reconstruction of deeper lesions or instances of fungal keratitis (**Fig. 13**).

Occasionally, corneal abscesses with an intact epithelium will be noted in the horse. Although technically nonulcerative at the time of diagnosis, there was likely an initial epithelial defect that permitted the invasion of the exposed stroma by a pathogen that subsequently reepithelialized. A corneal abscess may develop after epithelial cells adjacent to a traumatic epithelial micropuncture divide and migrate over the exposed stroma to enclose infectious agents or foreign bodies in the stroma. Reepithelialization forms a barrier that protects the pathogen from topically administered antimicrobial medications. Most cases of corneal abscesses in the horse are fungal in origin (**Fig. 14**).[51] Although abscesses do not exhibit the same degree of collagenolysis as seen in ulcerative disease, the pathogens do elaborate enough proteases to enable their posterior migration in the cornea. These enzymes may also facilitate damage to Descemet's membrane, which can result in rupture of the abscess and introduction of the organism into the anterior chamber. This

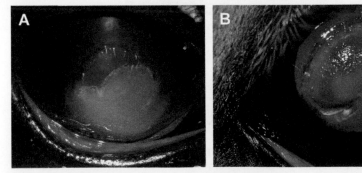

Fig. 11. (*A*) Fungal keratitis in a Quarter Horse. In addition to the cellular infiltrate present, note the deeper areas along the periphery of the lesion. This is a site of increased enzymatic destruction of corneal extracellular matrix. (*B*) Another example of a peripheral furrow or groove surrounding another lesion in a case of fungal keratitis.

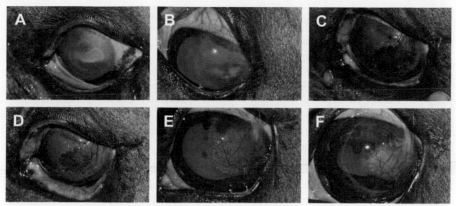

Fig. 12. (*A*) A case of fungal keratitis in a pony. Note the cellular infiltrate, irregular corneal stroma, and the early vascular invasion. (*B*) Same eye 3 days after initial presentation. The cellular infiltrate has begun to dissipate, indicating that the infection is improving, but the stroma has become more malacic and the periphery of the wound is beginning to get deeper, which suggests that proteases are causing continued destruction of host tissue. (*C*) The same eye immediately after keratectomy and placement of a conjunctival flap. (*D*) The same eye 5 days postoperatively. (*E*) The same eye 3 weeks post-operatively. Note the incorporation of the conjunctiva into the cornea. (*F*) The same eye 6 weeks postoperatively. Wound maturation, fibrosis, and contraction and remodeling have begun.

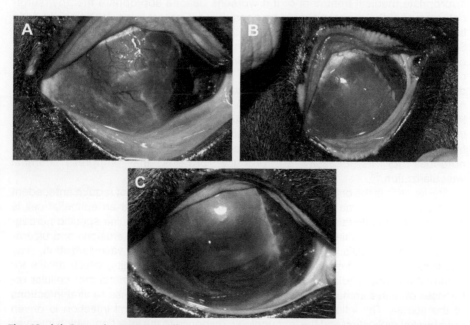

Fig. 13. (*A*) Corneal squamous cell carcinoma (SCC) in a pony before keratectomy. (*B*) Same eye as (*A*) immediately after removal of the SCC and coverage of the resultant wound bed with amniotic membrane. (*C*) Same eye 1 month after amniotic membrane transplantation (AMT) for reconstruction of the ocular surface. AMT can improve corneal clarity compared with other types of grafts. AMT is not recommended for the treatment of fungal keratitis.

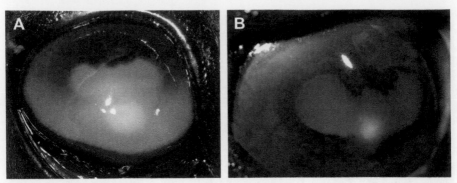

Fig. 14. (*A*) Deep stromal abscess (DSA) in an aged Thoroughbred. (*B*) Another example of a DSA with minimal vascular response. This abscess was caused by *Aspergillus*, which can elaborate antiangiogenic factors.

process usually exacerbates anterior uveitis, and can put the eye at risk for endophthalmitis.

Medical therapy for stromal abscesses consists of aggressive use of topical antifungals and antibiotics, and symptomatic therapy for the associated iridocyclitis. Unfortunately, owing to the presence of an intact epithelium, antimicrobial penetration is limited, which results in extended healing times or necessitates surgical removal of the nidus. If the iridocyclitis does not improve within a few days of appropriate medical treatment or if it worsens despite appropriate therapy, surgical removal of the abscess should be considered. Corneal transplantation via deep lamellar, posterior lamellar, or penetrating keratoplasties is recommended.[55] Surgical removal and corneal replacement eliminates sequestered microbial antigens, and removes necrotic debris, cytokines, and toxins from degenerating leukocytes in the abscess. If the abscess has not ruptured into the anterior chamber, drug delivery to the site may be improved with intrastromal injection with a microneedle.[56] Voriconazole is the most common antifungal used with this method. Interestingly, many cases of fungal keratitis (ulcerative and nonulcerative) fail to initiate an appropriate inflammatory vascular response in the cornea, possibly from the elaboration of antiangiogenic factors by the organism.[57] Aspergillus is notorious for its capacity to produce proteins that suppress corneal vascularization.[48]

Viral keratitis is the only form of infectious keratitis that does not require antecedent trauma or microtrauma to the cornea to establish itself. Once an epithelial cell is infected with an offending viral particle, most commonly an equine-specific herpesvirus, it replicates within and results in lysis of the cell causing erosions and ulcerations. Stromal keratitis, manifesting with cellular infiltrate and vascularization, may occur as well, likely from alteration of stromal cells' antigenicity, which allows for recurrent immune-mediated bouts of inflammation.[48] Both humoral and cellular responses of active immunity are responsible for the host response to viral infections of the cornea. The inflammatory response associated with viral infection is driven both by viral replication and the immunologic response to the infection, which involves the recruitment and activation of lymphocytes, PMNs, serum complement, and antiviral antibodies.[14,15] The abilities of viruses to replicate within epithelial cells and establish latency are virulence factors that contribute to persistence and recrudescence of disease.

Refractory Sterile Superficial Ulcers

Superficial ulcers that fail to reepithelialize in a timely fashion may have a variety of excuses for their refractory nature. It is important to rule out the presence of a mechanical irritant (cilia, foreign body, corneal degeneration, corneal exposure owing to an eyelid defect, neuroparalytic keratitis, or tear film deficiency) or a subclinical infection. Metabolic derangements, particularly pars pituitary intermedia dysfunction (equine Cushing's disease), may also contribute to impaired epithelial wound healing. In the absence of these predisposing origins, an aberration of the adhesion complexes that keep the epithelium adhered to its underlying basement membrane or a deviation of the normal healing response may be at play. A dearth of fibronectin, which plays an important role in the adhesion of cells, may contribute to delayed healing.[22-24] Persistent expression of tissue plasminogen activator results in prolonged activation of plasmin, which can contribute to the degradation of fibronectin and fibrin, and to stromal degradation.[49] Elevated levels of MMPs may also be present, causing degradation of the epithelial basement membrane or the adhesion complexes of the epithelial cells themselves.[27-30,52-54] For these reasons, the use of endogenous inhibitors of plasmin, plasminogen activators, and MMPs is indicated. Autologous serum or plasma contains alpha-2 macroglobulin, which is capable of inhibiting the lot. Additional helpful therapies include hypertonic saline, which exerts an osmotic effect to keep the superficial cornea dehydrated to minimize lifting of the epithelium, and bandage contact lenses, which relieve pain and protect loosely adherent epithelium from the abrasive effects of the eyelids. Surgical intervention with cotton-tipped applicator or diamond burr debridement may facilitate exposure of the epithelial basement membrane or underlying stroma by removing any surface membranes and exudate, and facilitating normal epithelial attachment and adhesion. Occasionally, superficial keratectomy to remove abnormal basement membrane is necessary.

Corneal Transplantation

In many instances of corneal disease, replacement of host tissue with that from a donor is necessary to maintain the structural integrity of the globe. Most corneal transplantations in horses are performed with frozen donor allografts, which act as space fillers to address and improve tectonic support. In these cases, the donor graft is not expected to maintain clarity. Live grafts, which provide viable keratocytes and endothelial cells, are not routinely used in equine ophthalmology owing to the logistical difficulties of acquiring and maintaining live grafts in culture.

Allograft rejection of corneal transplants is not nearly as much of a problem for the eye as it is for solid organ transplants elsewhere in the body. This is due in large part to the anterior chamber–associated immune deviation and a variety of soluble and cell membrane-bound immunosuppressive factors in the anterior segment that lend immune privilege to the eye.[15,25] That said, graft rejection does occur, especially when the circumstances of the underlying disease process (typically an infectious etiology) prevent the application of topical immunosuppressant therapy that would prevent corneal vascularization and introduction of Langerhans cells into the donor graft. Allograft rejection is an active cell-mediated immune response effected by T cells.[15] In the postoperative period, rejection is typically recognized clinically as swelling of the donor graft, usually 5 to 7 days after introduction of the allograft, which may exert considerable pressure or strain on the sutures holding the graft in place (**Fig. 15**).[55] This strain may induce structural failure and perforation of the repair and leakage of aqueous through a resultant rent. If the surgical

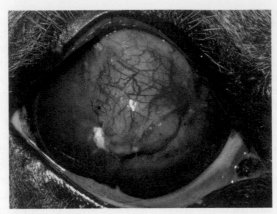

Fig. 15. Swelling of the corneal graft owing to rejection reaction 1 week after penetrating keratoplasty surgery has caused premature retraction of its overlying protective conjunctival flap.

site remains intact through this period, the routine cascade of healing responses proceeds and fibrosis of the graft and its juncture with the host tissue occurs (**Fig. 16**).

Immune-Mediated Keratitis

Nonulcerative keratitis is a recognized primary corneal disease syndrome with variable subsets of clinical appearance and etiology. Within this clinical diagnosis exists a group of inflammatory conditions that are seemingly immune-mediated in origin or progression referred to as IMMK.[58–60] There is considerable variation in the clinical appearance and response to therapy and subsets of disease are usually classified based on the depth of the lesions within the cornea (**Fig. 17**). In all types of IMMK, signs of significant discomfort are not usually observed.

Superficial IMMK is characterized by a nonpainful subepithelial, superficial, white to yellow infiltrate surrounded by superficial branching corneal vascularization that

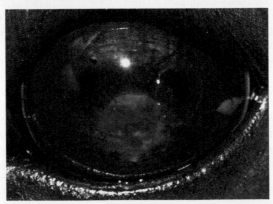

Fig. 16. Corneal fibrosis as the endpoint of healing 2 years after penetrating keratoplasty (PK). In most cases, it is recommended to cover a PK site with a conjunctival flap or amniotic membrane transplantation to protect the site from secondary infection, graft failure, and rejection.

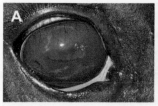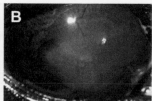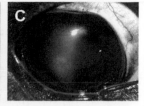

Fig. 17. (A) Superficial immune-mediated keratitis (IMMK). (B) Stromal IMMK. (C) Endothelial IMMK.

follows a waxing and waning course. This form can usually be controlled with topical steroids or cyclosporine. Superficial keratectomy seems to be useful to decrease antigen or autoantigen load and decrease recurrence.

The stromal form appears as a midstromal cellular infiltrate with surrounding corneal edema and vascularization. The cellular infiltrate is deeper and denser than the superficial form and the cornea is generally more opaque. Occasionally pockets or lacunae of green-tinged fluid and infiltrate are appreciated. Medical therapy is the same as for superficial IMMK; however, the stromal forms tend to be less responsive to intervention.

Deep or endothelial disease is also referred to as endotheliitis. This form is characterized by a chronic, slowly progressive, nonpainful focus of dense corneal edema with cellular infiltrate that accumulates at the level of the endothelium. Disruption of the function of the endothelium results in the accumulation of fluid in the stroma. Bullous keratopathy may also occur and result in secondary superficial focal or multifocal ulcerations. This form of IMMK may emerge as a precursor to a form of refractory anterior uveitis and secondary glaucoma. Endothelial disease is the least amenable to therapy, but some response may be seen with topical steroids and nonsteroidal antiinflammatory drugs such as bromfenac and systemic flunixin. Topical hypertonic saline may help to decrease the accumulation of microbullae.

Differences in the clinical appearance and response to therapy may vary depending on the geographic location of the affected patient. This finding suggests that different populations have different genetic predispositions or that different environmental factors influence or precipitate the disease process. The underlying etiology of IMMK in any form is unknown; however, the clinical signs suggest the natural healing process is attempting to respond to what the body presumes is a focus of disease or infection. IMMK may be the manifestation of an aberrant or deviant response to insult. Evidence for the involvement of a pathogen is lacking to date; however, it may be that such a pathogen has just yet to be identified.

Goals of therapy for corneal disease

1. Address any primary underlying etiology if one can be identified.

2. Treat or prevent infection.

3. Slow the breakdown/dissolution of corneal collagen.

4. Address secondary uveitis.

5. Provide structural support, if necessary; prevent self-trauma.

6. Analgesia.

When is surgical intervention indicated?
1. Corneal rupture or impending loss of integrity of the globe.
2. Progression of the condition of the cornea despite appropriate medical therapy.
3. Lack of response or progression of anterior uveitis despite appropriate medical therapy.
4. Targeted removal of diseased or infected tissue (remove offending organism, antigen, inflammatory products, cellular and ECM debris, and cytokine signals).

Anticollagenase medications and their actions	
Equine serum[a]	Alpha-2 macroglobulin and alpha-1 protease inhibitor; MMP, serine protease inhibitor; entrapment of protease
EDTA (0.17% in sterile water)[a]	Chelating agent (Ca and Zn); MMP inhibitor
N-Acetylcysteine (5% in artificial tears)[a]	Chelating agent (Ca and Zn); MMP inhibitor
Ilomostat (Galardin)	Competitive inhibition of MMP; direct inhibition of MMP; inhibits release of TNF-alpha
Doxycycline[a]	Competitive inhibition of MMP
Minocycline[a]	Competitive inhibition of MMP
Alpha-1 proteinase inhibitor	Serine protease inhibitor; entrapment of protease
Aprotinin	Serine protease inhibitor; entrapment of protease
Tissue inhibitor of metalloproteinase	Direct inhibition of MMPs
Amniotic membrane (tissue and homogenate)[a]	Direct inhibition of MMP; inhibits release of TNF-alpha
Tetanus antitoxin[a]	Competitive inhibition of MMP

Abbreviations: EDTA, ethylenediaminetetraacetic acid; MMP, matrix metalloproteinase; TNF, tumor necrosis factor.
[a] Available commercially or easily compounded.

REFERENCES

1. Gilger BC. Equine ophthalmology. In: Gelatt KN, Gilger BC, Kern TJ, editors. Veterinary ophthalmology. 5th edition. Ames (IA): Wiley-Blackwell; 2013. p. 1560–609.

2. Neaderland MH. Healing of experimentally induced corneal ulcers in horses. Am J Vet Res 1987;148:427–30.

3. Andrew SE, Ramsey DT, Hauptman JG, et al. Density of corneal endothelial cells and corneal thickness in eyes of euthanatized horses. Am J Vet Res 2001;62:479–82.

4. Ramsey D, Hauptmann J, Petereson-Jones S. Corneal thickness, intraocular pressure and optical corneal diameter in Rocky Mountain horses with cornea globosa or clinically normal corneas. Am J Vet Res 1999;60:1317–21.

5. Duane TD, Jaeger EA, Tasman W. Duane's foundations of clinical ophthalmology. Revised edition. Philadelphia: Lippincott; 1995.

6. Komai Y, Ushiki T. The three-dimensional organization of collagen fibrils in the human cornea and sclera. Invest Ophthalmol Vis Sci 1991;32:2244–58.

7. Meek KM, Fullwood NJ. Corneal and scleral collagens–a microscopist's perspective. Micron 2001;32:261–72.

8. Meek KM, Leonard DW, Connon CJ, et al. Transparency, swelling and scarring in the corneal stroma. Eye (Lond) 2003;17:927–36.
9. Takahashi T, Cho HI, Kublin CL, et al. Keratan sulfate and dermatan sulfate proteoglycans associate with type VI collagen in fetal rabbit cornea. J Histochem Cytochem 1993;41:1447–57.
10. Linsenmayer TF, Gibney E, Igoe F, et al. Type V collagen: molecular structure and fibrillar organization of the chicken alpha 1(V) NH2-terminal domain, a putative regulator of corneal fibrillogenesis. J Cell Biol 1993;121:1181–9.
11. Jester JV. Corneal crystallins and the development of cellular transparency. Semin Cell Dev Biol 2008;19:82–93.
12. Marfurt CF, Murphy CJ, Florczak JL. Morphology and neurochemistry of canine corneal innervation. Invest Ophthalmol Vis Sci 2001;42:2242–51.
13. Hogan MJ, Alvarado JA, Weddell JE. Histology of the human eye; an atlas and textbook. Philadelphia: Saunders; 1971.
14. Rich R. Clinical immunology principles and practice. St. Louis (MO): Mosby; 2001.
15. Bouchard CS. The ocular immune response. In: Krachmer J, Mannis M, Holland E, editors. Cornea. 2nd edition. Philadelphia: Elsevier; 2005. p. 59–93.
16. Pflugfelder SC. Tear fluid influence on the ocular surface. Adv Exp Med Biol 1998; 438:611–7.
17. Wilson SE, Chaurasia SS, Medeiros FW. Apoptosis in the initiation, modulation and termination of the corneal wound healing response. Exp Eye Res 2007;85: 305–11.
18. Zieske JD, Guimaraes SR, Hutcheon AE. Kinetics of keratocyte proliferation in response to epithelial debridement. Exp Eye Res 2001;72:33–9.
19. Wilson SE, Mohan RR, Ambrosio R Jr, et al. The corneal wound healing response: cytokine-mediated interaction of the epithelium, stroma, and inflammatory cells. Prog Retin Eye Res 2001;20:625–37.
20. Gan L, Fagerholm P, Kim H. Effect of leukocytes on corneal cellular proliferation and wound healing. Invest Ophthalmol Vis Sci 1999;40:5752–81.
21. Adler FH, Hart WM. Adler's physiology of the eye: clinical application. 9th edition. St Louis (MO): Mosby Year Book; 1992.
22. Wang X, Kamiyama K, Iguchi I, et al. Enhancement of fibronectin-induced migration of corneal epithelial cells by cytokines. Invest Ophthalmol Vis Sci 1994;35: 4001–7.
23. Mooradian DL, McCarthy JB, Skubitz AP, et al. Characterization of FN-C/H-V, a novel synthetic peptide from fibronectin that promotes rabbit corneal epithelial cell adhesion, spreading, and motility. Invest Ophthalmol Vis Sci 1993;34:153–64.
24. Watanabe K, Nakagawa S, Nishida T. Stimulatory effects of fibronectin and EGF on migration of corneal epithelial cells. Invest Ophthalmol Vis Sci 1987;28: 205–11.
25. Cameron JD. Corneal reaction to injury. In: Krachmer J, Mannis M, Holland E, editors. Cornea. 2nd edition. Philadelphia: Elsevier; 2005. p. 115–31.
26. Schermer A, Galvin S, Sun TT. Differentiation-related expression of a major 64K corneal keratin in vivo and in culture suggests limbal location of corneal epithelial stem cells. J Cell Biol 1986;103:49–62.
27. McLellan GJ. Deep and progressive corneal ulcers in horses: Inhibiting proteinase activity, controlling uveitis, and evaluating response to therapy. Comp Cont Ed Pract Vet 2004;26(12):972–5.

28. Ollivier FJ, Brooks DE, Kallberg ME, et al. Evaluation of various compounds to inhibit activity of matrix metalloproteinases in the tear film of horses with ulcerative keratitis. Am J Vet Res 2003;64:1081–7.
29. Ollivier FJ, Brooks DE, Van Setten GB, et al. Profiles of matrix metalloproteinase activity in equine tear fluid during corneal healing in 10 horses with ulcerative keratitis. Vet Ophthalmol 2004;6:397–406.
30. Sakimoto T, Sawa M. Metalloproteinases in corneal diseases: degradation and processing. Cornea 2012;31(Suppl 1):S50–6.
31. Myrna KE, Mendonsa R, Russell P, et al. Substratum topography modulates corneal fibroblast to myofibroblast transformation. Invest Ophthalmol Vis Sci 2012;53:811–6.
32. Myrna KE, Pot SA, Murphy CJ. Meet the corneal myofibroblast: the role of myofibroblast transformation in corneal wound healing and pathology. Vet Ophthalmol 2009;12(Suppl 1):25–7.
33. Jester JV, Ho-Chang J. Modulation of cultured corneal keratocyte phenotype by growth factors/cytokines control in vitro contractility and extracellular matrix contraction. Exp Eye Res 2003;77:581–92.
34. Jester JV, Petroll WM, Cavanagh HD. Corneal stromal wound healing in refractive surgery: the role of myofibroblasts. Prog Retin Eye Res 1999;18:311–56.
35. Wilson SE. Corneal myofibroblast biology and pathobiology: generation, persistence, and transparency. Exp Eye Res 2012;99:78–88.
36. Jester JV, Petroll WM, Barry PA, et al. Expression of alpha-smooth muscle (alpha-SM) actin during corneal stromal wound healing. Invest Ophthalmol Vis Sci 1995; 36:809–19.
37. Mulholland B, Tuft SJ, Khaw PT. Matrix metalloproteinase distribution during early corneal wound healing. Eye (Lond) 2005;19:584–8.
38. Brown D, Chwa M, Escobar M, et al. Characterization of the major matrix degrading metalloproteinase of human corneal stroma. Evidence for an enzyme/inhibitor complex. Exp Eye Res 1991;52:5–16.
39. Jester JV, Petroll WM, Barry PA, et al. Temporal, 3-dimensional, cellular anatomy of corneal wound tissue. J Anat 1995;186(Pt 2):301–11.
40. Dupps WJ Jr, Wilson SE. Biomechanics and wound healing in the cornea. Exp Eye Res 2006;83:709–20.
41. Fini ME, Stramer BM. How the cornea heals: cornea-specific repair mechanisms affecting surgical outcomes. Cornea 2005;24:S2–11.
42. Netto MV, Mohan RR, Sinha S, et al. Stromal haze, myofibroblasts, and surface irregularity after PRK. Exp Eye Res 2006;82:788–97.
43. Kawashima M, Kawakita T, Higa K, et al. Subepithelial corneal fibrosis partially due to epithelial-mesenchymal transition of ocular surface epithelium. Mol Vis 2010;16:2727–32.
44. Jester JV, Moller-Pedersen T, Huang J, et al. The cellular basis of corneal transparency: evidence for 'corneal crystallins'. J Cell Sci 1999;112:613–22.
45. Olson EA, Tu EY, Basti S. Stromal rejection following deep anterior lamellar keratoplasty: implications for postoperative care. Cornea 2012;31:969–73.
46. Foroutan A, Tabatabaei SA, Behrouz MJ, et al. Spontaneous wound dehiscence after penetrating keratoplasty. Int J Ophthalmol 2014;7:905–8.
47. O'Brien TP, Li Q, Ashraf MF, et al. Inflammatory response in the early stages of wound healing after excimer laser keratectomy. Arch Ophthalmol 1998;116: 1470–4.
48. Norlund ML, Pepose JS. Corneal response to infection. In: Krachmer J, Mannis M, Holland E, editors. Cornea. 2nd edition. Philadelphia: Elsevier; 2005. p. 95–114.

49. Tuli S, Goldstein M, Schultz GS. Modulation of corneal wound healing. In: Krachmer J, Mannis M, Holland E, editors. Cornea. 2nd edition. Philadelphia: Elsevier; 2005. p. 133–50.
50. Plummer CE, Ollivier FJ, Kallberg ME, et al. The use of amniotic membrane transplantation for ocular surface reconstruction: a review and series of 58 equine clinical cases (2002-2008). Vet Ophthalmol 2009;12(1):17–24.
51. Henriksen M, Andersen PH, Plummer CE, et al. Equine corneal stromal abscesses: an evolution in the understanding of pathogenesis and treatment during the past 30 years. Equine Vet Educ 2012. http://dx.doi.org/10.1111/j.2042-3292.2012.00440.x.
52. Ben-Shlomo G, Brooks DE, Plummer CE. In vitro efficacy and antiprotease activity of an antimicrobial ophthalmic drug combination against corneal pathogens of horses. Vet Med Anim Sci 2013;1:2, pp1-4.
53. Clode AB. Therapy of equine infectious keratitis: a review. Equine Vet J Suppl 2010;37:19–23.
54. Baker A, Plummer CE, Szabo N, et al. Doxycycline levels in preocular tear film of horses following oral administration. Vet Ophthalmol 2008;11(6):381–5.
55. Brooks DE, Plummer CE, Kallberg ME, et al. Corneal transplantation for inflammatory keratopathies in the horse: visual outcome in 206 cases (1993-2007). Vet Ophthalmol 2008;11(2):123–33.
56. Tsujita H, Plummer CE. Corneal stromal abscessation in two horses treated with intracorneal and subconjunctival injection of 1% voriconazole solution. Vet Ophthalmol 2013;16(6):451–8.
57. Welch PM, Gabal M, Betts DM, et al. In vitro analysis of antiangiogenic activity of fungi isolated from clinical cases of equine keratomycosis. Vet Ophthalmol 2000;3:145–52.
58. Matthews A, Gilger BC. Equine immune-mediated keratopathies. Vet Ophthalmol 2009;12(Suppl 1):10–6.
59. Gilger BC, Michau TM, Salmon JH. Immune-mediated keratitis in horses: 19 cases (1998-2004). Vet Ophthalmol 2005;8:233–9.
60. Pate DO, Clode AB, Olivry T, et al. Immunohistochemical and immunopathologic characterization of superficial stromal immune-mediated keratitis in horses. Am J Vet Res 2012;73(7):1067–73.

Medical and Surgical Management of Equine Recurrent Uveitis

Richard Joseph McMullen Jr, Dr med vet[a],*,
Britta Maria Fischer, DVM[b]

KEYWORDS

- Equine recurrent uveitis • Cyclosporine implant • Vitrectomy • Intravitreal injection
- Gentamicin

KEY POINTS

- Primary uveitis (isolated bouts of inflammation) must be differentiated from recurrent uveitis (multiple bouts of inflammation interrupted by periods of quiescence).
- Medical therapy/management alone leads to severe loss of vision or blindness in greater than 50% of all affected horses.
- There is a breed predilection for ERU in Appaloosa, draft, Knabstrupper, Icelandic, and warmblood breeds.

INTRODUCTION

Equine recurrent uveitis (ERU) is a widely recognized, complicated, multifaceted disease that is characterized by multiple, recurrent bouts of inflammation interrupted by variable periods of quiescence.[1–6] True recurrences of inflammation occur following complete elimination of inflammatory signs (eg, keratic precipitates [KPs], aqueous flare, miosis, cortical [equatorial] cataracts, vitreal opacification, fundus or optic nerve head [ONH] lesions) via topical and systemic antiinflammatory and immunosuppressive medication.[1,5,6] When medical therapy is withdrawn too soon, it may appear as if the inflammation returns within a short period of time (often 2–6 weeks). However, in many cases the signs associated with ERU had not been completely eliminated, but merely suppressed, giving the appearance that the eye had reached a stage of

Disclosure: The authors have nothing to disclose.
[a] Department of Clinical Sciences, Auburn University, Auburn University College of Veterinary Medicine, JT Vaughan Large Animal Teaching Hospital, 1500 Wire Road, Auburn, AL 36849-5540, USA; [b] Large Animal Internal Medicine, Auburn University, Auburn University College of Veterinary Medicine, JT Vaughan Large Animal Teaching Hospital, 1500 Wire Road, Auburn, AL 36849-5540, USA
* Corresponding author.
E-mail address: rjm0040@auburn.edu

Vet Clin Equine 33 (2017) 465–481
http://dx.doi.org/10.1016/j.cveq.2017.07.003
0749-0739/17/© 2017 Elsevier Inc. All rights reserved.

vetequine.theclinics.com

quiescence. This premature cessation of medications often occurs if the eyes become comfortable and subtle signs of inflammation (eg, KPs, aqueous flare, vitritis, inflammation of the ONH [optic neuritis]) are missed during reexamination (**Fig. 1**). This situation is referred to as a pseudorecurrence and can lead to a misdiagnosis or, worse, to progressive intraocular changes resulting in decreased vision or blindness if it goes undetected.[2]

A recent study from western Canada reported that 12 out of 32 (38%) horses with ERU were bilaterally blind on presentation and 20 out of 26 (76.9%) were bilaterally blind at the last follow-up, and 17 out of 20 (85%) of these blind horses were euthanized.[7] In another study from the southeastern United States, 96 out of 338 (28%) of the eyes presenting with ERU were blind on initial presentation.[8] Forty-one out of 338 (12.1%) eyes were enucleated and 29 out of 224 (14.9%) of the horses were euthanized.[8] Both of these studies reveal that too many horses are being referred far too late in the disease process (**Fig. 2**).[7,8] Therefore, it is essential that horses showing subtle clinical signs that are not immediately associated with ERU (intermittent redness [conjunctival hyperemia], tearing [epiphora], squinting [blepharospasm]) should be thoroughly examined for additional signs associated with chronic or recurrent uveitis (KPs, aqueous flare, miosis, decreased intraocular pressure [IOP]). This approach will allow for targeted therapy to be administered early in the disease process, which may prevent more severe secondary complications from developing, and will initiate a reevaluation pattern by owners, referring or primary veterinarians, and veterinary ophthalmologists alike, which may increase the likelihood of preserving vision.

There are several alternative treatment approaches that may prove useful in the earlier stages of intervention and may result in fewer horses losing vision or requiring more invasive surgical intervention to control inflammation caused by ERU. Such treatment options include intravitreal gentamicin (IVG) injections,[9–11] intravitreal triamcinolone injections,[12] intravitreal rapamycin injections,[13] suprachoroidal space injections of triamcinolone,[14] surgical placement of suprachoroidal cyclosporine sustained-release devices (cyclosporine implants),[15,16] and pars plana vitrectomy.[17–19] Diagnosing ERU and selecting the most appropriate treatment option is tedious, difficult, and riddled with setbacks. Conservative medical therapy provides the foundation of therapy and should be initiated in every case

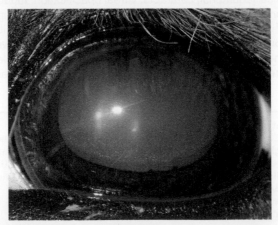

Fig. 1. Although the eye is open and comfortable, a moderate number of endothelial KPs remain visible during direct retroillumination. The dark, pinpoint KPs appear refractile during retroillumination. The pupil has been pharmacologically dilated.

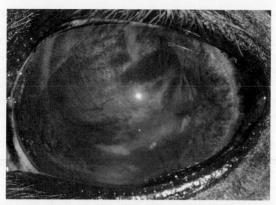

Fig. 2. Chronic and insidious panuveitis with corneal fibrosis and neovascularization, a shallow anterior chamber, rubeosis iridis (vascular engorgement of the iris vessels), and a ventrally displaced pupil (corectopia). The anteriorly displaced lens is entrapped posterior to the dorsal iris (note the spherical anterior protrusion in the dorsal portion of the iris).

of uveitis. Once all signs of inflammation have resolved, medical therapy can be discontinued. It is important that the antiinflammatory and immune-suppressive drugs are tapered off over a prolonged course of treatment (generally, 6–8 weeks) for 2 reasons. First, if the inflammation is not well controlled, clinical signs may worsen during the slow tapering of drugs, allowing for prompt increases in medication frequencies to again quickly suppress the inflammation. Second, stopping topical and systemic antiinflammatory and immunosuppressive therapy after 14 to 21 days, when subtle signs of inflammation (aqueous flare, pinpoint KPs) may be overlooked without careful examination, leads to the development of pseudorecurrences.[2] The return of bouts of inflammation in these situations is not caused by a new round of active uveitis but by a slow resurfacing of clinical signs of uveitis associated with the previous bout of insufficiently suppressed inflammation (**Fig. 3**).

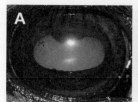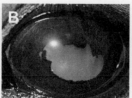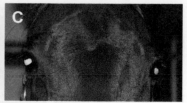

Fig. 3. (A) Right eye (oculus dexter [OD]) of a 20-year-old thoroughbred mare with chronic ERU 2 weeks following bilateral low-dose intravitreal injections of preservative-free gentamicin (4 mg) and topical and systemic antiinflammatory and immunosuppressive treatment. The pupil is only midrange, despite topical treatment with atropine. Note the degeneration of the corpora nigra and focal pigment deposition along the anterior lens capsule. Peripheral corneal neovascularization remains present, but is difficult to see because of the darkly pigmented iris. (B) Left eye (oculus sinister [OS]) of the horse from (A). The pupil is irregularly shaped (dyscoria), the corpora nigra show moderate degeneration, and there are focal adhesions between the pupil and anterior lens capsule (posterior synechiae) at both the 2:30 and 8:00 o'clock positions. Peripheral corneal neovascularization is present, but difficult to visualize, in this eye too. (C) A view of the same mare from the front reveals a yellow tapetal reflex, indicating that there is still significant inflammation present in both the anterior chamber and vitreous of both eyes (oculus uterque [OU]).

That is, these eyes never reach a true state of quiescence (periods without inflammation between separate bouts of active inflammation). Unrecognized pseudorecurrences may be mistaken for recurrent bouts of inflammation, suggesting that the underlying inflammation is more severe than may be the case. However, the development of pseudorecurrences can prove to be just as serious, if not more so, as a recurrent bout of inflammation recurring after a longer period of quiescence because the increased signs associated with the recurrences cause repeated and amplified damage to an already vulnerable eye.[2] Ensuring that a true state of quiescence is reached by gradually tapering medications over a prolonged period of time helps to accurately assess the horse's underlying state of inflammation. Recurrences that occur frequently (every 3–4 months, or less), and require longer durations of treatment before the signs of inflammation subside, are more likely to develop debilitating ocular complications associated with ERU (marked aqueous flare, fibrin accumulation in the anterior chamber [**Fig. 4**], posterior synechia [**Fig. 5**], vitritis, retinal folds or degeneration [**Fig. 6**], optic neuritis [**Fig. 7**]) or go blind than eyes with annual recurrent bouts of inflammation associated with minimal signs of disease (trace to mild flare, fine KPs [see **Fig. 1**], and miosis [**Fig. 8**]). Presently, there are several treatment options to reduce or prevent recurrent inflammation and that help to maintain vision in horses with ERU.[9–19]

PATIENT EVALUATION OVERVIEW

A detailed history is essential and can help to identify initial and mild recurrences, which often go unnoticed. Episodes of conjunctival hyperemia (redness), tearing (epiphora), and/or squinting (blepharospasm) that wax and wane are often reported by owners as being present before any so-called real eye problems develop. Many horses with ERU have 1 or several of the episodes described earlier during the years before clinical presentation. A heightened awareness or sensibility for the findings described earlier may lead to earlier recognition, earlier diagnosis, and ultimately to the earlier implementation of targeted treatment (**Table 1**).

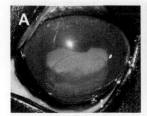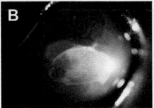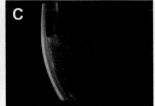

Fig. 4. (*A*) The left eye (OS) of a quarter horse yearling with a large fibrin clot in the anterior chamber. Note the other signs of severe uveitis: marked rubeosis irides, iris depigmentation and corpora nigra degeneration, and murky yellow tapetal reflex consistent with moderate aqueous flare and vitreal opacification. (*B*) Using tangential illumination (light directed obliquely from the temporal limbus) the superficial iris vessels (rubeosis irides) and the fibrin clot can be visualized with much more detail. Note the fibrin adhered to the corpora nigra along the dorsal edge of the pupil. (*C*) This handheld slit lamp image shows the thickened ventral cornea and partial adhesion of the fibrin to the corneal endothelium. Also note the smooth surface of the corpora nigra, which is visible just above the dorsal aspect of the fibrin clot occupying the entire depth of the anterior chamber (yellowish material between the white corneal light reflex and light brown slit of light along the surface of the iris).

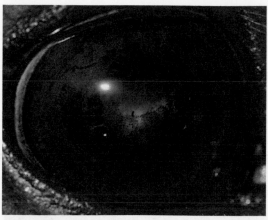

Fig. 5. Chronic recurrent panuveitis with predominantly anterior signs. Note the small tuft of fibrin near the iridocorneal angle of the anterior chamber at 8:30 o'clock. There is also marked posterior synechiae and diffuse pigment deposition along the anterior lens capsule. Note the thin, white, membranous veil containing pigment (fine punctate spots) spanning the ventral width of the pupil.

- ERU may also be further differentiated according to stages of chronicity, with cases being labeled as active (**Fig. 9**), quiescent (**Fig. 10**), or end stage (**Fig. 11**).
- The following anatomic diagnoses may make differentiation easier: panuveitis; panuveitis with predominant posterior signs; panuveitis with predominant anterior signs; anterior uveitis; posterior uveitis (**Fig. 12**); and heterochromic iridocyclitis with secondary keratitis (**Fig. 13** and **Table 2**).[20]

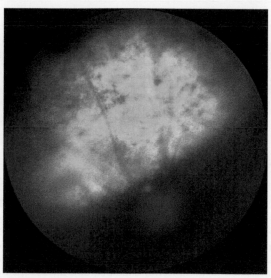

Fig. 6. The tapetal fundus of this 8-year-old quarter horse mare is markedly and diffusely hyperreflective, and there are multiple retinal folds manifest as linear bands extending radially from the ONH. This clinical presentation is very severe. Note the small area of subretinal cellular infiltrate along the 12:00 o'clock edge of the ONH.

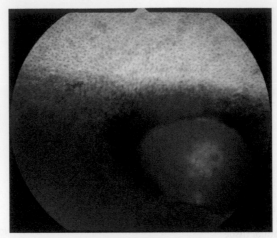

Fig. 7. The ONH in this horse with chronic recurrent panuveitis is moderately edematous and hyperemic. During binocular indirect ophthalmoscopy the anterior displacement of the thickened (edematous) peripapillary retina can be readily appreciated.

- With chronicity, regardless of which type of ERU is present, corneal vascularization, endothelial degeneration resulting in persistent corneal edema, linear corneal calcification (especially within and parallel to the palpebral margins), posterior (occasionally anterior) synechiae, cataract formation, and alterations in iris color and surface appearance commonly occur. Secondary glaucoma and phthisis bulbi can occur, ultimately resulting in irreversible blindness in many cases of ERU.

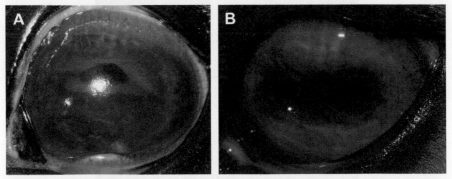

Fig. 8. (A) Miosis in the left eye (OS) of a 6-year-old quarter horse gelding. This active bout of inflammation recurred following early cessation of topical and systemic medications. This pseudorecurrence presented with marked blepharospasm, corneal neovascularization, and a shallow anterior chamber, with hypopyon (ventral iridocorneal angle), miosis, fibrin accumulation in the anterior chamber, and diffuse iris hypopigmentation. The corpora nigra are also atrophied (this is easier to visualize in the infrared image [B]). (B) Infrared image of OD from (A). Note that the pupil, degenerative/atrophied corpora nigra, and the fibrin veil in the anterior chamber are easier to visualize in the infrared image.

Table 1
Classification of equine recurrent uveitis

Categories of ERU	Description	Tissue Affected	Anatomic Diagnosis	Breed Predisposition

Classic	• Active bouts of inflammation
	• Followed by variable periods of quiescence
		Primary:
		  Uvea (iris, ciliary body, choroid)
		Secondary:
		  Cornea, anterior chamber, lens, vitreous, retina
			• Panuveitis
			• Panuveitis (anterior)
			• Panuveitis (posterior)
			• Anterior uveitis
			• HIK
				Warmblood
				Icelandic horses

Insidious	• Low-grade intraocular inflammation • Not outwardly painful • Gradual tissue destruction • Degeneration of multiple intraocular structures	• Posterior segment inflammation initially • Anterior segment inflammation follows • End-stage eyes globally affected	• Panuveitis • Panuveitis (anterior) • Panuveitis (posterior) • HIK	Appaloosa Draft breeds Knabstrupper
Posterior	• Acute bouts of inflammation are severe and respond slowly to medical therapy	• Predominantly posterior segment inflammation • Mild anterior inflammation is common	• Posterior uveitis • Panuveitis (posterior) • Panuveitis	Warmblood

Abbreviation: HIK, heterochromic iridocyclitis with secondary keratitis.

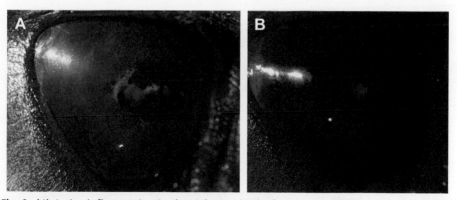

Fig. 9. (*A*) Active inflammation in the right eye (OD) of an 8-year-old bay warmblood mare with chronic recurrent panuveitis with predominantly anterior segment involvement. There is circumferential superficial corneal neovascularization and diffuse corneal haze, as well as a very shallow anterior chamber with complete miosis and fibrin and hyphema within the pupil. The iris is diffusely hyperpigmented and the posterior segment could not be visualized clinically. On ocular ultrasonography, only minimal vitreal hyperechogenicity could be appreciated. (*B*) Digital infrared image of the eye from (*A*). Despite the iris hyperpigmentation, a much better appreciation for the iridocorneal angle and pupil margin can be obtained with this method of clinical imaging.

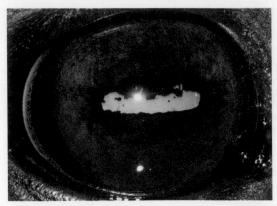

Fig. 10. Quiescent stage in the right eye (OD) from an 11-year-old bay warmblood gelding with a 3-year history of chronic recurrent inflammation that was only controlled while on high levels of immunosuppressive medications. He was ultimately treated with an intravitreal injection of low-dose gentamicin (4 mg). Although his eye had significant chronic signs of inflammation and secondary complications from ERU (he had significant discomfort, marked corneal vascularization, diffuse corneal fibrosis, complete miosis, and a mature cataract at the time of injection), he has remained free from recurrent bouts of inflammation for more than 602 days postinjection.

- It is important to consider/remember that current classifications of equine uveitis and ERU do not specifically differentiate between anatomic location (eg, anterior uveitis, posterior uveitis, and panuveitis) or clinical manifestation, but combine several potentially different clinical presentations into broader disease syndromes that are essentially a combination of several different individual classifications.

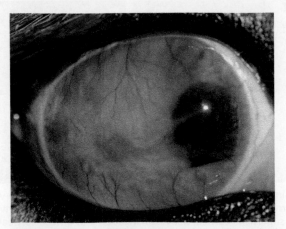

Fig. 11. End-stage uveitis. Phthisis bulbi (shrunken globe) with marked corneal vascularization, linear corneal fibrosis (representing folds in the cornea as a consequence of extremely low intraocular pressure), complete loss of anterior chamber depth, secluded pupil, and marked depigmentation of the iris. The posterior segment was not visible clinically, but ocular ultrasonography revealed moderate vitreal opacification and retinal detachment.

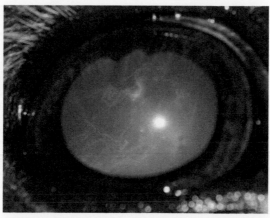

Fig. 12. Chronic, recurrent posterior uveitis in a 9-year-old Icelandic horse gelding. There is significant vitreal inflammation (vitritis) present, which can be readily identified through the pharmacologically dilated pupil. There are small, focal, anterior cortical cataracts associated with focal pigment deposition from recurrent bouts of inflammation but a relative lack of anterior segment signs.

PHARMACOLOGIC TREATMENT OPTIONS
Conventional Medical Therapy

Details of conventional medical therapy are given in **Tables 3–5**.

Long-term Control and/or Prevention of Recurrent Bouts of Inflammation

Conventional antiinflammatory and immunosuppressive medical therapy is necessary to reduce/eliminate inflammation and indirectly minimizes secondary ocular damage occurring as a result of each recurrent bout of inflammation. However, even when effective, conventional medical therapy cannot prevent recurrent bouts of inflammation. There are several other treatment options available that may effectively postpone or prevent such recurrences.

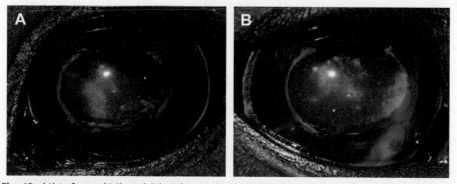

Fig. 13. (A) Left eye (OS) and (B) right eye (OD). Heterochromic iridocyclitis with secondary keratitis (HIK; endotheliitis) in a 12-year-old, bay warmblood gelding. Note the fine punctate (OS) and larger focal (OD) corneal opacifications and ventromedial areas of focal corneal edema. These findings, along with the diffuse depigmentation and iris atrophy/degeneration, are characteristic of this type of anterior uveitis.

Table 2
Clinical signs associated with equine recurrent uveitis

Categories of ERU	Clinical Signs		Sequelae
	Acute	Chronic	
Classic	• Increased lacrimation • Blepharospasm • Miosis • Photophobia • Aqueous flare • Intraocular fibrin • Hyphema • Hypopyon	• Miosis • Low IOP • Cataract formation/ progression • Phthisis bulbi	• Posterior synechiae • Misshapen pupil • Intermittent increases in IOP with chronicity • Severe vision loss and/ or blindness

Insidious	• Not outwardly painful
	  ○ Generally not detected until later stages of disease
	• Conjunctival and episcleral vascular hyperemia
	• Mild to moderate blepharitis
	• Aqueous flare
		• Focal or diffuse corneal edema (dull or lackluster appearance)
		• Iris atrophy/corpora nigra degeneration
		• Iris discoloration
		  ○ Hyperpigmentation
		  ○ Hypopigmentation
		• Lens subluxation or luxation
		  ○ Anterior or posterior
		• Shallow anterior chamber
			• Absent or sluggish pupillary light reflexes
			• Posterior synechiae
			• Pigment on anterior lens capsule
			• Pupillary occlusion
			• Focal/diffuse cataracts obscure visualization of the posterior segment
			• IOP generally low
			  ○ <12 mm Hg
			• Secondary glaucoma is common
			  ○ Grave prognosis for maintaining vision

Posterior	• Vitritis
	• Chorioretinal scarring
	• Retinal degeneration
	• Optic neuritis
	• Subtle anterior segment signs:
	  ○ KPs
	  ○ Aqueous flare
	  ○ Miosis
	  ○ Blepharospasm
		• Active/inactive chorioretinitis
		• Focal or diffuse retinal detachments
		  ○ Peripapillary retinal folds
		• Vitreous: cloudy/hazy appearance
		• ONH and surrounding retina may appear congested
			• Bullet-hole lesions
			• Butterfly lesions
			  ○ Prevalence associated with ERU unknown: lesions not commonly seen with ERU

NONPHARMACOLOGIC TREATMENT OPTIONS
Leptospira Vaccination

Leptospirosis, the intraocular (vitreous) sequestration of leptospiral antibodies, or the organism itself has been associated with ERU for decades.[21–28] Despite this fact, there is little known on the pathophysiology of leptospiral-induced ERU. Because leptospiral detection (antigen or antibodies) is not routinely performed, the prevalence of leptospiral-induced ERU remains enigmatic. A study from Zurich, Switzerland, described a useful protocol for ERU patient selection to better determine which horses are the best candidates for vitrectomy surgery.[29] A recent study from Germany, evaluating the use of low-dose IVG (4 mg) in which each horse was evaluated for the presence of leptospiral and equine herpesvirus (EHV) DNA (aqueous humor) and leptospiral antibody titers (serum and aqueous humor), showed that the overall exposure to leptospiral organisms is high (63 out of 79 eyes; 79.75%; C-value, 0–3), but that the presence of a C-value greater than 3 (indicating intraocular antibody production)

Table 3
Topical medications for equine recurrent uveitis

Drug Class	Medications	Frequency	Pros	Cons
Corticosteroid	Prednisolone acetate 1%	q 4–6 h	Potent Excellent ocular penetration	Immunosuppressive, predisposes to secondary corneal fungal infections
	Dexamethasone 0.1%	q 4–6 h	Potent Excellent ocular penetration	Immunosuppressive, predisposes to secondary corneal fungal infections
NSAIDs	Flurbiprofen, diclofenac, suprofen, or bromfenac	q 8–24 h	Good additional antiinflammatory medication alone or in conjunction with corticosteroids May be used when a corneal ulcer is present	May not be as effective as corticosteroids in acute phase of disease
Mydriatic	Atropine HCl 1%	q 4–24 h	Decreases iris muscle spasm (cycloplegia), induces mydriasis, minimizes synechia formation, stabilizes blood-ocular barriers	May decrease gut motility Monitor for signs of colic Pupil remains dilated for up to 21 d in normal eyes

Abbreviation: q, every.

was seen in only 16 out of 79 eyes (20.25%) of the horses tested.[11] The roe of EHV in ERU remains to be determined, but preliminary evaluation of the data mentioned earlier indicate that EHV-2 or EHV-5 DNA can be simultaneously detected in severe cases of ERU.[11] This information may become useful in the future when trying to determine the significance of leptospiral titers, especially in the context of vaccination. In addition, leptospiral vaccination in dogs can result in seroconversion, leading to increased titers from serovars other than Pomona.[30] If this occurs in horses, it will

Table 4
Subconjunctival medications for equine recurrent uveitis

Drug Class	Medications	Frequency	Pros	Cons
Corticosteroids	Methylprednisolone acetate (40 mg)	q 1–3 wk	Duration of action, 7–10 d	Markedly increased risk of secondary infections (fungal or bacterial) Cannot be removed once administered
	Triamcinolone acetonide (1–4 mg)	q 1–3 wk	Duration of action, 7–10 d	Markedly increased risk of secondary infections (fungal or bacterial) Cannot be removed once administered

Table 5
Systemic medications for equine recurrent uveitis

Drug Class	Medications	Frequency	Pros	Cons
NSAIDs	Flunixin meglumine (0.25–1.1 mg/kg IV, PO)	q 12–24 h	Potent and effective: ophthalmic disease	Chronic use may lead to gastric and renal toxicity
	Phenylbutazone (2.2–4.4 mg/kg IV, PO)	q 12–24 h	Moderately potent: ophthalmic disease	Chronic use may lead to gastric and renal toxicity Less effective than flunixin meglumine
Corticosteroids	Dexamethasone (6–10 mg/500 kg, PO or 2.6–6 mg/ 500 kg, IM)	q 24 h	Potent antiinflammatory	Use with caution and monitor for laminitis
	Prednisolone (100–300 mg/ 500 kg, IM, PO)	q 24 h	Potent antiinflammatory	Use with caution and monitor for laminitis

Abbreviations: IM, intramuscular; IV, intravenous; NSAIDs, nonsteroidal antiinflammatory drugs; PO, by mouth.

confuse things further. Therefore, it will become even more important in the future to evaluate both serum and aqueous humor for leptospiral titers and DNA and to correlate these results with the disease history and clinical signs present on presentation.[11,29]

COMBINATION THERAPIES

Intravitreal injections are routinely used in human ophthalmology to manage various forms of uveitis, and several medications have recently been evaluated in horses.[9–13] The data pertaining to the use of IVG injections have been anecdotal, and long-term follow-up data are presently not available.[9–11] A recent retrospective case series evaluating the efficacy of the IVG injections for various types and stages of ERU has been conducted and has influenced the way equine uveitis cases are managed.[11] The authors use a standard diagnostic protocol consisting of a complete and thorough ophthalmic examination by a board-certified veterinary ophthalmologist, which includes examination with a slit lamp biomicroscope, indirect ophthalmoscopy, tonometry, fluorescein staining of the external ocular structures, and color and infrared digital images, at a minimum. Ocular ultrasonography and fundus photography are performed as deemed necessary. Following examination and establishing a clinical diagnosis, the affected horses are sedated, local eyelid blocks are performed, and IVG 4-mg injections and aqueocentesis are performed.[11] The number of recurrences post-IVG injection is less than 15%. Therefore, the number of horses requiring surgical intervention or intensive long-term medical management is low. The complication rates associated with the injections are also low, but do consist of mature cataract formation/progression (5 out of 59 eyes; 8.5%) and/or retinal degeneration (3 out of 5 eyes; 5.1%).[11] Additional research and more long-term follow-up from a large number of treated horses will help to determine the true prevalence.[11]

Because aqueous paracentesis and IVG injections are performed under sedation, all risks associated with general anesthesia can be avoided, unless a horse requires additional treatment because it has not responded to the initial IVG injection, and surgical placement of a cyclosporine implant or pars plana vitrectomy are deemed necessary.[15–19] This logical step-by-step approach has reduced the number of horses requiring surgery, while simultaneously decreasing the number of recurrent bouts of inflammation in our study population.[11] Anecdotally, it is common to inject gentamicin and triamcinolone intravitreally as a combination, but we have refrained from doing so in order to gain an appreciation of the efficacy of gentamicin in controlling ERU and preventing recurrent bouts of inflammation, as well as to minimize/eliminate the complications that may occur when using intravitreal corticosteroids. Within our study population, the use of triamcinolone acetonide has not been deemed necessary (**Table 6**).[11]

Another promising technique is the injection of triamcinolone acetonide into the suprachoroidal space.[14] This technique requires specially machined microneedles to perform, and potentially eliminates the secondary complications (corneal ulceration, secondary infection, corneal mineralization [**Fig. 14**], and endophthalmitis) associated with intravitreal triamcinolone injections.[13]

SURGICAL TREATMENT OPTIONS

There are currently 2 surgical options to treat ERU: suprachoroidal placement of sustained-release cyclosporine devices and dual-port pars plana vitrectomy.[15–19] It is commonly inferred that ERU in Europe is different from ERU seen in the United States.[1–4] Although there are geographic and breed-related differences that are more pronounced on either side of the Atlantic Ocean, there are more similarities than is generally supposed.[31,32]

Table 6
Medications for intravitreal and suprachoroidal space injections for equine recurrent uveitis

Route of Administration	Medications	Frequency	Pros	Cons
Intravitreal injection	Gentamicin (4 mg, preservative free)	Once	Potential to interrupt and stop recurrent bouts of inflammation	Mechanism of action unknown May cause cataract formation/maturation or retinal degeneration
	Triamcinolone acetonide (2.5–5.0 mg)	As necessary based on clinical response	Duration of action, 4–9 mo (monitor intravitreal crystals)	Markedly increased risk of secondary infections (fungal or bacterial) and corneal degeneration Cannot be removed once administered
Suprachoroidal space injection	Triamcinolone acetonide (5.0 mg)	As necessary based on clinical response	Corneal drug concentration eliminated: drastically reduced risk of secondary infection	Special needles required (not commercially available)

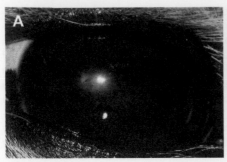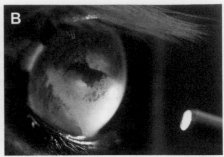

Fig. 14. (*A*) Diffuse corneal mineralization associated with intravitreal triamcinolone acetonide injection. This type of corneal mineralization is often anecdotally associated with the chronic use of topical corticosteroids (especially dexamethasone) as well. (*B*) Using oblique (or tangential) lighting as the sole source of illumination, the corneal mineralization of the cornea from (*A*) can be highlighted for better visualization.

Some of the misconceptions about ERU are linked to the simultaneous development of the pars plana vitrectomy[17–19] and intravitreal and subsequently suprachoroidal cyclosporine implants[15,33,34] in Germany and North Carolina, respectively. There is a greater population of Appaloosa and western sport horses in the United States compared with Germany's more dominant warmblood population. Coupled with the different examination techniques routinely used in each country, this accounts for some of the misconceptions. The many types and stages of ERU can be seen in both Europe and the United States, just at variable frequencies.

Suprachoroidal Cyclosporine Implants

Horses with documented recurrent bouts of inflammation that are well controlled with conventional medical therapy (eg, topical and systemic antiinflammatory medication effectively leading to a period of quiescence that remains even after medications are discontinued) are excellent candidates for suprachoroidal cyclosporine implantation.[33,34]

Inflammation can be well controlled and recurrences all but eliminated following placement of suprachoroidal cyclosporine implants.[34]

Pars Plana Vitrectomy

The pars plana vitrectomy, both single port and dual port, has been well described, and has seen widespread use, especially in Europe.[17–19,29,35] It is an intraocular procedure that is used primarily to remove the core of the vitreous with the horse under general anesthesia. The procedure is not routinely performed under an operating microscope and direct visualization of the vitrector (cutting instrument) is achieved using an indirect ophthalmoscope. Without the use of a condensing lens there is limited depth perception and extreme care must be taken not to inadvertently damage the posterior lens or retina. Although the procedure has seen widespread use in Europe, there are few studies evaluating the long-term surgical results following vitrectomy.[19,29,36] Reported postsurgical complications include transient hypopyon, vitreal and/or retinal hemorrhage, retinal detachment, and cataract formation.[1,19] Horses with *Leptospira*-associated uveitis (C-value >4), and moderate to severe vitreal inflammation (membranes) are considered good surgical candidates.[29]

EVALUATION OF OUTCOME AND LONG-TERM RECOMMENDATIONS

Conservative medical management is, and should be, the first line of treatment to stop active uveitis and to slow down or prevent recurrent bouts of inflammation. Once a horse has been diagnosed with ERU, it requires diligent and lifelong monitoring and care and the owners should be prepared for this.[8] If recurrences occur despite appropriate medical therapy,[6–8] then additional treatment modalities should be considered.

In these situations, intravitreal and suprachoroidal injections provide an effective alternative to surgery, and can be performed under sedation, at the same time as diagnostic aqueous paracentesis.[11–14,29] If the horse does not respond favorably to conservative medical or injection therapy, the best surgical option for each individual horse can be made based on the clinical signs that are still present, the anatomic diagnosis, and the laboratory results.[1,11,29,35]

SUMMARY

ERU is a complex and challenging disease, but clinicians are currently in a position to improve the long-term results with early intervention, making a proper diagnosis, and selecting the most appropriate treatment option for the individual horse. The reality is that more horses will go blind or experience debilitating ocular damage long term with medical therapy alone than with any other form of intervention.[1,7,8] Although the risks associated with the various injections and surgical options (cataract formation, retinal degeneration, retinal detachment, intraocular hemorrhage) remain present, the likelihood of their occurring can be dramatically reduced.[10,11,16,19,29,36]

REFERENCES

1. Gilger BC, Hollingsworth SR. Diseases of the uvea, uveitis, and recurrent uveitis. In: Gilger BC, editor. Equine ophthalmology. 3rd edition. Ames (IA): John Wiley; 2017. p. 369–415.
2. Lowe RC. Equine uveitis: A UK perspective. Equine Vet J 2010;(Suppl 37):46–9.
3. Spiess BM. Equine recurrent uveitis: the European viewpoint. Equine Vet J 2010;(Suppl 37):50–6.
4. Gilger BC. Equine recurrent uveitis: the viewpoint from the USA. Equine Vet J 2010;(Suppl 37):57–61.
5. Gilger BC, Michau TM. Equine recurrent uveitis: new methods of management. Vet Clin North Am Equine Pract 2004;20:417–27.
6. Allbaugh RA. Equine recurrent uveitis: a review of clinical assessment and management. Equine Vet Educ 2016. http://dx.doi.org/10.1111/eve.12548.
7. Sandmeyer LS, Bauer BS, Feng CX, et al. Equine recurrent uveitis in western Canada: a retrospective study. Dorothy Havemeyer Equine Ophthalmology Symposium. Malahide (Ireland). June 2–4, 2016. p. 20.
8. Gerding JC, Gilger BC. Prognosis and impact of equine recurrent uveitis. Equine Vet J 2016;48:290–8.
9. Pinard C. Gentamicin injection. American College of Veterinary Ophthalmologists Annual Conference. Nashville (TN). October 12–15, 2005.
10. Kleinpeter A. Intravitreale Gentamicin-Injektion zur Therapie der equinen rezidivierender Uveitis – Methode und Fallauswertung. Leipzig (Germany): Leipziger Tierärztekongress; 2014. 7.
11. Fischer BM, Brehm W, McMullen Jr RJ. Treatment of recurrent uveitis in horses with intravitreal low-dose gentamicin injection. Dorothy Havemeyer Equine Ophthalmology Symposium. Malahide (Ireland). June 2–4, 2016. p. 22.

12. Yi NY, Davis JL, Salmon JH, et al. Ocular distribution and toxicity of intravitreal injection of triamcinolone acetonide in normal equine eyes. Vet Ophthalmol 2008; 11(Suppl 1):15–9.
13. Douglas LC, Yi NY, Davis JL, et al. Ocular toxicity and distribution of subconjunctival and intravitreal rapamycin in horses. J Vet Pharmacol Ther 2008;31:511–6.
14. Gilger BC. Use of suprachoroidal injection of triamcinolone acetonide for treatment of non-responsive active uveitis. Dorothy Havemeyer Equine Ophthalmology Symposium. Malahide (Ireland). June 2–4, 2016. p. 24.
15. Gilger BC, Salmon JH, Wilkie DA, et al. A novel bioerodible deep scleral lamellar cyclosporine implant for uveitis. Invest Ophthalmol Vis Sci 2006;47:2596–605.
16. Gilger BC, Wilkie DA, Clode AB, et al. Long-term outcome after implantation of a suprachoroidal cyclosporine drug delivery device in horses with recurrent uveitis. Vet Ophthalmol 2010;13:294–300.
17. Werry H, Gerhards H. Möglichkeiten und Indikationen zur chirurgischen Behandlung der equinen rezidivierender Uveitis (ERU). Pferdeheilk 1991;7:321–31.
18. Werry H, Gerhards H. The surgical therapy of equine recurrent uveitis. Tierärztl Prax 1992;20:178–86.
19. Fruhauf B, Ohnesorge B, Deegen E, et al. Surgical management of equine recurrent uveitis with single port pars plana vitrectomy. Vet Ophthalmol 1998;1:137–51.
20. Pinto NI, McMullen RJ Jr, Linder KE, et al. Clinical histopathological and immunohistochemical characterization of a novel equine disorder: heterochromic iridocyclitis with secondary keratitis in adult horses. Vet Ophthalmol 2014. http://dx.doi.org/10.1111/vop.12234.
21. Davidson MG, Nasisse MP, Roberts SM. Immunodiagnosis of leptospiral uveitis in two horses. Equine Vet J 1987;19:155–7.
22. Dwyer AE, Crockett RS, Kalsow CM. Association of leptospiral seroreactivity and breed with uveitis and blindness in horses: 372 cases (1986-1993). J Am Vet Med Assoc 1995;207:1327–31.
23. Brem S, Gerhards H, Wollanke B, et al. Demonstration of intraocular *Leptospira* in 4 horses suffering from equine recurrent uveitis (ERU). Berl Münch Tierärztl Wochenschr 1998;111:415–7.
24. Brem S, Gerhards H, Wollanke B, et al. Leptospira isolated from the vitreous body of 32 horses with recurrent uveitis (ERU). Berl Münch Tierärztl Wochenschr 1999; 112:390–3.
25. Wollanke B, Rohrbach BW, Gerhards H. Serum and vitreous humor antibody titers in and isolation of *Leptospira interrogans* from horses with recurrent uveitis. J Am Vet Med Assoc 2001;219:795–800.
26. Faber NA, Crawford M, LeFebvre RB, et al. Detection of *Leptospira* spp. in the aqueous humor of horses with naturally acquired recurrent uveitis. J Clin Microbiol 2000;38:2731–3.
27. Halliwell RE, Brim TA, Hines MT, et al. Studies on equine recurrent uveitis. II: The role of infection with *Leptospira interrogans* serovar Pomona. Curr Eye Res 1985; 4:1033–40.
28. Gilger BC, Salmon JH, Yi NY, et al. Role of bacteria in the pathogenesis of recurrent uveitis in horses from the southeastern United States. Am J Vet Res 2008;69: 1329–35.
29. Tömördy E, Hässig M, Spiess BM. The outcome of pars plana vitrectomy in horses with equine recurrent uveitis with regard to the presence or absence of intravitreal antibodies against various serovars of *Leptospira interrogans*. Pferdeheilk 2010;26:251–4.

30. Barr SC, McDonough PL, Scipioni-Ball RL, et al. Serologic responses of dogs given a commercial vaccine against *Leptospira interrogans* serovar Pomona and *Leptospira kirschneri* serovar Grippotyphosa. Am J Vet Res 2005;66:1780–4.
31. Fritz KL, Kaese HJ, Valberg SJ, et al. Genetic risk factors for insidious equine recurrent uveitis in Appaloosa horses. Anim Genet 2014;45:392–9.
32. Kulbrock M, Lehner S, Metzger J, et al. A genome-wide association study identifies risk loci to equine recurrent uveitis in German warmblood horses. PLoS One 2013;8:e71619.
33. Gilger BC, Malok E, Stewart T, et al. Effect of an intravitreal cyclosporine implant on experimental uveitis in horses. Vet Immunol Immunopathol 2000;76:239–55.
34. Gilger BC, Wilkie DA, Davidson MG, et al. Use of an intravitreal sustained-release cyclosporine delivery device for treatment of equine recurrent uveitis. Am J Vet Res 2001;62:1892–6.
35. Dorrego-Keiter E, Tóth J, Dikker L, et al. Detection of *Leptospira* by culture of vitreous humor and detection of antibodies against *Leptospira* in vitreous humor and serum of 225 horses with equine recurrent uveitis. Berl Münch Tierärztl Wochenschr 2016;129:209–15.
36. Winterberg A, Gerhards H. Long-term results of pars plana vitrectomy in equine recurrent uveitis. Pferdeheilk 1997;4:377–83.

Disease and Surgery of the Equine Lens

Wendy M. Townsend, DVM, MS

KEYWORDS

• Lens • Cataract • Intraocular lens • Phacoemulsification

KEY POINTS

• Examination of the lens is a key portion of the ophthalmic examination.
• Pharmacologic dilation is necessary to adequately evaluate the lens.
• Phacoemulsification is the only treatment option for cataracts impairing vision.

INTRODUCTION

The lens is a transparent, biconvex structure positioned behind the iris and anterior to the vitreous. The lens fine focuses light on the retina.[1] The lens is suspended by zonular fibers that extend from the lens equator to the ciliary body. The equator is the outer edge of the lens hidden by the iris, whereas the lens axis is directed anterior to posterior. The lens is surrounded by an external capsule that encloses a peripheral cortex and inner nucleus.[1] If the lens is imagined as a hard-boiled egg, the shell would be the capsule, the egg-white would be the cortex, and the yolk would be the nucleus. The lens capsule is the basement membrane of the single, outer layer of lens epithelial cells. At the equator of the lens, epithelial cells elongate to form lens fibers. The lens fibers stretch from anterior to posterior and meet to form the anterior and posterior sutures.[1] The anterior suture is Y-shaped to slightly irregular, the posterior suture is Y to triradiate in shape, and both can normally be visualized.[2] The lens fibers form the lens cortex. As each new layer forms, the lens fibers are pushed centrally. The mature fibers form the adult portion of the nucleus. The central portion of the nucleus formed during embryologic development.[1,3] With age, the continual addition of new lens fibers compresses the nucleus and changes the degree that light is bent while passing through the lens. The nucleus becomes visible as a grayish, central sphere. This normal aging change is termed nuclear or lenticular sclerosis.[2]

Disclosure Statement: The author has nothing to disclose.
Department of Veterinary Clinical Sciences, Purdue University, 625 Harrison Street, West Lafayette, IN 47907-2026, USA
E-mail address: townsenw@purdue.edu

Vet Clin Equine 33 (2017) 483–497
http://dx.doi.org/10.1016/j.cveq.2017.07.004
0749-0739/17/© 2017 Elsevier Inc. All rights reserved.

Differentiating nuclear sclerosis from a cataract
Retroilluminate the eye from a distance.
Nuclear sclerosis DOES NOT block the tapetal reflection.
A cataract DOES block the tapetal reflection.

PATIENT EVALUATION OVERVIEW
Assess Vision

A complete ophthalmic examination is needed to accurately identify cataracts and determine their significance. Before administration of any type of sedation, vision should be assessed using the menace response:

- Ensure the horse has a positive palpebral reflex.
- Be sure not to touch the vibrissae or create air currents that could results in a false-positive response while performing the menace test.
- Move a hand from several directions to appraise the entire visual field.

The horse can be observed navigating a maze test constructed of straw bales, shavings bags, or other obstacles to further evaluate vision. In the author's experience, horses with partial vision loss may spook or be more distressed than horses with complete vision loss on 1 or both sides. The owner should be questioned about specific visual or behavioral concerns, such as spooking or shying on a particular side or in certain situations. For the remainder of the examination, a darkened area facilitates visualization of focal or subtle lesions.

Assess Pupillary Light Reflexes

The pupillary light reflexes (PLRs), both direct and consensual, are then evaluated using a Finoff transilluminator. If a transilluminator is not available, an LED or halogen penlight can be used. A bright, focused light source is needed to ensure adequate retinal stimulation to cause pupillary constriction. No matter the size or density of the cataract, the pupil should constrict. Absence of a PLR should prompt further examination to identify other ocular pathology. If the pupil is dilated and nonresponsive, but the eye is visual and/or a consensual PLR is present, the owner should be questioned about potential administration of topical mydriatics, such as atropine.

Dilate the Pupil

The intraocular pressures (IOPs) should then be assessed. As long as the IOP is within the normal range (see Tammy Miller Michau's article, "Glaucoma," in this issue for further details), the pupil should be pharmacologically dilated to allow maximal visualization of the lens and retina. Tropicamide 1% ophthalmic solution should be applied topically to both eyes. Mydriasis occurs within 20 minutes to 30 minutes.[3] Tropicamide is used instead of atropine because of tropicamide's faster onset and shorter duration of action.[3]

Sedation

Once mydriasis occurs, the examination can proceed. Depending on a horse's temperament, sedation may be required to fully assess the globe. Xylazine is typically sufficient, but detomidine or romifidine alone or in combination with butorphanol may be necessary in some horses. If blepharospasm is significant, an auriculopalpebral nerve block can be performed to facilitate opening of the eyelids.

Distant Direct Examination

Initially stand at arm's length from the globe and direct the light from a Finoff trans-illuminator or halogen penlight into the eye.[4] The direct illumination causes opacities in the lens to appear white (**Fig. 1**). Redirecting the light to obtain a bright tapetal reflection retroilluminates lens opacities, causing them to appear black. In older horses, a concentric cortical lamination, or onion ring appearance, can be noted within the cortex but does not represent a cataract and is of no clinical significance.[2]

Magnified Examination

After opacities have been identified with distant direct illumination, closer inspection is warranted. Magnification is helpful to identify focal opacities. Ideally, a slit-lamp biomicroscope is used, but 3.5-times to 5-times magnification head loupes and a trans-illuminator or direct ophthalmoscope also work well. The size, shape, and location of opacities should be carefully noted. Lesions can be axial or equatorial and further described as capsular, subcapsular, cortical, perinuclear, or nuclear (**Fig. 2**). Focal lesions along the visual axis, particularly in the posterior cortex or capsule, cause more visual difficulties than those in the lens periphery due to greater interference with the focusing of light on the retina.[5] Cataracts should be documented with photographs or detailed drawings.

Additional Examination Components

The cornea should be examined for evidence of previous penetrating injury or trauma. Aqueous flare, if present, denotes active inflammation. The anterior lens capsule should be closely examined for posterior synechia or pigment clumps; both suggest

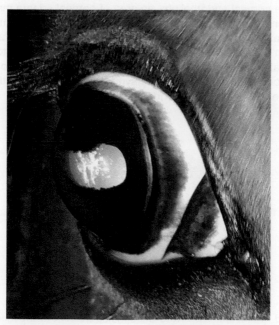

Fig. 1. The incipient cataracts appear white with direct illumination. The pupil has not yet been dilated. Visual deficits were not noted.

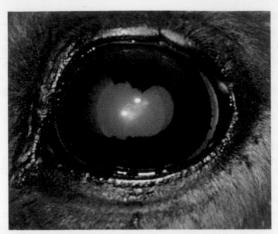

Fig. 2. Nuclear cataract in an older-grade gelding. Vision was not appreciably impaired.

previous bouts of inflammation. Clumped and atrophied corpora nigra and/or a fibrous or fibrovascular membrane spanning the anterior capsule can occur secondary to chronic inflammation.

The position of the lens should be assessed. Chronic inflammation can cause destruction of the lens zonules leading to lens luxation or subluxation.[6] Visualization of the lens' equator is not normal and means the lens is either no longer correctly positioned or the lens is malformed (lens coloboma). If the lens remains behind the iris within the patellar fossa but has shifted, this is a lens subluxation (**Fig. 3**). If the lens has come forward into the anterior chamber, this is an anterior lens luxation. If the lens contacts the corneal endothelium, an area of corneal edema may be present. If the lens has fallen back into the vitreous, this is a posterior lens luxation. Even if clear at the time of luxation, chronically luxated lenses often become cataractous.[7] Shifts in lens position can cause elevations in IOP or can occur secondary to glaucoma and resultant buphthalmos. Lens subluxation and cataract formation also occur with multiple congenital ocular anomalies (MCOA) syndrome associated with the silver coat dolor dilution, previously termed anterior segment dysgenesis.[8–11]

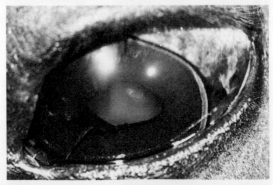

Fig. 3. Subluxated cataractous lens. Note the aphakic crescent in the medial aspect of the pupil. Several strands of vitreous extend through the pupil nasally into the anterior chamber.

The vitreous should be examined, if possible, for liquefaction (syneresis) or collagen clumping, which can occur secondary to inflammation or as an aging change.[12] A cellular infiltrate within the vitreous denotes active inflammation. Vitreous within the anterior chamber can occur with syneresis alone, but close inspection of the lens position is warranted because vitreal prolapse can also occur with zonular rupture.

Unless the cataract precludes their visualization, the retina and optic nerve should be examined. Indirect ophthalmoscopy is typically less affected by lens opacities and allows better visualization of the retina in their presence. The ability to visualize the retina suggests the degree of visual impairment the cataract should be causing, that is, if the retina and optic nerve are easily visualized, the cataract is unlikely to be causing significant visual dysfunction.

Classification of Cataracts

Cataracts can be classified based on the amount of the lens that is involved (incipient, immature (**Fig. 4**), mature, or hypermature) (**Table 1**); age of onset (congenital, juvenile, or senile); or cause. Mature cataracts involve 100% of the lens, completely block the tapetal reflection, and cause blindness (**Fig. 5**). Hypermature cataracts have sparkly appearing lens material due to liquefaction and resorption of lens proteins, causing subsequent shrinking and wrinkling of the lens capsule. Lens-induced uveitis can occur as lens proteins leak through the lens capsule and stimulate an immune response.[13] Significant shrinking of the lens capsule can cause tearing of the zonules and allow the lens to subluxate or luxate. Although cataracts diagnosed in foals and in horses with equine recurrent uveitis (ERU) are the most likely to progress,[2] any cataract has the potential to progress, and therefore close monitoring for cataract progression and for lens-induced uveitis is important in any horse with cataracts. Poor control of uveitis in horses with ERU may be associated with more rapid progression of cataracts. Location of the cataract within the lens also has implications for likelihood of progression, with cataracts located in the most metabolically active portion of the lens (ie, the equator or the anterior cortex) more likely to progress.

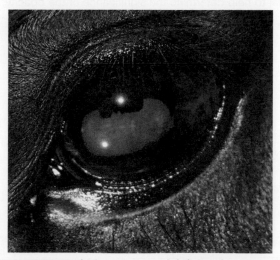

Fig. 4. Late immature cataract, which caused visual deficits. The eye is otherwise normal.

Table 1		
Classification of cataracts by percentage of lens involved		
Stage	**% Lens Involved**	**Visual Status**
Incipient	<15%	Visual
Immature	<15% to 99%	Visual to impaired
Mature	100%	Blind
Hypermature	100%, now resorbing	Blind unless marked resorption

Causes of Cataracts

Cataracts are the most common congenital ocular finding in foals and occur in 35% of foals with ocular lesions.[14,15] Cataracts may be seen in otherwise normal eyes or may be associated with other ocular anomalies, such as microphthalmia, anterior segment dysgenesis, persistent pupillary membranes, aniridia (absence of the iris), lens coloboma, posterior lenticonus, persistent hyaloid artery, and persistent hyperplastic primary vitreous.[3,16,17] Cataracts are inherited as a dominant trait in certain Belgian, quarter horse, and Thoroughbred bloodlines.[2,17,18] The Belgians and quarter horses may have aniridia, associated with the cataracts.[17,18] Owners should be counseled regarding the heritable nature of these cataracts. Morgan horses have a dominantly inherited, nonprogressive, nuclear, congenital cataract.[19,20] Nuclear and perinuclear cataracts typically do not progress and become smaller over time in relation to the rest of the lens as the lens fibers are compressed.[2,3] Congenital cataracts occur in horses with MCOA syndrome, which is inherited as an incompletely dominant trait and is due to a mutation at the *PMEL17* locus (**Fig. 6**).[8–11]

In adult horses, cataracts are most commonly caused by ERU.[2,3,21] ERU is estimated to affect 8% to 25% of the equine population and almost all of those horses develop some degree of cataract.[21] The cataracts associated with ERU are also likely to progress unless the inflammation can be completely controlled. Other causes for cataracts in adult horses include trauma, whiplash injury, neoplasia, and retinal detachment.[22,23] Cataracts have also been noted in 5% to 7% of horses with otherwise normal ophthalmic examinations.[2,24] Therefore, close inspection of the rest of the globe is critical to help determine the significance of the opacity.

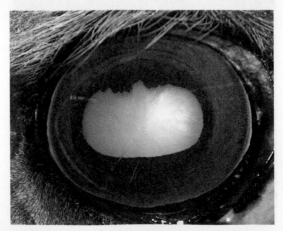

Fig. 5. Mature cataract. Note complete lack of tapetal reflection. This eye was not visual.

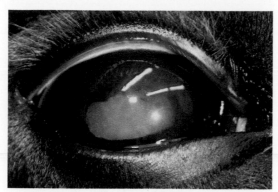

Fig. 6. Hypermature cataract in an eye with MCOA syndrome. Note the abnormal pupillary margin, clumped corpora nigra, and miotic pupil.

Senile cataracts may occur in horses over 18 years of age but rarely are they significant enough to interfere with vision.[2] Senile cataracts are typically bilateral, although not necessarily symmetric. In 1 survey, 58% of geriatric horses had cataracts.[25] Senile cataracts are often located along the suture lines or as focal opacities within the anterior and/or posterior cortex.[2] A yellowing of the lens, brunescence, may also occur in older horses.

PHARMACOLOGIC TREATMENT OPTIONS

Currently no therapies exist that dissolve cataracts. The only treatment option for vision-impairing cataracts is surgical removal. Any inflammation should be controlled with either topical or systemic anti-inflammatory medications. If the cataracts are focal or nuclear, pupillary dilation with 1% atropine ophthalmic solution might help to improve vision by widening the visual axis.[19,22,26] The atropine is applied once daily until pupillary dilation occurs and the effects on vision are then evaluated. The mydriasis could also cause photophobia, blepharospasm, and epiphora.

SURGICAL TREATMENT OPTIONS
Phacoemulsification

The only true therapy for vision impairing cataracts is surgical removal. The preferred method for surgical removal is phacoemulsification.[22,27–30] Phacoemulsification allows a small incision, which is associated with a minimal risk of iris prolapse intraoperatively and postoperative inflammation that can typically be controlled with routine medical therapy for uveitis. Ultrasonic energy breaks up the lens fibers while simultaneously aspirating fragments and providing an in-flow of fluid to keep the anterior chamber inflated. Due to the large size of equine eyes, phacoemulsification handpieces designed specifically for horses should be used, rather than handpieces designed for humans (**Fig. 7**).[13,31,32]

Equine cataract surgery does raise some ethical and philosophic concerns.[3] Even after placement of an intraocular lens (IOL), the vision of a horse after cataract surgery cannot be considered completely normal.[3] Therefore, if a rider were injured by an aphakic (without a lens) or pseudophakic horse, questions regarding liability may be raised.[3] The vision of aphakic horses is markedly hyperopic (far-sighted).[33,34] Some owners have reported their horse's vision seemed normal, but others noted differences in vision, particularly at night.[27,28,33–36]

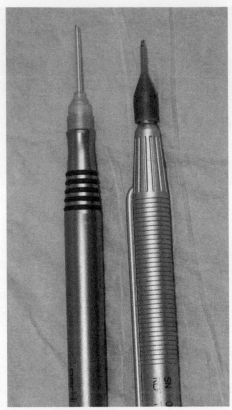

Fig. 7. Phacoemulsification needle for the equine eye on the left versus the standard needle on the right. Note the increased length of the equine needle. (*Courtesy of* Oertli Instrumente AG, Berneck, Switzerland; with permission.)

Key components of equine cataract surgery are proper patient selection and owner education. Owners need to understand the commitment in terms of both time and money. For at least 1 month to 2 months postoperatively, frequent topical medications are required. Horses must be on stall rest for at least a month. If complications occur, they often result in a loss of vision and may necessitate removal of the eye as well.

Patients should be halter-broken and easily handled. Struggling to apply medications postoperatively increases the risk of suture rupture. Weaning of foals can allow them to be handled more easily but is not essential. Foals with congenital cataracts should have cataract surgery performed within the first 6 months of life to ensure normal development of the visual pathways.[29,37] After birth, formation of images on the retina stimulates further development of the brain and associated visual pathways. In humans and cats, if visual stimuli are not received during the critical period for the development of visual pathways, the eye remains blind even after the opacity is removed, a condition termed deprivation amblyopia.[37–39] Because this critical period has not been determined for horses, it is safest to take a conservative approach by assuming it occurs early in life and remove cataracts as soon as is reasonable.

The globe should be otherwise normal on ophthalmic examination. The presence of marked corneal opacities, anterior or posterior synechia, miosis, ocular hypotony, lens capsule rupture, lens instability, extensive capsular fibrosis, and/or herniation of vitreous into the anterior chamber precludes surgery.[3,13] Horse with ERU must have their inflammation well controlled. An electroretinogram should be performed to rule out congenital stationary night blindness and ensure normal retinal function, particularly in horses with a history of ERU.[40-44] Ocular ultrasonography should be performed to rule out retinal detachment, persistent hyaloid arteries, vitreal abnormalities, and posterior lens capsule rupture, any of which would preclude surgery.

A complete physical examination, complete blood cell count, fibrinogen level, and serum biochemistry panel should be performed to ensure the absence of systemic disease. The stress of general anesthesia can cause aggravation of any smoldering conditions. In foals, particular concern is paid to potential *Rhodococcus equi* or other respiratory infections to prevent postoperative endophthalmitis.[27-30,35,45] Thoracic auscultation, including a rebreathing examination, thoracic radiographs, and or thoracic ultrasonography, is highly recommended to screen for potential pathology. If disease is detected, aggressive therapy should be instituted and surgery should be delayed until several weeks past resolution of all clinical signs.

Preoperative therapeutic protocol
The preoperative therapeutic protocol is critical to controlling postoperative inflammation and minimizing the risk of postoperative intraocular infection. A subpalpebral lavage (SPL) system can be placed the day prior to surgery or sedation administered to facilitate the frequent application of topical medications required in the 2 hours prior to surgery. A typical protocol is outlined in **Table 2**.

Operative protocol
Phacoemulsification is performed under general anesthesia. Use of an operating microscope is critical for proper visualization of intraocular structures. A systemic neuromuscular blocking agent or retrobulbar local anesthesia is used to facilitate globe positioning and prevent contraction of the extraocular muscles, which decreases the risk for anterior movement of the vitreous, posterior lens capsule, and iris.[13,31,32] The horse is positioned in lateral recumbency if only 1 eye is to be operated or dorsal recumbency if both eyes are having surgery performed under the same episode of

Table 2
Typical preoperative medication profile for phacoemulsification

Drug	Dose and Route of Administration	Frequency	Duration
Penicillin	22,000 IU/kg, intravenous	q6h	48 h
Gentamicin	6.6 mg/kg, intravenous	q24h	48 h
Flunixin meglumine	1.1 mg/kg intravenously or orally, then 0.5 mg/kg intravenously or orally	q12–24h	10–14 d
Omeprazole	1 mg/kg orally	q24h	14–28 d
Prednisolone acetate or neomycin–polymyxin B–dexamethasone	0.1 mL via SPL	q6h q30min	24 h before surgery 2 h before surgery
Ofloxacin	0.1 mL via SPL	q6h q30min	24 h before surgery 2 h before surgery
Flurbiprofen	0.1 mL via SPL	q6h q30min	24 h before surgery 2 h before surgery
Tropicamide 1% or atropine 0.5%–1%	0.1 mL via SPL	q30min only once	2 h before surgery

general anesthesia. Typically, surgery is only performed on both eyes if the patient is a foal or small pony due to concerns about ventilation when in dorsal recumbency. The head is positioned with sand bags or wedges so that the corneal surface is parallel to the surgical table.[46] A topical ocular anesthetic is applied to decrease the corneal reflex and decrease postoperative inflammation.

The eye is routinely prepared for surgery using a 1:50 povidone iodine solution diluted in saline. A lateral canthotomy may be performed to improve exposure of the globe. A 2-step or 3-step clear corneal incision or subconjunctival, scleral-based incision is created and the anterior chamber carefully entered taking care to avoid damaging the iris.[3,13,31,32,47] The anterior chamber is then reformed with a highly cohesive viscoelastic material to maintain a formed anterior chamber. An anterior capsulotomy is performed using either a small gauge hypodermic needle and modified (lengthened) Utrata forceps or a high-frequency diathermy probe customized for the equine eye.

The phacoemulsification needle is then used to emulsify the nuclear material within the capsular bag (**Fig. 8**). Great care is taken to avoid damage to the posterior lens capsule, which is very thin and becomes highly mobile as the lens material is removed.[13] Remaining cortical material is then removed using an irrigation/aspiration tip, preferably customized for use in horses. Potential intraoperative complications include prolapse of the iris or corpora nigra through the incision, miosis, hemorrhage, posterior capsular tears, loss of lens material into the vitreous, vitreal prolapse through posterior capsular tears, and retinal swelling.[3,13,31]

Once all lenticular material has been removed, an IOL can be implanted into the eye if desired (**Fig. 9**). The anterior chamber and capsular bag are inflated with viscoelastic material. The corneal incision is elongated. The IOL is folded and inserted through the corneal incision and into the capsular bag using a lens-folding forceps.

If an IOL is not placed due to preexisting conditions or intraoperative complications, some surgeons elect to perform a posterior capsulorrhexis. The posterior capsulorrhexis may decrease migration of lens epithelial cells across the visual axis, thereby ensuring maintenance of a clear visual pathway (**Fig. 10**).[46] The cornea is then closed with the suture pattern of choice using 8-0 or 9-0 absorbable suture. Before the final suture is secured, the surgeon may choose to remove any remaining viscoelastic material with the irrigation/aspiration device, although in equine eyes many surgeons elect not to remove the viscoelastic material.

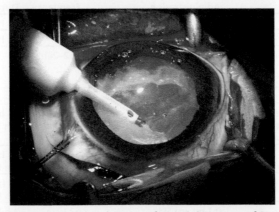

Fig. 8. Phacoemulsification procedure being performed. (*Courtesy of* Oertli Instrumente AG, Berneck, Switzerland; with permission.)

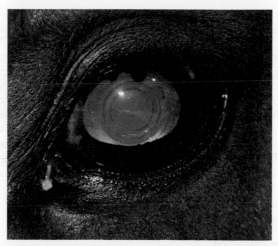

Fig. 9. Pseudophakic eye with mild capsular opacification. The horse was visual.

Intraocular lenses

Placement of an IOL after cataract extraction restores the normal refractive state (emmetropia) in which distant objects are focused clearly on the retina. Without placement of an IOL, the equine globe is severely hypermetropic (far-sighted).[33,34] Although aphakic horses seem to perform well after surgery, owners must be counseled that the horse's vision is not normal. Therefore, horses undergoing cataract extraction likely benefit from the placement of an IOL.

Currently 3 dioptric strengths are currently available for equine lenses: +14, +18, and +21.[3] The +14 diopter lens is available with an optic diameter of 12 mm and overall length of 21 mm or an optic diameter of 13 mm and overall length of 22 mm. These lenses are typically placed in foals or ponies.[3,48] The +18 diopter lens has an overall length of 24 mm. For adult horses both the +14 lens and the +18 diopter lens have been recommended.[30,32,49] As more IOLs are placed, more specific recommendations regarding the dioptric strength of the IOL will become available.

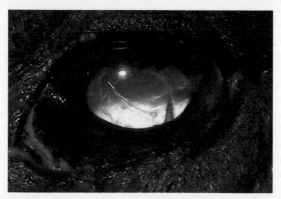

Fig. 10. Postoperative appearance of an aphakic eye. The surgical incision is visible temporally. Wrinkling of the capsular bag and capsular opacities are visible within the pupil. The horse was visual.

Postoperative care

Topical corticosteroids, topical antibiotics, and topical nonsteroidal anti-inflammatory medications are continued for 2 months to 3 months postoperatively depending on healing of the incision, degree of postoperative inflammation, and surgeon preference. The initial frequency is typically every 6 hours and the medications are tapered as the inflammation resolves. Development of a corneal ulcer precludes the use of topical corticosteroids. SPL systems are typically placed to facilitate application of topical medications without placing undue pressure on the globe. Systemic antibiotics are continued for 2 days to 7 days postoperatively to decrease the risk of endophthalmitis. Flunixin meglumine is continued as needed to control inflammation, typically for 2 weeks to 4 weeks after surgery. Gastric protectants are typically administered concurrently with flunixin meglumine, particularly in foals. Often masks with eye cups are placed to prevent rubbing on the eye and rupture of the corneal sutures. Horses are restricted to hand-walking only until the corneal incision has completely healed in 3 weeks to 4 weeks.

Intracapsular Lens Extraction

If a lens has luxated anteriorly, the cause must be determined. If traumatic in nature, the significant forces required to luxate the lens often cause significant intraocular damage and result in phthisis bulbi. If secondary to ERU, the prognosis for vision is poor due to previous retinal damage and the high likelihood for future bouts of inflammation. Particularly in a blind eye, enucleation or evisceration with placement of an intraocular prosthesis is likely the most appropriate therapeutic option.

In a potentially visual eye, an intracapsular lens extraction is typically required if it is decided to remove the lens. A very long corneal incision is required due to the large size of the equine lens. Significant complications, such as incisional dehiscence, corneal ulceration, iridal prolapse, marked uveitis, hyphema, glaucoma, and retinal detachment, occur frequently.[50] The prognosis for vision is guarded. The procedure is rarely performed due to the poor outcome.[50] Attempts to perform phacoemulsification on luxated lenses have been equally unrewarding.[50]

EVALUATION OF OUTCOME AND LONG-TERM RECOMMENDATIONS

Postoperative complications can occur days to years after cataract surgery. The success rate for vision in the first month postoperatively is 88%.[13] At 6 months to 12 months postoperatively, only 35% of horses retained vision in a study by Brooks and colleagues.[13] At 2 years postoperatively, only 26% of horses retained vision.[13] In a separate study performed over a similar time period, 58% of horses remained visual after 1 year.[31] Many horses in the study, however, were lost to follow-up. The complications after surgery can also result in loss of the globe.[13,31,36]

Potential complications include corneal edema, corneal ulceration, incision dehiscence, fibrin within the anterior chamber, hyphema, endophthalmitis, anterior or posterior synechia, iris bombé, postoperative ocular hypertension, glaucoma, persistent uveitis, retained lens material, posterior capsular opacification, decreased menace response, vitreal prolapse, retinal detachment, retinal degeneration, and phthisis bulbi.[3,13,31,32,36] Glaucoma and endophthalmitis most often result in enucleation.[13,31,32]

Previously foals were thought to have higher success rates than adult horses. A recent study per Edelmann and colleagues,[31] however, did not find age to be a factor in postoperative success. The recent customization of instruments for the adult equine eye likely contributed to the increased success rates in adult horses. Placement of an

IOL did not significantly influence the long-term success rate either positively or negatively.[31] Horses with ERU were less likely to maintain vision long term even if a cyclosporine implant had been placed previously or at the time of surgery. The causes of vision loss included retinal detachment, endophthalmitis, glaucoma, chronic uveitis, extensive posterior synechia, globe rupture, and phthisis bulbi.[13,31]

SUMMARY

Examination of the lens is critical, particularly when evaluating horses with visual impairment or performing prepurchase examinations. To adequately evaluate the lens, the pupil must be pharmacologically dilated. A cataract is any lens opacity. The size, density, and position of a cataract determine the impact on vision. Cataracts may be congenital or inherited or occur secondary to trauma or ERU. Surgical removal is the only treatment option for vision-impairing cataracts, but careful selection of surgical candidates is critical for successful outcomes.

REFERENCES

1. Beebe D. The lens. In: Kaufman P, Alm A, editors. Adler's physiology of the eye. 10th edition. St Louis (MO): Mosby; 2003. p. 117–58.
2. Matthews AG. The lens and cataracts. Vet Clin North Am Equine Pract 2004;20: 393–415.
3. Colitz CMM, McMullen RJ. Diseases and surgery of the lens. In: Gilger B, editor. Equine ophthalmology. 2nd edition. Maryland Heights (MO): Elsevier Saunders; 2011. p. 282–316.
4. Gilger BC, Stoppini R. Equine ocular examination: routine and advanced diagnostic techniques. In: Gilger BC, editor. Equine ophthalmology. 2nd edition. Maryland Heights (MO): Elsevier Saunders; 2011. p. 1–51.
5. Lambert SR, Drack AV. Infantile cataracts. Surv Ophthalmol 1996;40:427–58.
6. Rebhun WC. Diagnosis and treatment of equine uveitis. J Am Vet Med Assoc 1979;175:803–8.
7. Turner LM, Whitley RD, Hager D. Management of ocular trauma in horses: part II. Orbit, eyelids, uvea, lens, retina, and optic nerve. Mod Vet Pract 1986;67:341–7.
8. Segard EM, Depecker MC, Lang J, et al. Ultrasonographic features of PMEL17 (Silver) mutant gene-associated multiple congenital ocular anomalies (MCOA) in Comtois and Rocky Mountain horses. Vet Ophthalmol 2013;16:429–35.
9. Ramsey DT, Ewart SI , Render JA, et al. Congenital ocular abnormalities of rocky mountain horses. Vet Ophthalmol 1999;2:47–59.
10. Komaromy AM, Rowlan JS, La Croix NC, et al. Equine multiple congenital ocular anomalies (MCOA) syndrome in PMEL17 (Silver) mutant ponies: five cases. Vet Ophthalmol 2011;14:313–20.
11. Andersson LS, Axelsson J, Dubielzig RR, et al. Multiple congenital ocular anomalies in Icelandic horses. BMC Vet Res 2011;7:21.
12. Chandler KJ, Billson FM, Mellor DJ. Ophthalmic lesions in 83 geriatric horses and ponies. Vet Rec 2003;153:319–22.
13. Brooks DE, Plummer CE, Carastro SM, et al. Visual outcomes of phacoemulsification cataract surgery in horses: 1990-2013. Vet Ophthalmol 2014;17:117–28.
14. Priester W. Congenital ocular defects in cattle, horses, cats, and dogs. J Am Vet Med Assoc 1972;160:1504–11.
15. Roberts SM. Congenital ocular anomalies. Vet Clin North Am Equine Pract 1992; 8:459–78.

16. Matthews AG, Barnett K. Lens. In: Barnett K, Crispin S, Lavach J, editors. Equine ophthalmology: an atlas and text. 2nd edition. Edinburgh (United Kingdom): Saunders Elsevier; 2004. p. 165–82.

17. Erikson R. Hereditary aniridia with secondary cataract in horses. Nord Vet Med 1955;7:773–9.

18. Joyce J. Aniridia in a quarter horse. Equine Vet J 1983;2:21–2.

19. Beech J, Aguirre G, Gross S. Congenital nuclear cataracts in the Morgan horse. J Am Vet Med Assoc 1984;184:1363–5.

20. Beech J, Irby N. Inherited nuclear cataracts in the Morgan horse. J Hered 1985; 76:371–2.

21. Abrams KL, Brooks DE. Equine recurrent uveitis: current concepts in diagnosis and treatment Uveite ricorrente equina: concetti attuali nella diagnosi e nella terapia. Ippologia 1992;3:37–41.

22. McLaughlin S, Whitley RD, Gilger B. Diagnosis and treatment of lens diseases. Vet Clin North Am Equine Pract 1992;8:575–85.

23. Matthews AG. Lens opacities in the horse: a clinical classification. Vet Ophthalmol 2000;3:65–71.

24. Rushton J, Tichy A, Brem G, et al. Ophthalmological findings in a closed herd of Lipizzaners. Equine Vet J 2013;45:209–13.

25. Ireland JL, Clegg PD, McGowan CM, et al. Disease prevalence in geriatric horses in the United Kingdom: veterinary clinical assessment of 200 cases. Equine Vet J 2012;44:101–6.

26. Latimer CA, Wyman M. Neonatal ophthalmology. Vet Clin North Am Equine Pract 1985;1:235–59.

27. Whitley RD, Moore C, Slone D. Cataract surgery in the horse: a review. Equine Vet J 1983;2:127–34.

28. Dziezyc J, Millichamp NJ, Keller CB. Use of phacofragmentation for cataract removal in horses: 12 cases (1985-1989). J Am Vet Med Assoc 1991;198:1774–8.

29. Brooks DE. Phacoemulsification cataract surgery in the horse. Clin Tech Equine Pract 2005;4:11–20.

30. McMullen RJ Jr, Utter ME. Current developments in equine cataract surgery. Equine Vet J 2010;37:38–45.

31. Edelmann ML, McMullen R Jr, Stoppini R, et al. Retrospective evaluation of phacoemulsification and aspiration in 41 horses (46 eyes): visual outcomes vs. age, intraocular lens, and uveitis status. Vet Ophthalmol 2014;17:160–7.

32. Townsend WM, Jacobi S, Bartoe JT. Phacoemulsification and implantation of foldable +14 diopter intraocular lenses in five mature horses. Equine Vet J 2012;44: 238–43.

33. Farral H, Handscombe M. Follow-up report of a case of surgical aphakie with an analysis of equine visual function. Equine Vet J 1990;10:91–3.

34. Millichamp NJ, Dziezyc J. Cataract phacofragmentation in horses. Vet Ophthalmol 2000;3:157–64.

35. Whitley RD, Meek LA, Millichamp NJ, et al. Cataract surgery in the horse: a review of six cases. Equine Vet J 1990;13:85–90.

36. Fife TM, Gemensky-Metzler AJ, Wilkie DA, et al. Clinical features and outcomes of phacoemulsification in 39 horses: a retrospective study (1993-2003). Vet Ophthalmol 2006;9:361–8.

37. Crewther SG, Crewther DP, Mitchell DE. The effects of short-term occlusion therapy on reversal of the anatomical and physiological effects of monocular deprivation in the lateral geniculate nucleus and visual cortex of kittens. Exp Brain Res 1983;51:206–16.

38. Birch EE, Stager DR. Prevalence of good visual acuity following surgery for congenital unilateral cataract. Arch Ophthalmol 1988;106:40–3.

39. Whitley RD. Diseases and surgery of the lens. In: Gilger B, editor. Equine ophthalmology. St Louis (MO): Elsevier Saunders; 2005. p. 269–84.

40. Joyce JR, Witzel DA. Equine night blindness. J Am Vet Med Assoc 1977;170: 878–80.

41. Witzel DA, Joyce JR, Smith EL. Electroretinography of congenital night blindness in an Appaloosa filly. J Equine Med Surg 1977;1:226–9.

42. Witzel DA, Riis RC, Rebhun WC, et al. Night blindness in the Appaloosa: sibling occurrence. J Equine Med Surg 1977;1:383–6.

43. Nunnery C, Pickett JP, Zimmerman KL. Congenital stationary night blindness in a thoroughbred and a paso fino. Vet Ophthalmol 2005;8:415–9.

44. Sandmeyer LS, Breaux CB, Archer S, et al. Clinical and electroretinographic characteristics of congenital stationary night blindness in the Appaloosa and the association with the leopard complex. Vet Ophthalmol 2007;10:368–75.

45. Brooks DE. Complications of ophthalmic surgery in the horse. Vet Clin North Am Equine Pract 2008;24:697–734.

46. Townsend WM. Intraocular surgery. In: Robinson N, Sprayberry K, editors. Current therapy in equine medicine. 6th edition. St Louis (MO): Saunders Elsevier; 2009. p. 659–63.

47. Millichamp NJ, Dziezyc J. Cataract surgery in horses. Invest Ophthalmol Vis Sci 1996;37:S763.

48. Townsend WM, Wasserman N, Jacobi S. A pilot study on the corneal curvatures and ocular dimensions of horses less than one year of age. Equine Vet J 2013;45: 256–8.

49. McMullen RJ, Davidson MG, Campbell NB, et al. Evaluation of 30- and 25-diopter intraocular lens implants in equine eyes after surgical extraction of the lens. Am J Vet Res 2010;71:809–16.

50. Brooks DE, Gilger BC, Plummer CE, et al. Surgical correction of lens luxation in the horse: visual outcomes. Vet Med Anim Sci 2014. Available at: http://www. hoajonline.com/vetmedanimsci/2054-3425/2/2. Accessed April 30, 2017.

The Equine Fundus

Gil Ben-Shlomo, DVM, PhD

KEYWORDS

- Fundus • Retina • Optic nerve head • Optic disc • Horse • Electroretinography
- Ophthalmoscopy

KEY POINTS

- The equine retinal blood vessels are limited to the direct surrounding of the optic disc (paurangiotic retina), and extend a short distance into the nerve fiber layer.
- Choroidal blood vessels can be seen in lightly pigmented fundi, and should not be confused with retinal blood vessels or hemorrhage.
- The equine optic disc is elliptical, orange-pink in color, and located in the nontapetum fundus; it is positioned slightly ventrolateral to the posterior pole of the globe.
- Fundoscopy should be performed in dim light, to reduce glare from the corneal surface, and help with mydriasis. To view the optic disc the examiner should stand slightly in front of the horse and look slightly down.
- Due to their wider field of view, Panoptic and indirect ophthalmoscopy are the preferred methods for screening for fundic lesions, while the greater magnification of the direct ophthalmoscope should be utilized for close examination of lesions.

Fundus is an anatomic term referring to the portion of an organ opposite from its opening, and the fundus of the eye is the back portion of the posterior segment of the globe, including the optic nerve, the retina, and the choroid. Clinically, the fundus can be visualized by means of direct and indirect ophthalmoscopy. Understanding the normal anatomy and appearance of the equine fundus is crucial for differentiating normal variations from abnormalities when performing an examination of the fundus. This article reviews the normal anatomy and appearance of the equine fundus and discusses basic and advanced examination techniques. It also discusses common findings in the equine fundus and their interpretation.

ANATOMY OF THE EQUINE FUNDUS
Retina and Optic Disc

The equine neural retina consists of 10 layers and, similar to other vertebrates, forms a fundamental, vertical, synaptic chain from the photoreceptors (rods and cones) to bipolar cells, to ganglion cells (**Fig. 1**). The axons of the ganglion cells bundle together to

The author does not have any commercial or financial conflicts of interest.
Department of Veterinary Clinical Sciences, College of Veterinary Medicine, Iowa State University, 1600 S 16th Street, Ames, IA 50011, USA
E-mail address: gil@iastate.edu

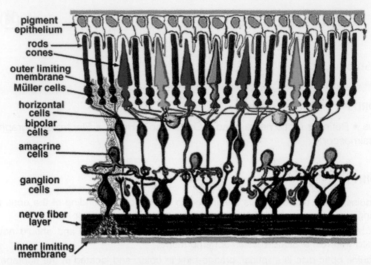

pigment
epithelium

rods
cones

outer limiting
membrane

Müller cells

horizontal
cells

bipolar
cells

amacrine
cells

ganglion
cells

nerve fiber
layer

inner limiting
membrane

Fig. 1. A simple diagram of the organization of the retina. (*Reproduced from* Webvision. The organization of the retina and visual system. Available at: www.webvision.med.utah. edu; with permission.)

form the optic nerve. In addition to the vertical pathway, the horizontal and amacrine cells form lateral connections within the retina.[1] The horizontal cells synapse with photoreceptors and bipolar cells in the outer plexiform layer, while the amacrine cells synapse with bipolar and ganglion cells in the inner plexiform layer (**Fig. 1**). The horizontal and amacrine cells are inhibitory in nature, and are crucial for the processing of visual stimuli in the retina.

The complex conversion of light energy into electrical signal (ie, phototransduction) takes place in the photoreceptors. Rods are the predominate photoreceptors in the equine retina, with a ratio of about 20 rods for every cone.[2] Whereas rods provide achromatic, low-acuity, scotopic (dim light) vision, cones provide color, high-acuity, photopic (bright light) vision. Two areas in the equine retina contain a higher concentration of cone photoreceptors, and hence are responsible for higher visual acuity. The first is the visual streak, which is a narrow horizontal area located immediately dorsal and lateral to the optic disc (also known as the optic nerve head; ONH), and in parallel to the ventral border of the tapetum. The horizontal visual streak correlates with the horizontal shape of the equine pupil. The second is the area centralis, a circular region located at the lateral end of the visual streak and measures 2 to 5 mm in diameter.[3,4] These 2 areas also contain the highest ganglion cell density, further demonstrating the importance of the visual streak and area centralis for high visual acuity.[3,5] Owing to the lateral position of horses' eyes, the visual streak contributes to monocular vision, while the more laterally located area centralis contributes to forward, binocular vision.[1] Lesions in these 2 areas are likely to have greater impact on vision and visual acuity compared with other areas of the retina.

The retinal pigment epithelium (RPE) is the outermost layer of the retina, and is an intrinsic component of the blood–retinal barrier.[1] The RPE consists of a single layer of cells overlying the photoreceptors, and is firmly attached to the underlying choroid (**Fig. 1**). When retinal detachment occurs, the RPE is separated from the underlying photoreceptors. Because the RPE cells provide nutrition and metabolic support to the photoreceptors, and have an important role in phototransduction (ie, regeneration of the photoreceptors' photopigment), a separation between the RPE and photoreceptors throughout the retina (complete retinal detachment) leads to blindness. The RPE cells contain a varying degree of melanin granules, and their appearance ranges from unpigmented, over the thickest portion of the tapetum (ie, at the visual streak area), to a gradual increase in pigmentation as the tapetum thickness tapers more peripherally (**Fig. 2**).[6] The lack of heavy RPE pigmentation over the tapetum allows passage of light through the RPE and its reflection by the tapetum back onto the photoreceptors. The amount of melanin in the nontapetal portion of the fundus may also vary, and usually fewer melanin granules are present in the RPE of horses with a light coat color, allowing partial view of the underlying choroid. In subalbinotic animals, the RPE may be unpigmented, allowing view of the entire choroidal vasculature (**Fig. 3**).

The vasculature pattern of the equine retina is paurangiotic (ie, it is limited to the direct surrounding of the optic disc). About 30 to 60 arterioles and venules, evenly spaced, radiate from the optic disc, and dividing a few times dichotomously, and extend a short distance (about 1–1.5 optic disc diameters) into the nerve fiber layer of the retina. These blood vessels serve inner retinal layers near the optic disc. Fewer and thinner retinal blood vessels are present at the ventral part of the optic disc at the 6 o'clock position, and in some cases are completely absent from this area. This area consists of a wedge-shaped notch, which is the region of the embryologic fetal fissure (**Fig. 3**).[1,7,8] The optic disc is horizontally elliptical, and orange-pink in color. It is located in the nontapetum, close to the tapetum–nontapetum junction, and is positioned slightly ventrolateral to the posterior pole of the globe. In the young foal, the normal optic disc is more round, and becomes more elliptical with maturation.

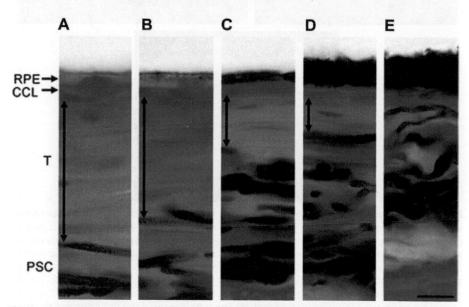

Fig. 2. Photomicrographs of the choroid and retinal pigment epithelium (RPE) in hematoxylin and eosin–stained vertical sections of a horse eye. The tapetal tissue (T) consists of eosinophilic layers between the choriocapillary layer (CCL) and the proper substance of the choroid (PSC), which includes the melanocytes. (*A*) Thick T area covered by unpigmented RPE. (*B*) Relatively thick T area covered by slightly pigmented RPE. (*C*) T area covered by moderately pigmented RPE. (*D*) Thin T area covered by heavily pigmented RPE. (*E*) Choroid without T tissue covered by heavily pigmented RPE. Scale bar: 10 μm (in (*E*); applies to [*A–E*]). (*Reproduced from* Shinozaki A, Takagi S, Hosaka YZ, et al. The fibrous tapetum of the horse eye. J Anat 2013;223(5):510; with permission.)

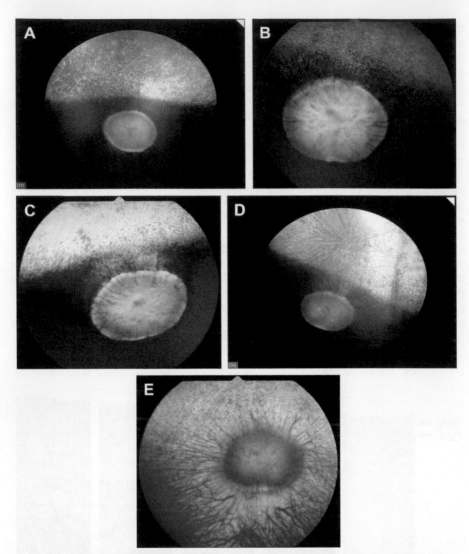

Fig. 3. Normal variations of the equine fundus. (*A*) Normal equine fundus. The tapetum is present and the nontapetum is heavily pigmented. The optic disc is pink in color, and it is located in the nontapetum, close to the tapetum–nontapetum junction. Multiple dark dots can be seen in the tapetum; these are small choriocapillaries viewed end on, and are also known as the "stars of Winslow." Note the view of a few choroidal blood vessels in the center of the tapetum and right above the optic disc this is a normal variation and should not be confused with retinal hemorrhages. Owing to the lower magnification of this picture, the retinal blood vessels cannot be seen clearly. (*B*) This is a close up of the optic disc and the peripapillary fundus. The equine retinal blood vessels are fine, present only in the direct area of the optic disc and cross its margin to extend a short distance into the retina. This vasculature pattern is called paurangiotic. Note the decreased number of blood vessels at the 6 o'clock position of the optic disc which is the region of the embryologic fetal fissure. (*C*) Normal fundus of a horse with dilute coat color. The fundus is lightly pigmented at the tapetum–nontapetum junction, allowing the view of choroidal blood vessels in these 2 areas, not to be confused with the retinal blood vessels that are crossing the optic disc margin, and extending a short distance into the retina. Note the red look of some of the stars of Winslow (*red dots*) owing to the lack

Choroid and Tapetum

The choroid is the posterior section of the uvea, and it is contiguous with the anterior uvea (the iris and ciliary body). The choroid predominantly consists of blood vessels and capillaries. It lies between the retina and the sclera, and it is the main provider of oxygen and nutrients to the equine retina. Although the choroid cannot be seen in heavily pigmented fundi, in lightly pigmented or subalbinotic fundi, the orange-red, dense, choroidal blood vessels can be seen and should not be confused with the retinal blood vessels or retinal hemorrhage (**Fig. 3**).

The choriocapillaries are arranged in a single layer, and are highly fenestrated. The capillaries in the tapetal area are more heavily fenestrated compared with the nontapetal area, further demonstrating the metabolic role of the choroid, supporting the relatively poorly vascularized tapetal area. Multiple, distinct, dark dots seen in the equine tapetal fundus are a series of small choriocapillaries viewed end on, and are known as the "stars of Winslow." In subalbinotic areas, the stars of Winslow appear as red dots[1,9] (**Fig. 3**).

The tapetum is located within the choroid, underneath the choriocapillary layer and on top of the choroid proper substance (substantia propria) (**Fig. 2**). Clinically, when viewed under bright light, the tapetum looks triangular to semicircular in shape, bluish-green to greenish-yellow in color,[6,10] and is located dorsal to the optic disc. However, when examined under dim light, it appears as a horizontal band, dorsal to the optic disc and is parallel to the visual streak (the visual streak is located in the ventral part of this horizontal band; **Fig. 4**). It has been suggested that the tapetal horizontal band is the only functional part of the tapetum under normal (day or night) light conditions.[6] The visual streak and the tapetal horizontal band, together with the horizontally shaped pupil, should provide horses good mesopic and scotopic vision in the horizontal visual field. The tapetal tissue extends further to the periphery to cover most of the ocular fundus, even underneath the pigmented RPE (**Fig. 2** and **Fig. 3**); hence, the pigmentation pattern of the RPE determines the macroscopic size and shape of the tapetum.[6] The tapetum is thickest over the horizontal band and gradually tapers as it extends to the periphery dorsally (**Fig. 2**). The equine tapetum consists of regularly arranged collagen fibrils (fibrous tapetum), similar to many ungulates.[6,11] The tapetum functions as a light reflector to increase the probability of light absorption by the photoreceptors, especially under dim light. Analysis of the collagen fibrils' diameter and intrafibrous distance revealed that the light wavelength reflected from the equine tapetum is approximately 468 nm, which is close to the peak absorption of the of the rod photoreceptors. It was speculated that, for this reason, the tapetal light reflection may not cause a significant visual blur under mesopic and photopic light conditions, as was previously thought.[6]

---

of pigment in this area. This is also a normal variation. (*D*) Another normal variation of a fundus of a horse with dilute coat color. In this case, a larger area of the tapetum is missing and the choroidal blood vessels can be easily seen in this region (*top left*). The nontapetum is very lightly pigmented except for a darker pigmented patch (*bottom right*). (*E*) Normal subalbinotic fundus. The tapetum is missing and the nontapetum lacks pigment, hence the choroidal blood vessels can be seen throughout the whole fundus. The stars of Winslow appear as multiple red dots dorsal to the optic disc. Retinal blood vessels can be seen crossing the optic disc margin, and should not be confused with choroidal blood vessels. Choroidal and retinal blood vessels should not be confused with retinal or choroidal hemorrhage. (*Courtesy of* [*B, C, E*] Dr Richard McMullen, Department of Clinical Sciences, College of Veterinary Medicine, Auburn University.)

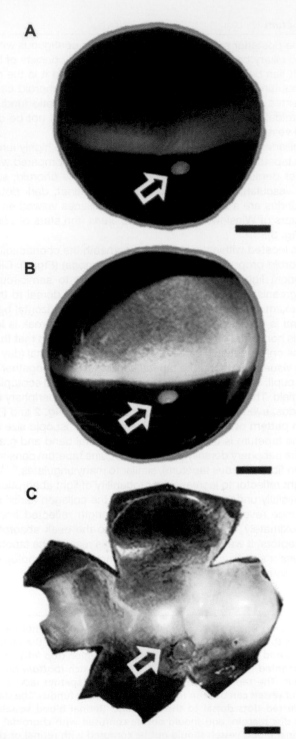

Fig. 4. Photographs of the horse's left ocular fundus under weak light (*A*), under a flash, that is strong light (*B*), and after the removal of the retinal pigment epithelium (*C*). The

EXAMINATION TECHNIQUES OF THE EQUINE FUNDUS

A complete eye examination should always include a thorough examination of the ocular fundus (fundoscopy or ophthalmoscopy) that, like the rest of the eye examination, is best performed in dim light (eg, a dark room, or shaded area), to reduce glare from the corneal surface and to aid with mydriasis. Although fundoscopy can be performed without pupil dilation, mydriasis provides better view of the fundus and facilitates a comprehensive examination. Mydriasis is achieved within 15 to 20 minutes of application of 1% tropicamide eye drops, and will last about 4 to 6 hours. In comparison, ophthalmic atropine takes about 1 hour to induce mydriasis and will last up to 2 weeks in the horse. As such, it is not recommended and it is impractical to use atropine as a mydriatic agent for the sole purpose of performing fundoscopy.

Fundoscopy should be performed systematically, and all components of the fundus should be screened: the tapetal fundus (dorsally), nontapetal fundus (ventrally), optic disc, and retinal blood vessels. The examiner should change her or his position according to the fundic region being screened. When attempting to examine the optic disc, one should keep in mind the slight ventrolateral position of the optic disc in the equine eye. Hence, to view the optic disc, the examiner should stand slightly in front of the horse, at approximately a 45° angle to the eye, and keep her or his head position at the eye level of the horse or slightly higher, looking slightly down so the midventral fundus, including the optic disc, can be viewed (**Fig. 5A**). When documenting fundic lesions or communicating with an ophthalmologist regarding fundic lesions, the size and location of the lesion should be described in reference to the optic disc, see the legend of **Fig. 6A** for an example.

Direct and Indirect Ophthalmoscopy

Both direct and indirect ophthalmoscopy can be used for fundic examination. Indirect ophthalmoscopy provides lower magnification and a wider field of view. As such, it provides the best method for routine screening of the fundus. A bright source of focused light such as the Finoff transilluminator, and a handheld lens are needed for indirect ophthalmoscopy. Other good sources of light for fundoscopy are the halogen-based otoscope head light and light-emitting diode (LED)–based penlights. Both 20-diopter (D) and 14-D converging lenses are useful for indirect ophthalmoscopy in horses. The 20-D lens, with a 0.79× lateral magnification,[12] provides a wider field of view, which is helpful for fundus screening, and is especially helpful when the pupil is not, or cannot, be dilated. The 14-D lens provides a higher lateral magnification of 1.18×,[12] and while allowing effective screening of the fundus, it also provides the examiner with greater details of the fundus and lesions, and it is this author's preferred lens for routine equine fundoscopy. Monocular indirect ophthalmoscopy is performed by holding the source of light close to the examiner's eye (eg, Finoff transilluminator), and the converging lens in front of the examined eye, about 5 to 7 cm from it (**Fig. 5A**). This technique can be mastered relatively quickly by the general practitioner, and allows effective and easy screening of the fundus. Binocular indirect ophthalmoscopy can be performed similarly, while an indirect ophthalmoscope headset is used instead of the handheld light source (**Fig. 5B**). The headset provides visual input to both of the

tapetum is metallic bluish green to blue in color. Under weak light, the tapetum appears as a horizontal band (A). The tapetum expands dorsally with increasing brightness of illumination (B). In (C), the tapetum is apparent over most of the ocular fundus, including the part ventral to the optic disc (arrow). The nasal direction is to the left. Scale bars: 1 cm. (Reproduced from Shinozaki A, Takagi S, Hosaka YZ, et al. The fibrous tapetum of the horse eye. J Anat 2013;223(5):512; with permission.)

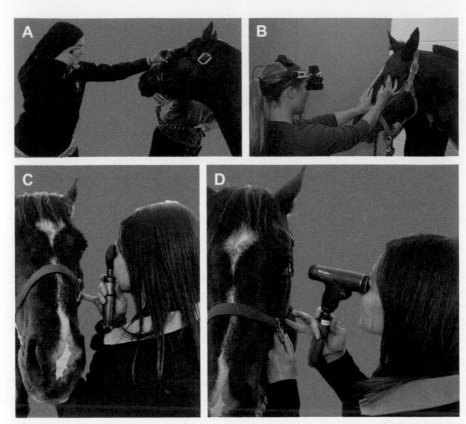

Fig. 5. Ophthalmoscopy. (*A*) Monocular indirect ophthalmoscopy is performed using a 14-diopter (D) lens and a Finoff transilluminator. To view the optic disc the examiner should stand slightly in front of the horse and look slightly down, owing to the ventromedial location of the optic disc in the equine eye. (*B*) An indirect ophthalmoscope headset and a 14-D lens are used to performed a binocular indirect ophthalmoscopy. Note the forward position of the examiner, allowing view of the optic disc. (*C*) Direct ophthalmoscopy. (*D*) Panoptic ophthalmoscope is used for fundoscopy in this horse.

examiner's eyes, allowing a 3-dimensional view of the fundus. In addition, because the indirect ophthalmoscope has an integral light, it frees 1 hand of the examiner that can be used to open the horse's eyelids and aid with the examination. Binocular indirect ophthalmoscopy is routinely used by veterinary ophthalmologists. The fundic image seen when performing indirect ophthalmoscopy is inverted and reversed (ie, up is down, and left is right), which is important to remember when documenting lesions in the medical records, or describing the lesions verbally.

The direct ophthalmoscope (**Fig. 5**C) allows monocular evaluation of the fundus, and provides 7.9× lateral magnification in the horse. Unlike the indirect ophthalmoscope, the direct ophthalmoscope provides upright image (not inverted or reversed), and it is probably the most popular ophthalmoscope among general practitioners owing to its relative ease of use. However, although a complete fundoscopy can be performed using a direct ophthalmoscope, it is more time consuming owing to its high magnification and its relative narrow field of view. It is also harder to use with an undilated pupil compared with indirect ophthalmoscopy or the Panoptic ophthalmoscope. Nonetheless, the indirect ophthalmoscope is an excellent tool for high magnification evaluation of fundic lesions. To examine the equine fundus the rotary lens setting should be set to 0, and the size of the circular light beam should be adjusted to the size of the pupil to reduce light reflection from the cornea.

The Panoptic ophthalmoscope is a patented direct ophthalmoscope (Welch-Allyn Inc, Skaneateles Falls, NY; **Fig. 5**D), with an intermediate lateral magnification between the direct and indirect ophthalmoscopes that makes it easier to view the fundus through an undilated pupil. Moreover, the Panoptic provides a field of view that is approximately 5 times greater than a standard direct ophthalmoscope, making it easier to use and more effective for screening of the fundus compared with a standard direct ophthalmoscope.

Smartphone Ophthalmoscopy (Smartphonoscopy)

The smartphone revolution that has started a decade ago is also affecting the field of veterinary ophthalmology! Specialized fundus cameras are expensive and usually wired, which make them a rare commodity in veterinary ophthalmology, and especially in equine ophthalmology. However, smartphones are equipped with high-resolution cameras and an LED–based, bright focused light, which turns them, with minor adjustments, into very effective and readily available fundic cameras. Smartphone photography and/ or videography can be used for both examining the fundus, and documenting findings. It can also be used for telemedicine consultation with a veterinary ophthalmologist.

Although some, usually expensive, adapters aiming to convert the smartphone into a fundic camera are available for purchase, high-quality fundic photography can be performed with a smartphone alone, without additional lenses or instruments. The proximity of the phone's light source to the lens of the camera allows the lens to overcome the optical power of the patient's lens, and captures the fundic image (**Fig. 6**). To take a fundic picture the flash of the smartphone should be kept on, and serves as the light source for the fundoscopy. Most phones do not allow keeping the phone light turned on when the phone is in camera mode. This issue can be resolved in one of two ways. A third-party camera app that allows keeping the phone's light on (such as the Camera+ app) can be installed, or the phone can be switched to video mode, which in most phones allows the phone's light to stay on. Then, both video and still pictures can be taken while the phone is in video mode. Moreover, even under sedated examination, horses usually keep moving their eyes, and the inherent delay of smartphone photography can make it challenging to capture a specific lesion in focus (or at all). Continuous videotaping of the fundus can help the examiner to capture fundic lesions more easily. Like with the use of ophthalmoscopes, an easier and better view of the fundus is achieved by inducing mydriasis. Another necessary adjustment is to the intensity of the smartphone's light. Although the features of some camera apps allow adjustment of light intensity, most camera apps do not. The very bright phone light may make the patient uncomfortable, and hence less cooperative. In addition, it will induce significant miosis or will interfere with mydriasis. Application of 1 or 2 layers of white medical tape (or more if needed) on top of the phone's light (**Fig. 7**) achieves both diffusion of the light (which decreases light reflection from the cornea, hence the flash artifact on the picture), and lowers its intensity. Additional reading and tips for the use of smartphone fundoscopy can be found at www.theeyephone.com.

ADVANCED EXAMINATION TECHNIQUES
Ultrasonography

Ultrasonography for retinal and fundus evaluation is usually performed when the optical media (cornea or lens) are opaque or hazy, blocking (partially or fully) the view of

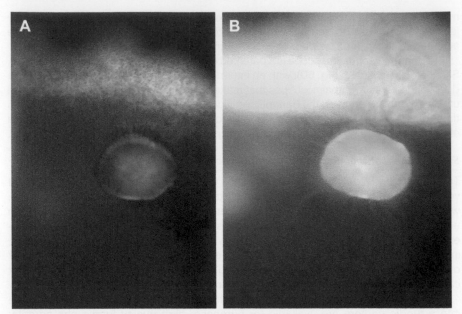

Fig. 6. Fundic pictures obtained by a smartphone photography with no adapters or additional lens. (*A*) A normal fundus. A hypopigmented streak is present adjacent to the optic disc at the 5 o'clock position, its width is approximately 20% of the optic disc diameter, and it is extending about 1 optic disc diameter into the nontapetal fundus. This is an incidental finding. (*B*) Retinal folds from previous retinal detachment that reattached are seen as pale gray streaks radiating from the optic disc. The hazy view is owing the uveitis present in this eye.

the fundus. Sedation and an auriculopalpebral nerve block allow easy, safe, and fast examination. Topical anesthesia (eg, proparacaine or tetracaine ophthalmic solutions) are needed if the ultrasound gel and probe are applied directly to the cornea, but is not required if a transpalpebral approach is elected. The latter approach should be selected to minimize the risk of corneal injury, contamination, or worsening of corneal lesions (eg, corneal ulcer, descemetocele), when applicable, although application of the transducer directly on the cornea (with gel) will provide better image of the posterior segment. A sterile ultrasound gel should be used for ocular imaging, especially when the gel is applied to the cornea (rather than the eyelids) and/or if the corneal surface is not intact. A 10-MHz transducer with a focal range of 3 to 4 cm is adequate for evaluation of the equine eye, including the fundus. A 5.0- or 7.5-MHz transducer can also be used for imaging of the fundus, with greater depth of penetration for imaging of the retrobulbar space.[13] The transducer should be placed in both horizontal and vertical orientations to image all areas of the posterior segment. This maneuver is important to identify focal lesions, such as focal retinal detachment. An oblique orientation of the transducer can provide imaging of additional regions of the eye and retina. The retina and choroid cannot be discriminated by ultrasonography of a normal fundus. However, retinal detachment is usually identified easily by ultrasound examination. It appears as a hyperechoic linear line in the vitreous. Complete retinal detachment has a typical shape of "seagull wings" on ultrasound imaging because the detached retina is usually still attached to the optic disc and ora ciliaris retinae (**Fig. 8**). Partial or rhegmatogenous retinal detachment can also be identified by ocular ultrasonography, as well as subretinal fluids/hemorrhage, choroidal and optic disc masses, and so on.

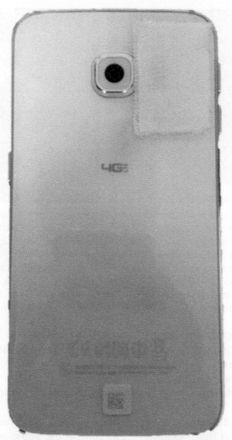

Fig. 7. White medical tape is applied to the phone's flash to diffuse the light and lower its intensity.

Electroretinography

Electroretinography (ERG) is an objective, noninvasive method used to evaluate retinal function. Full field ERG (also known as flash ERG [fERG]) is the most common electroretinographic test, and it is the only type of ERG routinely used for evaluation of retinal function in veterinary patients. Before ERG testing, pupils should be fully dilated with 1% tropicamide eye drops. For fERG recording, light stimuli are projected on the tested eye, and the electrical changes generated by the retina in response to these stimuli are recorded and analyzed. A Ganzfeld half-sphere bowl light stimulator is preferred for fERG recordings because the half-sphere bowl distributes the light stimulus homogeneously to the eye. Handheld mini-Ganzfeld stimulators can be easily used for equine ERG (**Fig. 9**B). Three electrodes are required for ERG recording. A signal-receiving electrode is placed on the corneal surface with the aid of viscous ophthalmic gel (**Fig. 9**A). Topical corneal anesthesia such as proparacaine or tetracaine should be applied to the cornea at least 1 minute before placement of the corneal electrode. Often, the signal-receiving electrode is referred to as an active electrode; however, this is a misnomer, because this electrode is used only for passive recording. A reference electrode is placed over the skin or subcutaneously (using a needle electrode), about 3 cm lateral to the lateral

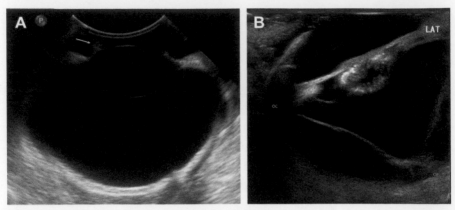

Fig. 8. Ocular ultrasonography in the horse. (*A*) Ultrasound imaging of a normal equine eye. The vitreal body is clear and the bottom of the eye is smooth. Note the corpora nigra in the anterior chamber, laying on the surface of the anterior lens capsule (*yellow arrow*). (*B*) Retinal detachment is demonstrated by ocular ultrasonography. The detached retina is clearly visible in the vitreous as a hyperechoic linear line. It is still attached around the optic disc (OP) and the ora ciliaris retinae (OC), giving it the typical look of seagull wings. The cataractous lens is clearly demonstrated (compare with the clear lens seen in [*A*]). The lens looks smaller in this image because the transducer is placed off-center.

canthus, over the zygomatic arch. A grounding electrode can be placed anywhere on the body, over the skin or subcutaneously; common locations for the ground electrodes are the forehead, the base of the ear, or the middle of the neck. The latter is this author's preference (**Fig. 9**). The purpose of the grounding electrode is to decrease noise interference from power lines, hence improving the quality of the recordings.

In older literature, it is stated that "proper ERG recording requires general anesthesia in animals," and that, "electroretinography in the standing horse can be frustrating because sedation will not eliminate the almost constant head movement."[14] In this author's experience, ERG can be performed easily and quickly when adequate technique is used. Sedation with detomidine (0.010–0.015 mg/kg intravenously) achieves appropriate sedation level for ERG testing, that lasts about 30 to 40 minutes, with minimal to no head movements. The head should be supported, either by a headrest or cross-ties, to minimize head movements. The electrodes and first stage amplifier should be taped to the halter, ensuring that the electrodes move with the horse head, if there are head movements, without being pulled off their insertion (**Fig. 9**C). In addition, an auriculopalpebral nerve block should be performed before ERG testing. Auriculopalpebral nerve block decreases or eliminates blinking, and thus prevents the horse from blinking out the corneal electrode and decreases the blinking artifact from the recordings.

The main contributor to the fERG is the outer retina (ie, rods and cones) and the trace recorded in response to light stimuli reflects the summation of activity of all retinal cells. Because the equine retina is rod dominant, the rod photoreceptors have the greatest effect on the equine ERG. A dark adaptation of at least 20 minutes is required to perform scotopic (dark-adapted) ERG in the horse.[15] Scotopic ERG evaluates rod or combined rod–cone responses; the intensity and frequency of the stimuli determine which subpopulation of photoreceptors will be stimulated. A 10-minute light adaptation is required to bleach all rod photoreceptors and record photopic (light-adapted) ERG, evaluating only cone function. It is important to

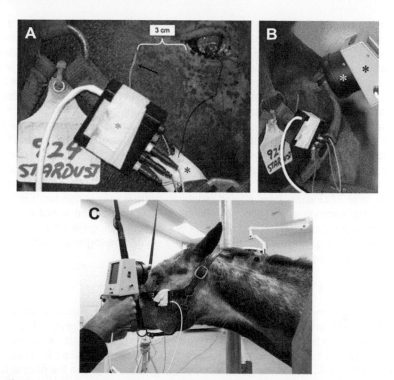

Fig. 9. Electroretinography. (*A*) The reference electrode (*blue arrow*) is placed subcutaneously approximately 3 cm posterior to the lateral canthus and the signal recording, contact lens electrode (*red arrow*) is placed on the corneal surface with viscous ophthalmic gel. Both electrodes (*red asterisk*) and first stage amplifier (*green asterisk*) were secured to the halter with medical tape (the grounding electrode is not shown in this picture). (*B*) The electrodes are connected to the handheld ERG machine (*black asterisk*) with a mini-Ganzfeld half-sphere bowl (*white asterisk*) that is used to apply the stimulation homogeneously to the eye. (*C*) The horse is sedated and the head is supported by 2 cross-ties. The corneal and reference electrodes are secured to the halter. The grounding electrode is placed subcutaneously in the middle of the neck. (*Reproduced from [A, B]* Ben-Shlomo G, Plummer C, Barrie K, et al. Characterization of the normal dark adaptation curve of the horse. Vet Ophthalmol 2012;15(1):43; with permission.)

remember that a normal ERG can be recorded from a blind animal if the blindness has originated from lesions in deeper retinal layers, the optic nerve, or the brain.[16] Retinal disease leading to alteration of retinal function are not common in the horse compared with canine patients. However, ERG is indicated in cases of visual impairment or blindness that cannot be explained by ophthalmic physical examination alone, that is, the funduscopic findings alone cannot explain the reason for such visual impairment,[17,18] and differentiation between retinal and central blindness is warranted. It is also indicated when evaluation of retinal function is desired but the retina cannot be viewed, such as before cataract surgery. When retinal lesions are observed on fundoscopy, fERG can be useful for quantitative assessment of the affected retina's function.[19] Suspected congenital stationary night blindness, hyphema owing to trauma, chorioretinal lesions (owing to equine recurrent uveitis or other causes), and glaucoma are some of the common indications for ERG in equine patients.

The 2 main components of the equine ERG are the a- and the b-waves. The a-wave is the first trough of the ERG trace, and it reflects photoreceptor function. The b-wave is the first peak of the trace, and it originates from the bipolar cells. The amplitude of the a-wave is measured from the prestimulus baseline to the a-wave trough, and the b-wave amplitude is measured from the a-wave trough to the b-wave peak. The a- and b-wave peak time (also known as implicit time) is measured from the time of the flash to the peak of the respective wave (**Fig. 10**). In unhealthy retinas, the fERG's implicit time usually increases, and the amplitude decreases. It is noteworthy that the amplitudes of the a- and b-waves may be affected by the type of ERG machine, type of electrodes, the anatomic position of the electrodes, state of dark or light adaptation, intensity and frequency of the light stimuli, averaging of traces, and the level of sedation (or lack thereof). As such, consistent technique should be applied for ERG recording, and ERG examiners should establish normal references for fERG amplitudes for their settings and technique. Although ERG equipment is not available to the general practitioner, all practicing veterinary ophthalmologists should be able to perform ERG testing, and referral to a veterinary ophthalmologist should be considered when ERG is indicated.

COMMON DISEASES OF THE EQUINE FUNDUS

In this section, the most common findings seen in the equine fundus are discussed. A comprehensive review of equine retinal and optic disc diseases is beyond the scope of this article and can be found elsewhere.[20,21] One should be familiar with the normal appearance of the fundus and its variations, which were discussed in detail at the beginning of this article, and demonstrated in **Fig. 3**. Familiarity with the normal fundus and its variations will prevent misdiagnosis, which may have significant implication (eg, a decision after a prepurchase examination, incorrect prognosis, unnecessary diagnostic testing or treatment).

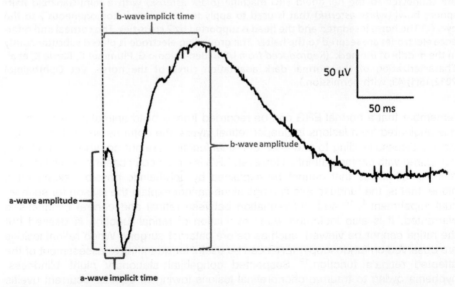

Fig. 10. A typical electroretinography trace of scotopic, combined rod–cone response in a horse.

Chorioretinal Lesions

Owing to the close proximity of the choroid and retina, inflammation in one usually leads to inflammation in the other. Any cause of uveitis can cause chorioretinitis, and some common causes of uveitis in horses include equine recurrent uveitis, trauma, leptospirosis, bacteremia, and septicemia. The inflammation usually starts in the vascular choroid, and progresses to affect the retina. Chorioretinal lesions are a relatively common finding in the horse. They can be active (ie, chorioretinitis) or inactive (ie, chorioretinal scars from historical chorioretinitis; **Fig. 11**). The inflammatory process is damaging to the neuroretina and may lead to loss of retinal function in the affected area. Horses usually compensate well for minor visual deficits. As such, when chorioretinal lesions are focal, they are not likely to cause noticeable visual deficits. However, the greater the extent of the lesion (active or scar), the more likely it is to cause visual impairment. In addition, lesions in the retinal area centralis may lead to greater effect on vision than peripheral lesions. Moreover, retinal lesions that affect

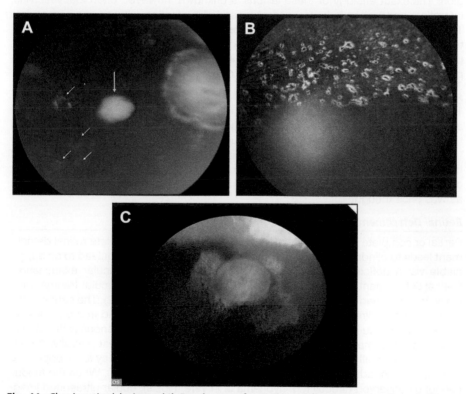

Fig. 11. Chorioretinal lesions. (A) Focal area of retinitis, with subretinal cellular infiltrate seen as a raised, yellowish lesion (*yellow arrow*). Multiple, greyish-white, flat, chorioretinal scars are scattered throughout the fundus (*white arrows*), and around the optic disc (on the *right*), as a result of previous chorioretinitis in these areas. (B) Multiple "bullet hole" chorioretinal lesions in the tapetum–nontapetum junction. Some of the lesions are extending into the tapetal fundus. A few retinal blood vessels can be seen on the left. (C) A typical "butterfly" lesion. In this horse, this was the result of peripapillary inflammation after ocular trauma. (*Courtesy of [A, B]* Dr Richard McMullen, Department of Clinical Sciences, College of Veterinary Medicine, Auburn University.)

only the outer retina may have a lesser effect on vision compared with deeper lesions that affect the inner retina and the nerve fiber layer, because the nerve fiber layer carries visual input from photoreceptors in other areas of the retina. The extent of the lesion, depthwise, cannot be determined without the advanced imaging technique of the ocular coherence tomography, which is rarely available to the veterinary ophthalmologist. Chorioretinal scars in the nontapetal fundus look like gray, depigmented lesions, whereas in the tapetal fundus they may look hyperreflective, owing to thinning of the retina and "overexposure" of the underlying tapetum. In both areas, pigment clumps may be seen within the lesion.

Focal chorioretinopathy ("bullet hole" lesions)
"Bullet hole" lesions can occasionally be found in the nontapetum, usually adjacent to the optic disc, and are considered incidental findings. These lesions appear as pinpoint, focal depigmentation of the nontapetum, with central hyperpigmentation, resembling bullet holes. The lesions may be a small cluster in a focal area, or more diffusely spread in the nontapetum. Rarely, they can also extend into the tapetal region. The exact etiology of these lesions is unknown; however, choroidal vasculitis, infarction, and ischemia have been proposed. An infection with equine herpesvirus 1 in utero has also been suggested as a possible etiology. A recent study has shown that even extensive bullet hole lesions occupying most of the nontapetal fundus (>"150 bullet holes") did not affect retinal function, as measured by fERG, and the reported horses did not seem to have visual deficits.[19]

Peripapillary chorioretinal scar ("butterfly" lesion)
This typical chorioretinal scar is located in the peripapillary (around the optic disc) area, and resembles butterfly wings, giving it its name (**Fig. 11C**). The depigmented "wings" may contain areas of pigment clumping and radiate medially and laterally from the optic disc. Peripapillary chorioretinal scars may extend to only one side of the optic disc, or appear linear. Any cause of uveitis with peripapillary involvement can lead to this type of lesion, and it is not pathognomonic to equine recurrent uveitis as was once thought.

Retinal Detachment

Partial or complete retinal detachment may occur. Whereas complete retinal detachment leads to blindness, partial or focal retinal detachment may not lead to an appreciable visual deficit, and may be an incidental finding during ocular examination. Retinal detachment is usually caused by inflammation (uveitis) or ocular trauma. Clinically, the detached retina looks like a gray, translucent veil (**Fig. 12**). The cause of the inflammation leading to retinal detachment should be identified and treated. If identified and successfully treated in a timely manner, a nonrhegmatogenous (with no tear) detached retina may reattach, and vision may be regained, at least partially. A reattached retina usually does not reattach perfectly and retinal folds may form, appearing as gray streaks radiating from the optic disc (**Figs. 6**B and **12**A, B). When the fundus cannot be observed directly (eg, hyphema or severe miosis), ocular ultrasound imaging can be used to assess the retina, as discussed (**Fig. 8**).

Senile Retinopathy

This condition is commonly seen in geriatric horses. Bilateral, irregular, hyperpigmented lines appear in the nontapetal fundus ventral to the optic disc, and a zone of depigmentation may be seen adjacent to the hyperpigmented lines (**Fig. 13**). The tapetum is not involved, and in the author's experience and others (Chandler and colleagues[22] 2003, Barnett[23] 1972) visual deficits are not appreciated. This condition is considered

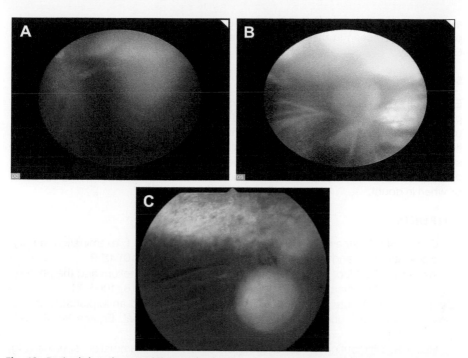

Fig. 12. Retinal detachment. (*A*) Detached retina that reattached. Multiple retinal folds are seen as pale-gray streaks radiating from the optic disc (the folds are not reattached). This picture was taken from a horse with active uveitis, hence the hazy view of the fundus. (*B*) Partial retinal detachment in the ventral fundus, appearing as gray veil ventral to the optic disc and partially over it. This eye has panuveitis, leading to the hazy view of the optic disc and retina. (*C*) Rhegmatogenous retinal detachment. The retina was torn from its dorsal insertion and has fallen like a veil over the optic disc and the ventral retina, leading to a hazy view of these areas. (*Courtesy of* [*C*] Dr Richard McMullen, Department of Clinical Sciences, College of Veterinary Medicine, Auburn University.)

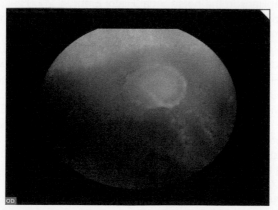

Fig. 13. Senile retinopathy. Irregular, linear, hyperpigmentation is seen mostly ventral to the optic disc. Depigmented areas are seen adjacent to the hyperpigmented lines. No visual deficits were noted by the owner of this horse, and this was an incidental finding.

a benign age-related retinopathy, and should not be confused with the honeycomb pigment pattern seen in the fundus of horses with motor neuron disease or vitamin E deficiency.

SUMMARY

Evaluation of the ocular fundus is a vital part of a complete eye examination. Although proper use of ophthalmic instruments and examination technique facilitates a thorough view of the fundus, knowing the normal appearance of the equine fundus, and its variations, ensures appropriate diagnosis and treatment. Advanced diagnostic instruments and skills can be used at the specialist level, and a referral to a veterinary ophthalmologist should be considered and offered to clients, in challenging cases or when in doubt.

REFERENCES

1. Crispin SM, Matthews AG, Parker J. The equine fundus. I: examination, embryology, structure and function. Equine Vet J Suppl 1990;(10):42–9.
2. Wouters L, De Moor A. Ultrastructure of the pigment epithelium and the photoreceptors in the retina of the horse. Am J Vet Res 1979;40(8):1066–71.
3. Harman AM, Moore S, Hoskins R, et al. Horse vision and an explanation for the visual behaviour originally explained by the 'ramp retina'. Equine Vet J 1999; 31(5):384–90.
4. Hebel R. Distribution of retinal ganglion cells in five mammalian species (pig, sheep, ox, horse, dog). Anat Embryol (Berl) 1976;150(1):45–51.
5. Guo X, Sugita S. Topography of ganglion cells in the retina of the horse. J Vet Med Sci 2000;62(11):1145–50.
6. Shinozaki A, Takagi S, Hosaka YZ, et al. The fibrous tapetum of the horse eye. J Anat 2013;223(5):509–18.
7. De Schaepdrijver L, Simoens P, Lauwers H, et al. Retinal vascular patterns in domestic animals. Res Vet Sci 1989;47(1):34–42.
8. Brooks DE. Equine Ophthalmology. 2nd edition. Jackson (WY): Teton Newmedia; 2008.
9. Altunay H. Fine structure of the retinal pigment epithelium, bruch's membrane and choriocapillaris in the horse. Anat Histol Embryol 2000;29(3):135–9.
10. Cutler TJ, Brooks DE, Andrew SE, et al. Disease of the equine posterior segment. Vet Ophthalmol 2000;3(2–3):73–82.
11. Ollivier FJ, Samuelson DA, Brooks DE, et al. Comparative morphology of the tapetum lucidum (among selected species). Vet Ophthalmol 2004;7(1):11–22.
12. Murphy CJ, Howland HC. The optics of comparative ophthalmoscopy. Vision Res 1987;27(4):599–607.
13. Williams J, Wilkie DA. Ultrasonography of the eye. Comp Cont Educ Pract 1996; 18(6):667.
14. Gilger BC, Stoppini R. Equine ocular examination: routine and advanced diagnostic techniques. In: Gilger BC, editor. Equine ophthalmology. 2nd edition. Maryland Heights (MO): Elsevier; 2011. p. 1–51.
15. Ben-Shlomo G, Plummer C, Barrie K, et al. Characterization of the normal dark adaptation curve of the horse. Vet Ophthalmol 2012;15(1):42–5.
16. Hepworth KL, Wong DM, Sponseller BA, et al. Survival of an adult quarter horse gelding following bacterial meningitis caused by Escherichia coli. Equine Vet Educ 2014;26(10):507–12.

17. Sandmeyer LS, Breaux CB, Archer S, et al. Clinical and electroretinographic characteristics of congenital stationary night blindness in the appaloosa and the association with the leopard complex. Vet Ophthalmol 2007;10(6):368–75.

18. Nunnery C, Pickett JP, Zimmerman KL. Congenital stationary night blindness in a thoroughbred and a paso fino. Vet Ophthalmol 2005;8(6):415–9.

19. Allbaugh RA, Ben-Shlomo G, Whitley RD. Electroretinogram evaluation of equine eyes with extensive 'bullet-hole' fundic lesions. Vet Ophthalmol 2014;17(Suppl 1): 129–33.

20. Nell B, Walde I. Posterior segment diseases. Equine Vet J Suppl 2010;(37):69–79.

21. Allbaugh RA, Townsend WM, Wilkie DA. Diseases of the equine vitreous and retina. In: Gilger BC, editor. Equine ophthalmology. 3rd edition. Ames (IA): Wiley & Son, Inc; 2017. p. 469–507.

22. Chandler KJ, Billson FM, Mellor DJ. Ophthalmic lesions in 83 geriatric horses and ponies. Vet Rec 2003;153(11):319–22.

23. Barnett KC. The ocular fundus of the horse. Equine Vet J 1972;4(1):17–20.

Equine Glaucoma

Tammy Miller Michau, DVM, MS, MSpVM[a,b,]*

KEYWORDS

- Equine • Glaucoma • Neurodegenerative • Surgery • Therapy • Tonometry

KEY POINTS

- Any horse that develops corneal edema, focal or diffuse, or that has a history of uveitis should be tested for glaucoma.
- Overall, the prognosis for vision in horses with glaucoma is poor. Lowering the IOP can improve vision in horses in the short term by clearing corneal edema and improving retinal and optic nerve vascular perfusion.
- Cyclophotocoagulation combined with medical therapy is the best current therapeutic option for maintaining vision long term.
- The limitations in controlling IOP in the horse, together with the concept that lowering IOP is not enough to prevent/slow down glaucomatous damage, highlights the importance of combining hypotensive treatment with new pharmacologic approaches aimed at increasing outflow and neuroprotection.

INTRODUCTION

Glaucoma is a multifactorial neurodegenerative ocular disease that leads to progressive loss of retinal ganglion cells (RGC) and their axons that form the optic nerve. The end result is blindness. Knowledge of the pathogenesis and development of equine glaucoma is still in its relative infancy compared with human glaucoma. The overall incidence of equine glaucoma has been reported to be less than 1%.[1–3] It is likely higher because it occurs most commonly secondary to uveitis and may be underdiagnosed or misdiagnosed in horses suffering from that disease. For example, horses with equine recurrent uveitis (ERU) that develop a cloudy eye are routinely treated for a "flare" instead of having their intraocular pressure (IOP) measured. A cloudy cornea eye that develops following trauma may be presumed to be from the trauma when the IOP may be elevated because of intraocular damage. The recognition and clinical diagnosis of glaucoma in the horse is improved with clinician awareness and the availability of handheld tonometers. Therapy for glaucoma is primarily aimed at decreasing aqueous humor production through medical and surgical means. Even

Disclosure Statement: None.
a BluePearl Veterinary Partners, 3000 Busch Lake Boulevard, Tampa, FL 33614, USA; b Brandon Equine Medical Center, 605 E. Bloomingdale Avenue, Brandon, FL 33511, USA
* 3000 Busch Lake Boulevard, Tampa, FL 33614.
E-mail address: Tammy.millermichau@bluepearlvet.com

with therapy, long-term prognosis for vision is poor. As more is learned about the underlying changes in glaucoma in the horse, it is hoped that other therapies, such as prevention of neurodegeneration, will become available.

ANATOMY AND PATHOPHYSIOLOGY

Elevated IOP is recognized as a significant risk factor for glaucoma. The IOP is a balance between aqueous humor production and outflow. Aqueous humor is produced primarily by continuous secretion from the ciliary body.[4–6] The enzyme carbonic anhydrase plays a role in this secretion by catalyzing the reaction transforming bicarbonate into carbon dioxide and water and is a target of therapy. Aqueous humor then exits the eye by either conventional or unconventional outflow. Conventional outflow occurs via the iridocorneal angle through the pectinate ligaments, trabecular meshwork, and then into the episcleral and conjunctival veins or scleral venous plexus and vortex veins via the angular aqueous plexus (**Fig. 1**). It is the predominant means of outflow in dogs and humans. Unconventional or uveoscleral outflow is not a distinctive pathway and occurs through means other than via the trabecular meshwork. Aqueous humor is absorbed by the iris, ciliary body, and suprachoroidal and supraciliary spaces (see **Fig. 1**). Unconventional or uveoscleral outflow is approximately 4% to 14%%, 15%, and 3% in humans, dogs, and cats, respectively.[7] Uveoscleral outflow may be extensive in the horse but the actual percentage is unknown.[5] Horses have robust pectinate ligaments that span the opening to the trabecular meshwork. Unlike the dog, these are easily visible as a gray line at the nasal and temporal limbus in most horses (**Fig. 2**).[5,8]

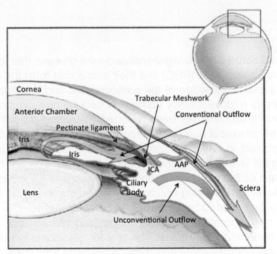

Fig. 1. Drainage of aqueous humour (AH) via the conventional and unconventional (uveoscleral) outflow pathways in the equine eye. Aqueous humour is produced by the nonpigmented epithelium of the ciliary body. It passes from the posterior chamber, through the pupil and into the anterior chamber. Conventional outflow occurs via the iridocorneal angle (ICA) through the pectinate ligaments, trabecular meshwork (uveal and corneoscleral), angular aqueous plexus (AAP), anteriorly to the episcleral and conjunctival veins, or posteriorly into the scleral venous plexus and vortex veins. In the unconventional outflow pathway, aqueous humor passes through the iris, ciliary body, and suprachoroidal and supraciliary spaces to eventually diffuse out the sclera. (*Adapted from* the National Eye Institute, National Institutes of Health. Available at: https://www.flickr.com/photos/nationaleyeinstitute/7544457582/in/album-72157646829197286/.)

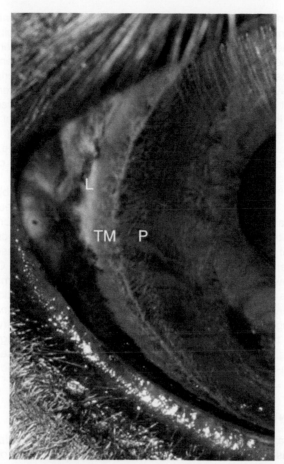

Fig. 2. Photograph of the iridocorneal angle of a normal horse with a pigmented iris. The conjunctiva transitions to the cornea at the limbus (L). The broad pectinate ligaments (P) extend from the iris base to the corneal endothelium and the attachments form the visible gray line seen at the nasal and temporal limbus in the horse. The trabecular meshwork is located in the area of the gray line. TM, trabecular meshwork.

The exact proportion of conventional versus unconventional outflow in the horse is unknown but uveoscleral outflow is extensive.[4,5] Outflow resistance, the resistance to the outflow of aqueous humor from the eye, is the primary determinant of IOP elevation and in humans, occurs primarily in the trabecular meshwork affecting conventional outflow.[9,10] The location of conventional outflow resistance in glaucomatous horses most likely occurs at the angular aqueous plexus and scleral venous plexus.[4–6,11] The location of unconventional/uveoscleral outflow resistance has not been definitively determined.[12]

Clinical changes, such as retinal degeneration and optic nerve cupping in the posterior segment of horses with glaucoma, are expected. These changes occur secondary to the elevated IOP and possibly primarily from abnormalities that develop in the optic nerve head (ONH) and its supporting structures. Horses have a large number of RGC in the retina.[12,13] These cells are a population of central nervous system neurons with their soma in the inner retina and axons in the optic nerve. The axons of the RGC converge and become arranged into optic nerve bundles in the pores of the lamina cribrosa of the ONH.[12] The lamina cribrosa is a specialized extracellular matrix of collagen fibers, like the trabecular meshwork, and supports and surrounds the optic nerve. The normal appearance of the ONH or disk in the horse is a result of myelin extending anterior to the lamina cribrosa to cover the surface of the nerve, the white peripapillary scleral ring (viewed easily at 6 o'clock), and retinal vessels fanning out a short distance from the ONH except ventrally.[12] The increase in IOP in glaucoma eventually disrupts axoplasmic flow in the axons of the optic nerve, displaces the scleral lamina cribrosa posteriorly, and results in the ONH cupping that is seen clinically (**Fig. 3**).[13]

Although elevated IOP is a major contributing factor in glaucoma, blindness can progress in the face of a normal IOP.[6,14] Also, ocular hypertension can occur when the IOP is elevated but does not damage the RGCs and optic nerve.[15,16] These findings support the theory that although IOP is currently the only modifiable clinical sign in glaucoma, other factors are influencing the progression of the neurodegenerative changes. In humans, glaucoma becomes more prevalent with aging, and predisposing epigenetic, genetic, and environmental factors also contribute to increased risk and eventual death of the RGCs.[17] Some of these factors include decreased ocular blood flow, extracellular matrix remodeling in the lamina cribrosa of the ONH and in the trabecular meshwork of the iridocorneal angle, subclinical inflammation, oxidative stress, glutamate toxicity, activation of intrinsic and extrinsic apoptotic signals, down-regulation of neuroprotective factors, mitochondrial dysfunction, axonal transport failure, misbehaving reactive glia, and loss of synaptic connectivity.[10,17–24] These changes occur through several pathways, including transforming growth factor (TGF)-β signaling, Rho kinase, nitric oxide/soluble guanylate cyclase/cGMP, adenosine A1, mitogen-activated proteinkinase, brain-derived neurotrophic factor, and potassium channels.[20,25,26]

CLINICAL PRESENTATION

Equine glaucoma is generally described as being primary or secondary in origin. Primary glaucoma is an elevated IOP and observation of characteristic optic neuropathy

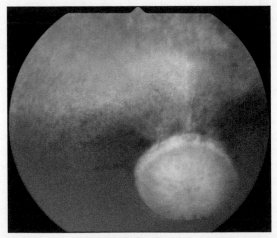

Fig. 3. Fundus photograph of a horse with glaucoma. The retinal vasculature is attenuated and the optic nerve head is cupped. Instead of myelin overlaying the optic nerve head, the scleral lamina cribrosa is visualized. (*Courtesy of* Dr Richard McMullen Jr, Drmedvet, DACVO, DECVO, CAQ Eq Ophth [Germany], Auburn, AL.)

with no distinguishable pathologic cause. Secondary glaucoma refers to an elevated IOP with an identifiable pathologic cause.

Congenital, primary, and secondary glaucoma occur in the horse.[1,27-30] Glaucoma has been reported in the American Paint, American Saddlebred, Appaloosa, Arabian, Draft (Percheron, other), Haflinger, Morgan, mule, Paso Fino, Percheron, Pony (Americas, Connemara, Shetland), Quarter Horse, Standardbred, Tennessee Walking Horse, Thoroughbred, and Warmbloods (ie, Trakehner, other).[2,8,13,27,31-33] Overall, the most common presenting breeds are the Appaloosa, Quarter Horse, and Thoroughbred.[32]

Glaucoma secondary to chronic uveitis, especially ERU, is the most commonly recognized form of glaucoma in the horse.[32,34] Clinical signs of ERU have been reported in 85% to 90% of cases.[32,33,35,36] Other causes of secondary glaucoma include trauma, hyphema, intraocular neoplasia, lens luxations, and postcataract surgery (Fig. 4).[2,12,37-46] Inflammation can lead to secondary glaucoma by causing preiridal fibrovascular membranes, anterior and posterior synechia, and pigment-laden, inflammatory, neoplastic, or red blood cell accumulation, all leading to blockage of the outflow pathways.

Primary glaucoma is infrequently reported but does occur, especially in older horses.[1,32,40] In humans, the most common form of primary glaucoma is classified as "open angle" and in the dog is "closed angle"; however, angle changes seen in horses with glaucoma are not well defined. Again, aqueous humor leaves the eye by conventional and uveoscleral outflow. Degeneration or genetic abnormalities can lead to obstruction of outflow. Uveoscleral outflow decreases with advancing age in humans, and this may also occur in the horse.[47] Congenital glaucoma is rare.[27,32,41] Although no breed disposition for congenital glaucoma has been established, it has been reported in Thoroughbred, Arabian, and Standardbred foals.[27,28,40,41,48,49]

Active, recurrent, and chronic/persistent uveitis, age (>15 years), and breed (Appaloosa) are the reported risk factors for the development of glaucoma.[2,12,32,35,41] The Appaloosa develops a particularly aggressive form of glaucoma, likely related to underlying ERU, which is poorly responsive to therapy.[50]

PATIENT EVALUATION OVERVIEW
Clinical Signs

The clinical signs in horses with glaucoma can vary widely depending on the underlying pathology, the stage of the glaucoma, and the severity of the IOP elevation

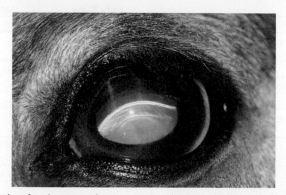

Fig. 4. Photograph of a horse with a posterior lens luxation and glaucoma following trauma. (Courtesy of Dr Richard McMullen Jr, Drmedvet, DACVO, DECVO, CAQ Eq Ophth [Germany], Auburn, AL.)

(**Table 1**). In the early stages the signs can be subtle and nonspecific. The reliable clinical signs seen in dogs, such as redness, pain, corneal edema, and blindness, may be absent. Corneal edema may not manifest at modest IOP elevations. In horses, corneal edema can sometimes be the only presenting sign. In contrast to dogs, it can also present as focal edema instead of diffuse, especially in the early stages (**Fig. 5**). Ocular discomfort characterized by blepharospasm and epiphora may or may not be present until later or with high IOPs.

If uveitis is the underlying cause of the glaucoma, all the clinical signs of uveitis may be present including blepharospasm, blepharoedema, photophobia, miosis instead of mydriasis, aqueous flare, keratic precipitates corpora nigra atrophy, posterior synechia, dyscoria, cataract, vitreal degeneration, retinal and optic nerve atrophy, and retinal detachment.[12] Clinical signs of corneal edema, chemosis, blepharospasm, blepharoedema and pain can also be confused with active uveitis, Descemet membrane detachment, heterochromic iridocyclitis, and endothelial immune mediated keratitis.[51–53] In a uveitic horse, the development of glaucoma can be mistaken as a uveitic flare that does not respond to routine uvetis therapy.

Clinical signs in the later stages of the disease include partial thickness breaks in Descemet membrane (corneal striae, Haab stria) from limbus to limbus (**Fig. 6**), worsening edema (**Fig. 7**), buphthalmos (**Fig. 8**), and progressive vision loss. Corneal striae may occur in the acute stage or chronic stage of glaucoma. The breaks may occur because of stretching from globe enlargement (buphthalmos) but the underlying pathogenesisis in the acute stage of glaucoma is unknown. These breaks can also be seen in normal horses (ie, band keratopathy) and horses following blunt trauma, and may not be signficant.[54] The presence of corneal stria should raise the suspicion of glaucoma and a complete ophthalmic examination and tonometry should be performed to rule out glaucoma.

The eye remains visual in the early stages of glaucoma and vision can still be retained once the globe is clinically buphthalmic. The equine eye seems to be more tolerant of elevations in IOP than other species, such as the dog. Some horses can remain visual when IOPs are 50 mm Hg for several days to weeks.[33,55,56] In contrast to dogs, buphthalmos may resolve in horses with lowering of the IOP. The ability to

Table 1
Clinical signs of early and late stage glaucoma in the horse

Clinical Signs	Early Stage	Late Stage
Redness	–/+	+
Pain (blepharospasm, photophobia, epiphora, eyelid swelling)	–/+	+
Chemosis	+	+/–
Corneal edema (focal or diffuse)	+	++
Corneal bullae	+/–	+/–
Breaks in Descemet membrane (corneal striae, Haab striae)	–/+	++
Mydriasis	+/–	+ (unless synechia present)
Buphthalmos	–	++
Optic nerve cupping, vascular attenuation	–	+
Absent menace, vision loss	–/+ (corneal edema can affect vision)	+

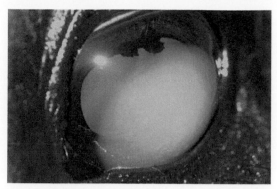

Fig. 5. Photograph of a horse with glaucoma and focal severe corneal edema.

retain vision in a buphthalmic globe and the resolution of buphthalmos is likely a result of greater elasticity of the equine fibrous tunic.[12] The large number of RGCs may also act as an anatomic reservoir that protects against vision loss.[12] Some RGCs may be more resistant to the elevated IOP.[12] In the early stages of glaucoma the salmon pink optic nerve begins to look pale. Progressive vision loss occurs as the RGCs die and optic nerve begins to lose axons. Eventually optic nerve cupping, retinal vascular attenuation, and visual deficits are clinically detected (see **Fig. 3**). Other clinical signs seen include bullous keratopathy and corneal ulceration secondary to the corneal edema (see **Fig. 7**; **Fig. 9**). Buphthalmos can also lead to ulcerative and nonulcerative exposure keratitis.

Diagnostics

The diagnosis of glaucoma in the horse is made based on the history, signalment, clinical signs, and documentation of an elevated IOP.[12] A potential drawback of current approaches to glaucoma diagnosis includes the inability to positively diagnose glaucoma before considerable damage to the retina has probably already occurred. In

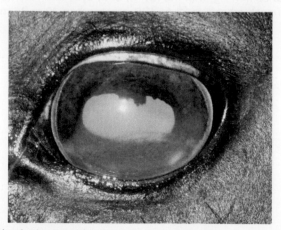

Fig. 6. Photograph of a horse with glaucoma. Corneal striae are seen traversing from the dorsal to ventral limbus nasally and nasal to temporal limbus ventrally. Corneal edema is predominantly ventral. The pupil is not mydriatic. The IOP was 40 mm Hg.

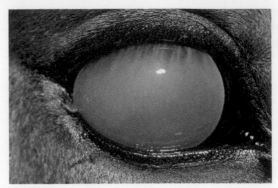

Fig. 7. Photograph of a horse with glaucoma and diffuse corneal edema. Punctate corneal bullae are appreciated ventral and temporal.

humans, RGC apoptosis has been identified as the earliest form of cell death. It is estimated that up to 40% of RGCs are lost before visual field defects are detected.[57] These data are not available for horses.

IOP, presently the only modifiable risk factor for glaucoma, is assessed using hand-held applanation or rebound tonometry (**Fig. 10**). Tonometry is indicated in horses for the following reasons[3,12]:

- Corneal edema (focal or diffuse)
- A red or painful eye
- A history of uveitis
- Recurrent epiphora
- Orbital trauma or blunt ocular trauma
- Hyphema
- A history of glaucoma in the opposite eye
- Lens luxation

The normal mean equine IOP is 21 to 23 mm Hg (**Table 2**).[58–61] The equine IOP ranges from 15 to 30 mm Hg, with the IOP of both eyes of an individual being within 5 to 8 mm Hg of each other.[58,62–66] An IOP greater than 32 to 35 mm Hg is usually

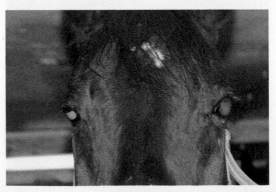

Fig. 8. Photograph of a horse with glaucoma of the left eye. Buphthalmos is appreciated when observing the horse from the front and comparing with the normal eye. (*Courtesy of* Dr Richard McMullen Jr, Drmedvet, DACVO, DECVO, CAQ Eq Ophth [Germany], Auburn, AL.)

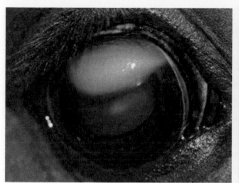
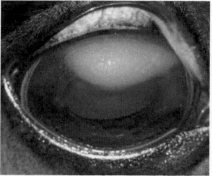

Fig. 9. Photograph of a horse with glaucoma. The edema is focal and severe and bullae are present. Fluorescein dye staining is positive in the photograph on the right. (*Courtesy of* Dr Richard McMullen Jr, Drmedvet, DACVO, DECVO, CAQ Eq Ophth [Germany], Auburn, AL.)

diagnostic, or at least suspicious of glaucoma. Horses with primary glaucoma and secondary glaucoma are reported to have IOPs of 35 to 80 mm Hg and 40 to 80 mm Hg, respectively.[67] Topical anesthetic is required for applanation tonometry but not rebound tonometry.

Obtaining an accurate IOP in the horse is challenging (**Table 3**). The same protocol should be used for repeated measurements (ie, sedation, tonometry method, head position, auriculopalpebral block or not). Comparison with the unaffected normal eye may be indicated. If significant corneal disease is present, the most normal part of cornea should be used to take readings. A fibrotic and edematous cornea may result in a falsely elevated IOP.[62] Diurnal variations in IOP have been reported in many species including the horse.[2,8,68,69] Normal horses have a peak IOP at the end of day and a trough during nightime.[68] The IOP in horses with glaucoma does not remain consistently elevated, which results in fluctuations in clinical signs and makes the diagnosis and therapy challenging in this species.[2,12] Frequent and repeated IOP measurements may be required to confirm the clinical suspicion.[70]

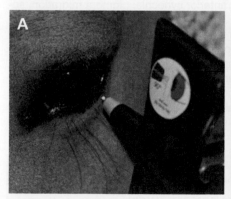
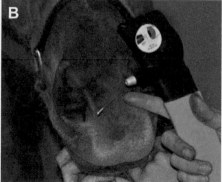

Fig. 10. Handheld applanation (Tonopen XL, Mentor, Norwell, Mass) or rebound tonometry (TonoVet, Tiolat Ltd, Helsinki, Finland) in the horse is necessary for the diagnosis of an elevated IOP. The TonoVet can be used without topical anesthetic and easily without sedation and manipulation of the eyelids (*A*). However, failure to keep the TonoVet at a 90° angle, which occurs easily when struggling with a horse, can result in loss of the preplaced probe (*B*).

Table 2
Mean intraocular pressure ± standard deviation for two applanation tonometers and a rebound tonometer in the horse

Tonometry Instrument	Applanation or Rebound	Intraocular Pressure (mm Hg)
Perkins	Applanation	23.4 ± 3.2 (range, 18–28)
Tonopen	Applanation	23.3 ± 6.9
TonoVet	Rebound	22.1 ± 5.9

The horse has a strong obicularis oculi and opening the eyelids in a painful horse can require the exertion of a significant amount of pressure. This compression may artificially increase IOP. The effect of an auriculopalpebral nerve block on IOP has had conflicting results. In two studies, horses that were not blocked showed an elevated IOP.[62,71] In two other studies, the results were comparable between horses with and without a block.[58,63] Performing an auriculopalpebral block is the best chance of obtaining an accurate IOP, especially when unsure of the diagnosis. IOP is also significantly increased when the horse's head position is below heart level.[72] The IOP should always be taken in a head up position. If sedated, the handler should support the horse's head.

Horses that require sedation for ocular examination may show dramatic decreases in IOP. Xylazine, acepromazine, detomidine, and romifidine have all been shown to decrease IOP.[63,73–77] Ketamine has been reported to both raise and lower IOP.[71,78] In one report in horses with an auriculopalpebral block, combined ketamine and xylazine decreased IOP but in other reports the combined drugs had no effect.[8,71]

Advanced Imaging

Gonioscopy, the use of a specialized lens to evaluate the iridocorneal angle, is not needed in the horse because the angle is visualized directly. Gonioscopic changes in horses have been reported and the angle can look normal, narrow, or closed.[2] Iridocorneal angle changes by direct observation in horses with glaucoma are infrequently reported, but abnormalities are identified (**Figs. 11** and **12**).[11,12,79] These abnormalities include narrowing, distortion, anterior synechia, pigment migration, solidification, and difficulty viewing.

Routine ultrasound is used to evaluate for signs of retinal detachment to help determine if uveitis is present. High-resolution ultrasonography or ultrasound biomicroscopy (20–60 MHz) can reveal changes in the iridocorneal angle consistent with outflow blockage and predisposing anatomic changes potentially identified.[80] High-frequency ultrasound changes have not yet been reported in horses with glaucoma. Ultrasound can also be used to evaluate globe size if unsure if buphthalmos is present. A globe size greater than 40 to 45 mm is consistent with globe

Table 3
Factors that can increase or decrease intraocular pressure in the horse

Increase Intraocular Pressure	Decrease Intraocular Pressure
Lowering the head below the heart No auriculopalpebral block (±) Fibrotic/edematous cornea External globe compression Sedation (ketamine) ±	Sedation (xylazine, acepromazine, romifidine, detomidine) Sedation (ketamine) ± (in combination with xylazine no effect)

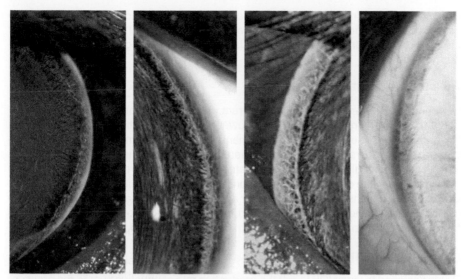

Fig. 11. The iridocorneal angle (ICA) is visualized directly in the horse. Photographs of normal-appearing ICAs in four horses without ocular disease. Broad pectinate ligaments from the iris span the iridocorneal angle to insert on the corneal endothelium. This is seen clinically as a gray line at the nasal and temporal limbus. Aqueous humor moves through the pectinate ligaments into the trabecular meshwork. The horse on the *right* has a blue iris and no pigment in the ICA.

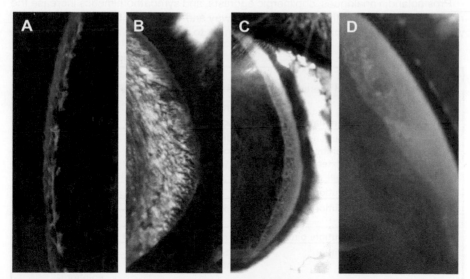

Fig. 12. The iridocorneal angle (ICA) is visualized directly in the horse. Photographs of abnormal-appearing ICAs in four horses with glaucoma. (*A*) Narrow ICA. (*B*) Narrowing and loss/inability to visualize the ICA. (*C*) More solid ICA. (*D*) Broad anterior synechia in the ICA following trauma.

enlargement.[67] The measurement of retinal nerve fiber layer thickness changes by optical coherence tomography and the assessment of structural changes at the site of the ONH by disk tomography (confocal laser-scanning tomography) are not yet reported in horses.

THERAPEUTIC TARGETS

Lowering the IOP represents the only current measurable component of equine glaucoma therapy. The goal of therapy is to lower the IOP to less than or equal to 20 mm Hg and includes medical and surgical management.[12] Determination of whether to pursue medical therapy alone, medical therapy and surgical therapy, or surgical therapy alone is primarily dependent on whether or not vision is present. The two main goals of therapy are either to salvage vision for as long as possible or provide comfort. Other factors to consider when choosing a course of therapy are concurrent disease (ie, ERU, lens luxation, intraocular tumor), age and purpose of the horse, economic factors, and ability of the owner to treat the horse as directed.[12]

PHARMACOLOGIC TREATMENT OPTIONS

Drugs designed to lower IOP target the production rate of aqueous humor, the pressure in the episcleral veins, and/or the drainage of aqueous humor through the trabecular or uveoscleral outflow pathways. The drugs used most effectively in equine glaucoma, β-adrenergic blockers and carbonic anhydrase inhibitors (CAIs), reduce aqueous humor production (**Table 4**). Initial glaucoma therapy in the horse should be a combination of the topical β-blocker 0.5% timolol and the topical CAI 2% dorzolamide, used every 8 to 12 hours.[12] The combination is more effective than when the two drugs are administered concomitantly versus alone.[81,82] Another CAI, brinzolamide, has also been shown to lower IOP in the horse.[83] No studies have evaluated the effects of oral CAIs in horses and with the possible systemic side effects, should be avoided.

Prostaglandin analogues, cholinergic agonists, and sympathomimetics increase the rate of outflow through the uveoscleral pathway and/or through the trabecular meshwork. Prostaglandin analogues are designed to increase uveoscleral outflow in

Table 4
The most commonly used pharmacologic agents for treating glaucoma in the horse

Drug	Formulation	Mechanism of Action	Frequency	Adverse Effects
Timolol 0.5%	Solution, ointment,[a] extended-release gel	β-Adrenergic blocker	BID	Miosis ±
Dorzolamide 2%	Solution, ointment[a]	CAI	BID-TID	
Dorzolamide 2%/ timolol 0.5%	Solution, ointment[a]	CAI/β-blocker	BID-TID	
Brinzolamide 1%	Solution, ointment	CAI	Q 24 h TID	
Latanoprost 0.005%	Solution	Prostaglandin analogue	Q 24 h	Blepharospasm, blepharoedema, epiphora, conjunctival hyperemia, miosis

[a] Compounded.

humans over time and with the horse's extensive uveoscleral outflow, theoretically should be effective. However, the prostaglandin analogue latanoprost resulted in substantial discomfort and prolonged miosis, with only a small IOP reduction, and is not recommended in horses.[84,85] Prostaglandin analogues may also worsen intraocular inflammation and should be used with caution in horses with underlying uveitis. Studies looking at other prostaglandin analogues for side effects and for longer periods of time may prove beneficial. Several animal studies have found neuroprotective effects and increased blood flow with the use of topical prostaglandin analogues independent of their IOP-lowering effects.[86] Medications that increase outflow through the iridocorneal angle, such as the parasympathomimetics, are not effective or have not been tested in horses.[12,87]

Medical therapy for glaucoma in horses should include topical steroids (dexamethasone 0.1%, prednisolone acetate 1%), nonsteroidals (diclofenac, flurbiprofen, bromfenac, ketorolac), and systemic suppression of inflammation with nonsteroidals (flunixin meglumine, firocoxib). Topical anti-inflammatories, especially steroids, should be used with care in horses with severe corneal edema that may form bullae and develop corneal ulcerations (see **Fig. 9**). Horses with uveitis may also benefit from placement of a suprachoroidal cyclosporine sustained-release implant.[34]

Atropine has been recommended to increase unconventional (uveoscleral) outflow of aqueous humor and thereby decrease the incidence of glaucoma in uveitis. However, published studies reflect a variable effect of atropine on IOP.[88,89] Use of atropine topically in horses with glaucoma is not recommended unless it is early in the therapy for uveitis and posterior synechia could be prevented.[12]

The initial response to medical therapy can be favorable, but long-term prognosis for maintaining vision with medical therapy alone is guarded.[12]

NOVEL TREATMENT OPTIONS

Novel therapeutic agents targeting factors influencing the progression of the neurodegenerative changes seen in glaucoma have shown preliminary success in animal models and even human trials, demonstrating that they may eventually be used to enhance outflow and preserve retinal neurons and vision. For example, Rho-associated coiled-coil forming protein kinase inhibitors improve ocular blood flow, prevent RGC death/increase RGC survival, and retard axonal degeneration or induce axonal regeneration.[90] Elevated levels of TGF-β are found in the aqueous humor and in reactive optic nerve astrocytes in patients with glaucoma.[91,92] Possible therapeutic strategies targeting TGF-β in the treatment of glaucoma are being investigated. Little is known about these changes in the horse and experimental treatment modalities directed at these abnormalities have not yet been reported. Further study is needed and the causes, clinical findings, and treatments may differ for horses with glaucoma compared with other species.

NONPHARMACOLOGIC/SURGICAL TREATMENT OPTIONS

Surgical therapy is indicated in eyes that are poorly or nonresponsive to medical therapy and the technique dependent on whether or not vision is present.

Surgical Treatment in Visual Eyes

Surgical therapy in visual eyes is divided into techniques directed at reducing aqueous humor production by the ciliary body (cyclocryosurgery, cyclophotocoagulation) and techniques directed at opening up an outflow pathway (gonioimplants). Cyclodestructive procedures have been described in horses using various techniques, including cyclocryotherapy, transcleral cyclophotocoagulation (TSCP), and endoscopic cyclo-photocoagulation. This is indicated in visual eyes and may provide the best chance for long term IOP control.[12] Cyclocryosurgery was performed historically, but because of its significant side effects, has been largely replaced by laser procedures.[93] TSCP has been accomplished using the neodymium:yttrium-aluminum-garnet laser and semiconductor diode lasers.[33,35,55,94,95] Vision was preserved in 58% to 60% of cases and TSCP is considered the therapy of choice for long-term IOP control in hors-es.[12,33,55] The diode laser is preferentially absorbed in pigmented tissue and may not be as effective in animals with decreased melanin (albino horses, palominos, blue-eyed horses). TSCP can be performed under general anesthesia or as a standing procedure where indicated. Laser settings (power and time), sites of application, and variations for visual versus nonvisual eyes have been reported.[12,35,67,96] Insufficient laser energy, insufficient sites, and ciliary body epithelial regrowth can result in a nega-tive result and need for further surgical intervention. Excessive laser energy or sites can result in hyphema, hypotony, severe intraocular inflammation, and phthisis bulbi. Globes that are affected with ERU are at increased risk and complete hyphema and blindness has occurred after application of laser energy to a single site by the author. Pre-existing ocular conditions, such as corneal ulceration and inflammation from uve-itis, should be controlled before laser therapy to minimize complications.[67] Cyclopho-tocoagulation is contraindicated in the presence of intraocular neoplasia.

Endoscopic cyclophotocoagulation, where the laser is introduced into the eye and the ciliary processes is visualized directly, has been reported in cadaver globes but no clinical studies in horses with glaucoma have been published to date.[97] The use of endoscopic versus TSCP minimizes collateral tissue damage but introduces the risks associated with intraocular surgery.[98] The formation of a cataract following endo-scopic cyclophotocoagulation may necessitate phacoemulsification of the lens concomitant with the laser procedure.[97]

Surgical techniques to increase outflow are limited to placement of a gonioimplant to shunt aqueous humor to the subconjunctival space. Gonioimplants have not been commonly performed in the horse. As in humans, fibrosis of the shunt footplate in the conjunctiva decreases its longevity and may necessitate further surgical intervention to deroof the footplate. A Baerveldt gonioimplant has been reported effective in a sin-gle horse with glaucoma for more than a year.[99] The use of Ahmed shunts has also been reported and lowered IOP for 28 days.[100] Complications following shunt place-ment include hypotony, fibrosis around the footplate of the implant, inflammation and occlusion of the shunt tip by fibrin, incarceration of the corpora nigra, a shallow/collapsed anterior chamber, keratitis, shunt migration, and dehiscence/extrusion of the footplate (**Fig. 13**).[100]

Surgical Treatment in Nonvisual Eyes

Surgical therapy for a chronic blind painful eye with glaucoma is directed at controlling pain via end-stage procedures (ie, destruction of the ciliary body/pharmacologic abla-tion, enucleation, or evisceration and intrascleral implant).[101–103] Surgery may decrease the frequency of medical therapy but does not preclude it in the absence of an end-stage procedure.

Pharmacologic ciliary body ablation (CBA) is performed by intravitreal injection of 25 to 30 mg of gentamicin with 1 mg of dexamethasone-SP. This can be performed in a standing horse with use of sedation and local blocks.[12] Gentocin concentration should be 100 mg/mL to minimize the volume, because this same volume of fluid plus slightly more (dependent on how high the preoperative IOP is) must be removed from the vitreous or anterior. Complications can include uveitis; pain; hyphema; and when

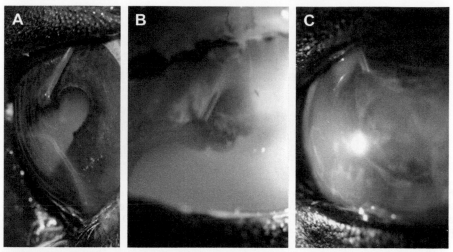

Fig. 13. Gonioimplant complications. (*A*) Shunt tip in contact with corneal endothelium and fibrosis. (*B*) Corpora nigra incarcerated in the shunt tip. (*C*) Extensive fibrin in the anterior chamber following cyclophotocoagulation sucked into and occluding the shunt tip. (*Courtesy of* Dr Richard McMullen Jr, Drmedvet, DACVO, DECVO, CAQ Eq Ophth [Germany], Auburn, AL.)

longer-term, cataract formation and phthisis bulbi. The appearance of the eye following a CBA cannot be predicted and the injection may not work and require repetition. The use of intravitreal cidofovir as an agent for pharmacologic CBA has not been evaluated in the horse.[104] A pharmacologic CBA should not be performed in horses with intraocular neoplasia or infection.

Enucleation provides the most conclusive therapy for the pain of glaucoma and is associated with minimal postoperative complications, but is cosmetically unappealing for the owner. Enucleation can be performed in the standing horse.[105,106] Mesh implants and intraorbital silicone or hydroxyapatite implants can minimize the depression following enucleation (**Fig. 14**).[12,107,108] Orbital implants may be associated with

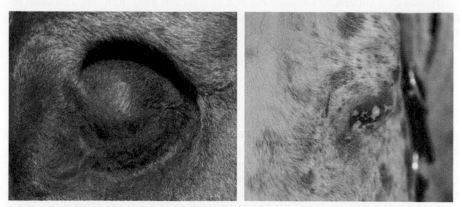

Fig. 14. Photographs of two horses with orbital implants following enucleation for glaucoma. The horse on the *left* still has sinking around and over a small implant. The horse on the *right* has a large enough orbital implant to prevent sinking and an improved aesthetic outcome.

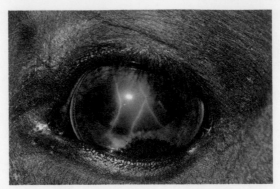

Fig. 15. Photograph of a horse with glaucoma and a Gunderson inlay flap ventrally. The flap was successful in improving corneal edema in this case. Multiple corneal striae are also apparent. (*Courtesy of* Dr Richard McMullen Jr, Drmedvet, DACVO, DECVO, CAQ Eq Ophth [Germany], Auburn, AL)

increased complications in the horse including wound dehiscence, draining tracts, and extrusion of the implant months to years following the procedure horse.[12,107,108] Alternatively, an evisceration of the intraocular contents and placement of intrascleral prosthesis may provide a more cosmetic outcome.[101,102] Complications of this procedure may include corneal ulceration and perforation in addition to infection.[12]

ADDITIONAL THERAPY

Significant corneal edema can result in the formation of bullae and subsequent ulceration and pain. Thermalkeratoplasty uses low-voltage cautery to induce fibrosis of the anterior stroma, forming a barrier against fluid uptake and it is hoped protection against or treatment of ulceration.[109] Thermalkeratoplasty can result in scarring that worsens vision, but can also improve vision by decreasing the edema. The visual outcome with this procedure cannot be guaranteed and may be less effective in horses with glaucoma compared with horses with uveitis.[54]

The use of a superficial keratectomy and Gunderson inlay graft has also been reported in three horses with possible glaucoma (**Fig. 15**).[110] This is a very thin permanent conjunctival graft placed in part of the cornea to reduce corneal edema, eliminate recurrent ulceration, and improve vision.[110] The Gunderson graft may be effective and result in improved corneal clarity but needs to be performed in more horses with glaucoma.

SUMMARY

Any horse that develops corneal edema, focal or diffuse, or that has a history of uveitis should be tested for glaucoma. Overall, the prognosis for vision in horses with glaucoma is poor. Lowering the IOP can improve vision in horses in the short term by clearing corneal edema and improving retinal and optic nerve vascular perfusion.[12] Cyclophotocoagulation combined with medical therapy is the best current therapeutic option for maintaining vision long term. The limitations in controlling IOP in the horse, together with the concept that lowering IOP is not enough to prevent/slow down glaucomatous damage, highlights the importance of combining hypotensive treatment with new pharmacologic approaches aimed at increasing outflow and neuroprotection.

REFERENCES

1. Cutler TJ. Ophthalmic findings in the geriatric horse. Vet Clin North Am Equine Pract 2002;18:545–74.
2. Miller TR, Brooks DE, Smith PJ, et al. Equine glaucoma: clinical findings and response to treatment in 14 horses. Vet Comp Ophthalmol 1995;7:170–82.
3. Brooks DE, Mathews AG. Equine ophthalmology. In: Gelatt KN, editor. Veterinary ophthalmology. 4th edition. Philadelphia: Saunders; 2007. p. 1233–43.
4. Smith PJ, Samuelson DA, Brooks DE, et al. Unconventional aqueous humor outflow of microspheres perfused into the equine eye. Am J Vet Res 1986;47: 2445–53.
5. Samuelson D, Smith P, Brooks D. Morphologic features of the aqueous humor drainage pathways in horses. Am J Vet Res 1989;50:720–7.
6. De Geest JP, Lauwers H, Simoens P, et al. The morphology of the equine irido-corneal angle: a light and scanning electron microscopic study. Equine Vet J Suppl 1990;(10):30–5.
7. Gum GG, MacKay EO. Physiology of the eye. In: Gelatt KN, Gilger BC, Kern TJ, editors. Veterinary ophthalmology. Ames (IO): Wiley-Blackwell; 2013. p. 171–207.
8. Smith PJ, Gum GG, Whitley RD, et al. Tonometric and tonographic studies in the normal pony eye. Equine Vet J Suppl 1990;(10):36–8.
9. Johnson M. What controls aqueous humour outflow resistance? Exp Eye Res 2006;82:545–57.
10. Braunger BM, Fuchshofer R, Tamm ER. The aqueous humor outflow pathways in glaucoma: a unifying concept of disease mechanisms and causative treatment. Eur J Pharm Biopharm 2015;95:173–81.
11. Utter ME, Brooks DE. Glaucoma. In: Gilger BC, editor. Equine ophthalmology. Maryland Heights (MO): Elsevier; 2011. p. 350–66.
12. Wilkie DA, Gemensky-Metzler AJ, Lassaline-Utter M, et al. Glaucoma. In: Gilger BC, editor. Equine ophthalmology. 3rd edition. Ames (IA): John Wiley & Sons, Inc.; 2017. p. 453–68.
13. Brooks DE, Blocker TL, Samuelson DA, et al. Histomorphometry of the optic nerves of normal horses and horses with glaucoma. Vet Comp Ophthalmol 1995;5:193–210.
14. Brooks DE, Strubbe DT, Kubilis PS, et al. Histomorphometry of the optic nerves of normal dogs and dogs with hereditary glaucoma. Exp Eye Res 1995;60: 71–89.
15. Smith PJ, Brooks DE, Lazarus JA, et al. Ocular hypertension following cataract surgery in dogs: 139 cases (1992-1993). J Am Vet Med Assoc 1996;209: 105–11.
16. Fife TM, Gemensky-Metzler AJ, Wilkie DA, et al. Clinical features and outcomes of phacoemulsification in 39 horses: a retrospective study (1993-2003). Vet Ophthalmol 2006;9:361–8.
17. Almasieh M, Wilson AM, Morquette B, et al. The molecular basis of retinal ganglion cell death in glaucoma. Prog Retin Eye Res 2012;31:152–81.
18. Levkovitch-Verbin H. Retinal ganglion cell apoptotic pathway in glaucoma: Initiating and downstream mechanisms. Prog Brain Res 2015;220:37–57.
19. Bradley JM, Vranka J, Colvis CM, et al. Effect of matrix metalloproteinases activity on outflow in perfused human organ culture. Invest Ophthalmol Vis Sci 1998;39:2649–58.

20. Gauthier AC, Liu J. Epigenetics and signaling pathways in glaucoma. Biomed Res Int 2017;2017:1–12.
21. Prendes MA, Harris A, Wirostko BM, et al. The role of transforming growth factor beta in glaucoma and the therapeutic implications. Br J Ophthalmol 2013;97: 680–6.
22. Davis BM, Crawley L, Pahlitzsch M, et al. Glaucoma: the retina and beyond. Acta Neuropathol 2016;132:807–26.
23. Gupta N, Yucel YH. Glaucoma as a neurodegenerative disease. Curr Opin Ophthalmol 2007;18:110–4.
24. Brooks DE, Garcia GA, Dreyer EB, et al. Vitreous body glutamate concentration in dogs with glaucoma. Am J Vet Res 1997;58:864–7.
25. Pascale A, Drago F, Govoni S. Protecting the retinal neurons from glaucoma: lowering ocular pressure is not enough. Pharmacol Res 2012;66:19–32.
26. Gauthier AC, Liu J. Neurodegeneration and neuroprotection in glaucoma. Yale J Biol Med 2016;89:73–9.
27. Halenda RM, Grahn BH, Sorden SD, et al. Congenital equine glaucoma: clinical and light microscopic findings in two cases. Vet Comp Ophthalmol 1997;7: 105–9.
28. Latimer CA, Wyman M. Neonatal ophthalmology. Vet Clin North Am Equine Pract 1985;1:235–59.
29. Malalana F. Ophthalmologic disorders in aged horses. Vet Clin North Am Equine Pract 2016;32:249–61.
30. Leiva M, Felici F, Carvalho A, et al. Benign intraocular teratoid medulloepithelioma causing glaucoma in an 11-year-old Arabian mare. Vet Ophthalmol 2013;16:297–302.
31. Pickett JP, Ryan J. Equine glaucoma: a retrospective study of 11 cases from 1988 to 1993. Vet Med 1993;88:56–63.
32. Curto EM, Gemensky-Metzler AJ, Chandler HL, et al. Equine glaucoma: a histopathologic retrospective study (1999-2012). Vet Ophthalmol 2014;17:334–42.
33. Annear MJ, Wilkie DA, Gemensky-Metzler AJ. Semiconductor diode laser transscleral cyclophotocoagulation for the treatment of glaucoma in horses: a retrospective study of 42 eyes. Vet Ophthalmol 2010;13:204–9.
34. Gerding JC, Gilger BC. Prognosis and impact of equine recurrent uveitis. Equine Vet J 2016;48:290–8.
35. Wilkie DA, Peckham ES, Paulic S, et al. Equine glaucoma and diode laser transscleral cyclophotocoagulation: 27 cases. Vet Ophthalmol 2001;4:294.
36. Gilger BC, Wilkie DA, Clode AB, et al. Long-term outcome after implantation of a suprachoroidal cyclosporine drug delivery device in horses with recurrent uveitis. Vet Ophthalmol 2010;13:294–300.
37. Wilkie DA, Gilger BC. Equine glaucoma. Vet Clin North Am Equine Pract 2004; 20:381–91.
38. Monk CS, Craft WF, Abbott JR, et al. Clinical behavior of intraocular teratoid medulloepithelioma in two-related Quarter Horses. Vet Ophthalmol 2016. [Epub ahead of print].
39. Davidson HJ, Blanchard GL, Wheeler CA, et al. Anterior uveal melanoma, with secondary keratitis, cataract, and glaucoma, in a horse. J Am Vet Med Assoc 1991;199:1049–50.
40. Cullen CL, Grahn BH. Equine glaucoma: a retrospective study of 13 cases presented at the Western College of Veterinary Medicine from 1992 to 1999. Can Vet J 2000;41:470–80.

41. Wilcock BP, Brooks DE, Latimer CA. Glaucoma in horses. Vet Pathol 1991;28: 74–8.
42. Millichamp NJ, Dziezyc J. Cataract phacofragmentation in horses. Vet Ophthalmol 2000;3:157–64.
43. McMullen RJ Jr, Utter ME. Current developments in equine cataract surgery. Equine Vet J Suppl 2010;(37):38–45.
44. McCluskie LK, Woodford NS, Carter WJ. Posterior lens luxation with associated glaucoma in a pony. Equine Vet Education 2009;21:228–31.
45. Edelmann ML, McMullen R Jr, Stoppini R, et al. Retrospective evaluation of phacoemulsification and aspiration in 41 horses (46 eyes): visual outcomes vs. age, intraocular lens, and uveitis status. Vet Ophthalmol 2014;17(Suppl 1): 160–7.
46. Brooks DE, Plummer CE, Carastro SM, et al. Visual outcomes of phacoemulsification cataract surgery in horses: 1990-2013. Vet Ophthalmol 2014;17(Suppl 1): 117–28.
47. Toris CB, Yablonski ME, Wang YL, et al. Aqueous humor dynamics in the aging human eye. Am J Ophthalmol 1999;127:407–12.
48. Barnett KC, Cottrell BD, Paterson BW, et al. Buphthalmos in a Thoroughbred foal. Equine Vet J 1988;20:132–5.
49. Gelatt KN. Glaucoma and lens luxation in a foal. Vet Med Small Anim Clin 1973; 68:261.
50. Dwyer AE, Crockett RS, Kalsow CM. Association of leptospiral seroreactivity and breed with uveitis and blindness in horses: 372 cases (1986-1993). J Am Vet Med Assoc 1995;207:1327–31.
51. Matas Riera M, Donaldson D, Priestnall SL. Descemet's membrane detachment in horses; case series and literature review. Vet Ophthalmol 2015;18:357–63.
52. Gilger BC, Michau TM, Salmon JH. Immune-mediated keratitis in horses: 19 cases (1998-2004). Vet Ophthalmol 2005;8:233–9.
53. Pinto NI, McMullen RJ Jr, Linder KE, et al. Clinical, histopathological and immunohistochemical characterization of a novel equine ocular disorder: heterochromic iridocyclitis with secondary keratitis in adult horses. Vet Ophthalmol 2015; 18:443–56.
54. Gilger BC. Diseases of the cornea. In: Gilger BC, editor. Equine ophthalmology. Ames (IA): Wiley-Blackwell; 2017. p. 252–368.
55. Whigham HM, Brooks DE, Andrew SE, et al. Treatment of equine glaucoma by transscleral neodymium:yttrium aluminum garnet laser cyclophotocoagulation: a retrospective study of 23 eyes of 16 horses. Vet Ophthalmol 1999;2:243–50.
56. Lassaline ME, Brooks DE. The enigma of equine glaucoma. In: Gilger BC, editor. Equine ophthalmology. 1st edition. St Louis (MO): Elsevier; 2005. p. 228–340.
57. Kerrigan-Baumrind LA, Quigley HA, Pease ME, et al. Number of ganglion cells in glaucoma eyes compared with threshold visual field tests in the same persons. Invest Ophthalmol Vis Sci 2000;41:741–8.
58. Miller PE, Pickett JP, Majors LJ. Evaluation of two applanation tonometers in horses. Am J Vet Res 1990;51:935–7.
59. Brooks DE. Hypertensive iridocyclitis and glaucoma of horses. Clinical techniques in equine practice. Elsevier Inc.; 2005. p. 72–80.
60. Andrade SF, Kupper DS, Pinho LF, et al. Evaluation of the Perkins handheld applanation tonometer in horses and cattle. J Vet Sci 2011;12:171–6.
61. Knollinger AM, La Croix NC, Barrett PM, et al. Evaluation of a rebound tonometer for measuring intraocular pressure in dogs and horses. J Am Vet Med Assoc 2005;227:244–8.

62. Severin GA. Veterinary ophthalmology notes. 3rd edition. Fort Collins (CO): Colorado State Univeristy; 1995.
63. van der Woerdt A, Gilger BC, Wilkie DA, et al. Effect of auriculopalpebral nerve block and intravenous administration of xylazine on intraocular pressure and corneal thickness in horses. Am J Vet Res 1995;56:155–8.
64. Dziezyc J, Millichamp NJ, Smith WB. Comparison of applanation tonometers in dogs and horses. J Am Vet Med Assoc 1992;201:430–3.
65. Ramsey DT, Hauptman JG, Petersen-Jones SM. Corneal thickness, intraocular pressure, and optical corneal diameter in Rocky Mountain Horses with cornea globosa or clinically normal corneas. Am J Vet Res 1999;60:1317–21.
66. Plummer CE, Ramsey DT, Hauptman JG. Assessment of corneal thickness, intraocular pressure, optical corneal diameter, and axial globe dimensions in Miniature Horses. Am J Vet Res 2003;64:661–5.
67. Gilger BC. Equine ophthalmology. In: Gelatt KN, Gilger BC, Kern TJ, editors. Veterinary ophthalmology. 5th edition. Ames (IO): Wiley-Blackwell; 2013. p. 1560–609.
68. Bertolucci C, Giudice E, Fazio F, et al. Circadian intraocular pressure rhythms in athletic horses under different lighting regime. Chronobiol Int 2009;26:348–58.
69. Wada S. Changes in intraocular pressure in uveitis horses. J Equine Vet Sci 2006;17:67–73.
70. Wilkie DA. Equine glaucoma: state of the art. Equine Vet J Suppl 2010;(37):62–8.
71. Trim CM, Colbern GT, Martin CL. Effect of xylazine and ketamine on intraocular pressure in horses. Vet Rec 1985;117:442–3.
72. Komaromy AM, Garg CD, Ying GS, et al. Effect of head position on intraocular pressure in horses. Am J Vet Res 2006;67:1232–5.
73. McClure JR Jr, Gelatt KN, Gum GG, et al. The effect of parenteral acepromazine and xylazine on intraocular pressure in the horse. Vet Med Small Anim Clin 1976; 71:1727–30.
74. Holve DL. Effect of sedation with detomidine on intraocular pressure with and without topical anesthesia in clinically normal horses. J Am Vet Med Assoc 2012;240:308–11.
75. Trbolova A, Selk Ghaffari M. Effects of intravenous detomidine on intraocular pressure readings obtained by applanation tonometry in clinically normal horses. J Equine Vet Sci 2013;33:182–5.
76. Stine JM, Michau TM, Williams MK, et al. The effects of intravenous romifidine on intraocular pressure in clinically normal horses and horses with incidental ophthalmic findings. Vet Ophthalmol 2014;17(Suppl 1):134–9.
77. Marzok MA, El-Khodery SA, Oheida AH. Effect of intravenous administration of romifidine on intraocular pressure in clinically normal horses. Vet Ophthalmol 2014;17(Suppl 1):149–53.
78. Ferreira TH, Brosnan RJ, Shilo-Benjamini Y, et al. Effects of ketamine, propofol, or thiopental administration on intraocular pressure and qualities of induction of and recovery from anesthesia in horses. Am J Vet Res 2013;74:1070–7.
79. Thomasy SM, Lassaline M. Equine glaucoma: where are we now? Equine Vet Education 2015;27:420–9.
80. Bentley E, Miller PE, Diehl KA. Use of high-resolution ultrasound as a diagnostic tool in veterinary ophthalmology. J Am Vet Med Assoc 2003;223:1617–22, 1599.
81. Willis AM, Robbin TE, Hoshaw-Woodard S, et al. Effect of topical administration of 2% dorzolamide hydrochloride or 2% dorzolamide hydrochloride-0.5% timolol maletae on intraocular pressure in clinically normal horses. Am J Vet Res 2001; 61:709–13.

82. Van Der Woerdt A, Wilkie DA, Gilger BC, et al. Effect of single- and multiple-dose 0.5% timolol maleate on intraocular pressure and pupil size in female horses. Vet Ophthalmol 2000;3:165–8.

83. Germann SE, Matheis FL, Rampazzo A, et al. Effects of topical administration of 1% brinzolamide on intraocular pressure in clinically normal horses. Equine Vet J 2008;40:662–5.

84. Willis AM, Diehl KA, Hoshaw-Woodard S, et al. Effects of topical administration of 0.005% latanoprost solution on eyes of clinically normal horses. Am J Vet Res 2001;62:1945–51.

85. Davidson HJ, Pinard CL, Keil SM, et al. Effect of topical ophthalmic latanoprost on intraocular pressure in normal horses. Vet Ther 2002;3:72–80.

86. Yamagishi R, Aihara M, Araie M. Neuroprotective effects of prostaglandin analogues on retinal ganglion cell death independent of intraocular pressure reduction. Exp Eye Res 2011;93:265–70.

87. van der Woerdt A, Gilger BC, Wilkie DA, et al. Normal variation in, and effect of 2% pilocarpine on intraocular pressure in female horses. Am J Vet Res 1998;59:1459–62.

88. Mughannam AJ, Buyukmihci NC, Kass PH. Effect of topical atropine on intraocular pressure and pupil diameter in the normal horse eye. Vet Ophthalmol 1999;2:213–5.

89. Herring IP, Pickett JP, Champagne ES, et al. Effect of topical 1% atropine sulfate on intraocular pressure in normal horses. Vet Ophthalmol 2000;3:139–43.

90. Van de Velde S, De Groef L, Stalmans I, et al. Towards axonal regeneration and neuroprotection in glaucoma: Rho kinase inhibitors as promising therapeutics. Prog Neurobiol 2015;131:105–19.

91. Wang J, Harris A, Prendes MA, et al. Targeting transforming growth factor-beta signaling in primary open-angle glaucoma. J Glaucoma 2017;26:390–5.

92. Michau TM, Salmon JH, English RV, et al. Transforming growth factor beta2 in the aqueous humor of normal dogs and dogs with glaucoma. Vet Ophthalmol 2007;10:404.

93. Frauenfelder HC, Vestre WA. Cryosurgical treatment of glaucoma in a horse. Vet Med Small Anim Clin 1981;76:183–6.

94. Cavens VJ, Gemensky-Metzler AJ, Wilkie DA, et al. The long-term effects of semiconductor diode laser transscleral cyclophotocoagulation on the normal equine eye and intraocular pressure(a). Vet Ophthalmol 2012;15:369–75.

95. Morreale RJ, Wilkie DA, Gemensky-Metzler AJ, et al. Histologic effect of semiconductor diode laser transscleral cyclophotocoagulation on the normal equine eye. Vet Ophthalmol 2007;10:84–92.

96. Gemensky-Metzler AJ, Wilkie DA, Weisbrode SE, et al. The location of sites and effect of semiconductor diode trans-scleral cyclophotocoagulation on the buphthalmic equine globe. Vet Ophthalmol 2014;17(Suppl 1):107–16.

97. Harrington JT, McMullen RJ Jr, Cullen JM, et al. Diode laser endoscopic cyclophotocoagulation in the normal equine eye. Vet Ophthalmol 2013;16:97–110.

98. Bras D, Maggio F. Surgical treatment of canine glaucoma: cyclodestructive techniques. Vet Clin North Am Small Anim Pract 2015;45:1283–305, vii.

99. Wilson R, Dees DD, Wagner L, et al. Use of a Baerveldt gonioimplant for secondary glaucoma in a horse. Equine Vet Education 2015;27:346–51.

100. Townsend WM, Langohr IM, Mouney MC, et al. Feasibility of aqueous shunts for reduction of intraocular pressure in horses. Equine Vet J 2014;46:239–43.

101. Meek LA. Intraocular silicone prosthesis in a horse. J Am Vet Med Assoc 1988;193:343–5.

102. Provost PJ, Ortenburger AI, Caron JP. Silicone ocular prosthesis in horses: 11 cases (1983-1987). J Am Vet Med Assoc 1989;194:1764–6.

103. Gilger BC, Pizzirani S, Johnston LC, et al. Use of a hydroxyapatite orbital implant in a cosmetic corneoscleral prosthesis after enucleation in a horse. J Am Vet Med Assoc 2003;222:343–5, 316.

104. Low MC, Landis ML, Peiffer RL. Intravitreal cidofovir injection for the management of chronic glaucoma in dogs. Vet Ophthalmol 2014;17:201–6.

105. Hewes CA, Keoughan GC, Gutierrez-Nibeyro S. Standing enucleation in the horse: a report of 5 cases. Can Vet J 2007;48:512–4.

106. Pollock PJ, Russell T, Hughes TK, et al. Transpalpebral eye enucleation in 40 standing horses. Vet Surg 2008;37:306–9.

107. Michau TM, Gilger BC. Cosmetic globe surgery in the horse. Vet Clin North Am Equine Pract 2004;20:467–84, viii-ix.

108. Hartley C, Grundon RA. Diseases and surgery of the globe and orbit. In: Gilger BC, editor. Equine ophthalmology. Ames (IA): Wiley-Blackwell; 2017. p. 151–96.

109. Bentley E, Murphy CJ. Thermal cautery of the cornea for treatment of spontaneous chronic corneal epithelial defects in dogs and horses. J Am Vet Med Assoc 2004;224:250–3, 224.

110. Scherrer NM, Lassaline M, Miller WW. Corneal edema in four horses treated with a superficial keratectomy and Gundersen inlay flap. Vet Ophthalmol 2017;20: 65–72.

Neuro-ophthalmology in the Horse

Kathern E. Myrna, DVM, MS

KEYWORDS

- Neuro • Facial nerve paralysis • Blindness • Neuro-ophthalmology
- Horner syndrome

KEY POINTS

- Neuro-ophthalmic disease is uncommon in the horse and requires a thorough examination to localize lesions.
- Visual deficits and pupillary size abnormalities must be approached in a systematic fashion to ensure proper diagnosis and treatment.
- Common neurologic abnormalities of the eye are discussed including facial nerve paralysis, strabismus, nystagmus, anisocoria, and blindness and their treatments.

Neuro-ophthalmic disease is relatively uncommon in horses and can prove a diagnostic challenge. In this review, the basics of the neuro-ophthalmic examination will be covered, and the most common abnormalities and their causes will be discussed with a focus on clinically relevant details.

The neuro-ophthalmic examination includes the portion of the cranial nerve examination associated with vision, pupillary light response, blink reflex, and eye position. Arguably the most important part of a neuro-ophthalmic assessment is an accurate neurologic examination. The thorough examination should start at a distance looking for asymmetries. Looking head on, the lashes of the upper lids should extend equally and laterally; downward directed lashes indicate enophthalmos, which can be associated with pain or other disorders. The nose and ears should be symmetric. As the patient is approached (before sedation), visual tracking can be observed. A menace response is assessed by making a menacing gesture with the hand toward the eye. It is important that this be silent and to ensure that air not be pushed toward the eye. The long lashes and periocular vibrissae are easy to inadvertently hit, which can result in a false-positive result. A positive menace is a blink in response to the

Disclosure Statement: The author does not have any relationship with a commercial company that has a direct financial interest in subject matter or materials discussed in article or with a company making a competing product.
Department of Small Animal Medicine and Surgery, Veterinary Medical Center, University of Georgia, 2200 College Station Road, Athens, GA 30602, USA
E-mail address: kmyrna@uga.edu

menacing gesture. The menace response in different regions of the visual field may be assessed by angling from the nasal portion of the eye and then the temporal. Differences in menace coming from either side suggest a deficit of the visual field. The palpebral reflex can then be assessed by touching the inner and outer corner of the eyelids and seeing that the eyelids close. Ocular position is then evaluated at rest and by gently grasping the head and rotating to the left and right followed by a dorsal and ventral flexion. A physiologic nystagmus should be apparent with the eye rotating to center, showing the oculocephalic reflex. After assessing symmetry of eyelid and globe position, and the menace response, palpebral reflex and oculocephalic reflex, sedation, and lid blocks can be administered if necessary to help with patient compliance for the remainder of the examination.

Resting pupil size should be evaluated to look for anisocoria (different-sized pupils). Pupillary light reflexes can be a challenge to assess, as the lateral position of the eyes makes it nearly impossible for a practitioner alone to assess the consensual pupillary light reflex (PLR). The direct PLR should be a moderate constriction of the pupil in response to direct bright focused light. The brightest light available, such as a halogen penlight or Finoff transilluminator (Welch Alyn Skaneateles Falls, New York), should be used for assessing the PLR. Traditional penlights are weak and have diffuse light, which is not as effective. A false-negative result may be obtained by holding the light too far from the eye or using a light that is too weak. In bright sun conditions, the pupil may already be constricted; thus, moving to a dimmer environment may be necessary to allow dilation before assessment. To assess the consensual PLR, an assistant should direct the bright light in the position for direct PLR assessment while the clinician illuminates the contralateral eye with the dimmest light possible that still allows a clear view of the pupil to assess the consensual PLR to that eye. Positioning the clinician low relative to the horse's eye and illuminating the eye such that the tapetal reflex is apparent aids in the assessment of the PLR. The clinician should look for constriction of the contralateral pupil while avoiding activating the direct PLR on that side.

After evaluation of the cranial nerves, the clinician should complete the ophthalmic examination including direct illumination of the eye, indirect illumination of the cornea and anterior chamber, retroillumination of the tapetal reflex, and an evaluation of the optic nerve head with a direct ophthalmoscope. Any opacities of the cornea or lens should be noted as well as flare in the anterior chamber or changes to the optic nerve head. A complete ophthalmic examination would then include diagnostic tests such as a Schirmer tear test, fluorescein stain, and tonometry if available.

Having evaluated the patient, any neuro-ophthalmic abnormalities are identified. What follows is a list of rule-outs for the most common abnormalities and appropriate subsequent diagnostics or treatments. Again, an emphasis is on clinically relevant disease.

FACIAL NERVE PARALYSIS

The facial nerve is predominantly a motor nerve that innervates the facial muscles, including ears, eyelids, lips, and nostrils as well as certain salivary glands and the lacrimal gland. Paralysis originates in the medulla oblongata at the facial nucleus and travels notably close to the tympanic cavity before coming to the superficial facial structures and splitting into the auricular, palpebral, and buccal superficial branches. Facial nerve paralysis is a common finding in the equine patient. Rather than the ocular signs, the most common clinical indicator is a deviation of the nose away from the side of facial nerve dysfunction. The loss of facial tone allows the nose to be pulled to the healthy side (**Fig. 1**). Ptosis, or dropping of the upper eyelid, is also a common presenting feature of facial nerve paralysis. Depending on the location of the facial nerve

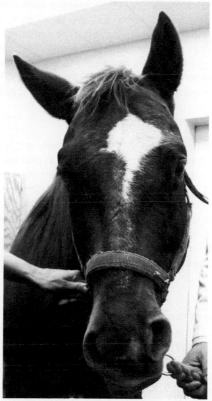

Fig. 1. A peripheral facial nerve paralysis in a horse. Note the deviation of the muzzle, the drooping of the ear, and the ptosis of the upper eyelid indicating that all 3 peripheral branches are affected.

lesion, you may see a deviated ear or complete or partial loss of the blink reflex. Ophthalmic presentations of complete or partial facial nerve paralysis may include a central corneal ulcer that will not heal in the typical 3 to 5 days. The outline of the ulcer correlates to the eyelid opening because the patient is unable to effectively blink and moisturize the central cornea.

Facial nerve paralysis may be subtle when the horse is alert and active and becomes more obvious with sedation. Once facial nerve disease is identified, the clinician should differentiate central (facial nucleus) from peripheral nerve disease if possible. Superficial branch damage is more likely to just affect one branch of cranial nerve (CN) VII, such as the buccal branch, easily damaged from pressure of a halter, that will result in lip and nasal changes. However, it is worth noting that central disease can involve only parts of the facial nucleus and mimic peripheral disease. Equine protozoal myeloencephalitis and listeriosis can present in this fashion. Central disease is far more likely to have concurrent signs from involvement of structures next to the facial nucleus. Ataxia, head tilt, and limb weakness may indicate more widespread disease of the medulla oblongata, whereas inner ear disease will present with vestibular signs in addition to the facial nerve paralysis. Additionally, central CN VII dysfunction may result in less facial droop and instead a grimacing appearance.

Peripheral facial nerve damage will often resolve with rest and the removal of compression to the nerves. Facial nerve damage associated with inner ear disease associated with temporohyoid osteoarthropathy or guttural pouch mycosis may improve with the resolution of the primary disease. If the blink function is impaired because of facial nerve paralysis, it is important to protect the corneal surface, as it is prone to drying. The placement of a temporary tarsorrhaphy (**Fig. 2**) to partially close the eyelid opening or the administration of lubricating ointments is indicated.

NEUROGENIC KERATOCONJUNCTIVITIS SICCA

Dry eye or keratoconjunctivitis sicca (KCS) is extremely uncommon in the horse, but when it occurs it can be a serious disorder resulting in corneal disease. KCS is characterized by a dull and lusterless corneal surface, associated conjunctivitis, and a low Schirmer tear test result (<15 mm/min). Facial nerve damage secondary to trauma such as mandibular fracture is arguably the most common cause of dry eye in the horse, although there are reports of KCS secondary to locoweed poisoning and hypothyroidism.[1,2] Treatment can be challenging and consists of tear supplementation combined with anti-inflammatories. A surgical correction in the form of a parotid duct transposition has been successfully performed in the horse.[3]

STRABISMUS

Strabismus, or deviation of the globe, can be observed at rest or may become more obvious during rotation of the head. Strabismus occurs with a loss of innervation to an extraocular muscle or with a fibrotic constriction of an extraocular muscle. The oculomotor nerve (CN III) innervates the ventral oblique, dorsal, medial, and ventral rectus muscles. The abducent nerve (CN VI) innervates the lateral rectus and retractor bulbi, and the trochlear nerve (CN IV) innervates the dorsal oblique. Loss of nerve function will result in deviation of the globe as follows: CN III dysfunction results in a laterally and lightly ventral strabismus, CN VI results in a prominent globe with a medial strabismus (**Fig. 3**), and a CN IV deficiency results in a dorsomedially rotated pupil. Restrictive strabismus is the result of fibrosis, often after an injury or associated with a mass effect. To differentiate denervation strabismus from restrictive, one must perform forced duction tests by grasping the globe with forceps and gently moving it. A globe with a restrictive strabismus will not be able to be manually deviated in

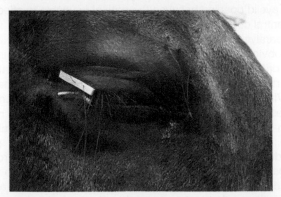

Fig. 2. A temporary tarsorrhaphy suture placed to close the lids and protect the corneal surface. This can be performed to mitigate damage as a consequence of facial nerve paralysis.

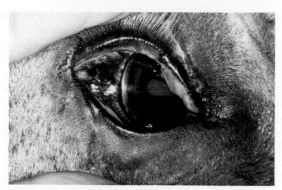

Fig. 3. A medial strabismus presumed to be related to cranial nerve VI dysfunction associated with equine protozoal meningoencephalitis.

the other direction, whereas a neurologic disorder should allow the eye to rotate normally.

Few specific diseases are associated with a strabismus as a presenting sign. Appaloosas with congenital stationary night blindness will often have a characteristic dorsomedial strabismus.[4] A dorsomedial rotation can also be seen with cerebellar abiotrophy, a genetic neurologic condition found almost exclusively in Arabian horses, owing to disruption of the vestibular tone.[5] Equine protozoal myeloencephalitis can result in selective loss of function of CN III, IV, or VI, and a full neurologic evaluation is warranted to look for other systemic signs. Restrictive strabismus is unlikely to resolve without surgical intervention, and neurologic strabismus response depends on the nature of the underlying disease process.

NYSTAGMUS

Spontaneous, continuous movement of the globe in a horizontal, vertical, or rotational direction would be termed a *nystagmus*. It is rare to have an ocular nystagmus without systemic signs of vestibular dysfunction such as staggering, swaying, leaning, or falling. A head tilt is typical of unilateral vestibular disease. Temporohyoid osteoarthropathy often presents with unilateral vestibular disease including nystagmus. Otitis media can present with a head tilt toward the lesion and nystagmus or ventral strabismus. Bilateral nystagmus is more likely to be induced by central cerebellar disease, and a transient nystagmus is common with general anesthesia.

ANISOCORIA

Anisocoria is the condition of having pupils of 2 different sizes. Because of the lateral positioning of the globes, it is difficult to assess both pupils simultaneously, so subtle differences can be missed. The most common source of anisocoria is an abnormally miotic pupil in one eye. If you cannot tell which eye is clinical (unable to decide if one pupil is abnormally small or abnormally large), observe pupil size in ambient light and then dim light. An abnormally miotic pupil will not dilate significantly or symmetrically in dim light. Similarly, an abnormally dilated pupil should not respond significantly or symmetrically to a bright light source.

Abnormal miosis (ie, pupil constriction not caused by bright light) is caused predominantly by ciliary spasm. Increased levels of aqueous humor prostaglandins will trigger a ciliary muscle constriction resulting in discomfort and a visibly reduced pupil size.

Common causes for miosis induced by inflammation include reflex uveitis from corneal disease and equine recurrent uveitis. Usually this is a straightforward diagnosis, as there will be other signs of ocular inflammation including red eye, discharge, aqueous flare, fluorescein-positive areas, or corneal infiltrate. Pharmacologic constriction is unlikely but can be associated with the use of latanoprost, a prostaglandin analogue used to treat glaucoma in dogs and people. Horner syndrome is another common cause of miosis.

Horner syndrome is the result of a loss of sympathetic innervation to the head. Manifestations include head sweating, upper eyelid ptosis (resulting in a downward deflection of the eyelashes), and mild miosis. Enophthalmos and elevation of the nictitating membrane are inconsistently found and can be subtle.[6] Horner syndrome can be anatomically localized based on the area of sweating rather than response to topical phenylephrine as is the case in dogs. Lesions at or distal to the guttural pouch will only exhibit sweating to the level of the atlas, whereas preganglionic lesions result in sweating down the neck (C2–C3), and cranial thoracic disease will result in sweating over the entire head and neck.[7,8] Because of the pathway of the sympathetic fibers in the equid, Horner syndrome is not associated with otitis media, rather it is more commonly associated with guttural pouch disease. Symptoms often persist for months to years and can impair athletic performance in the horse.

Mydriasis can be the result of either afferent or efferent defects. Ascending defects indicate problems along the light pathway including retina, optic nerve, and optic tracts and is typically associated with blindness and pupil dilation. Descending defects should not have visual deficits and can include structural problems with the iris such as pharmacologic dilation or adhesions to the lens (posterior synechiae) preventing free movement of the iris. Efferent neurologic defects are uncommon and involve dysfunction of the oculomotor nerve (CN III). Isolated CN III dysfunction resulting in a visual eye with a fixed and dilated pupil with no extraocular muscle dysfunction is referred to as *internal ophthalmoplegia* and is exceedingly rare. Systemic and topical administration of toxins with atropinelike action (the belladonna alkaloids) can result in dilation. Thorough questioning of the client before examination of the patient may reveal that they have medication in a container with a red cap (indicating that it functions to dilate the pupil).

BLINDNESS

Vision assessment in all animals, because they are nonverbal, is substantially hindered relative to patients who can provide verbal reports of what they see; therefore, subtle deficiencies can be difficult to identify. For this reason, the client's assessment of the visual status of the patient must be incorporated into our own. If a menace response is inconsistent, suggesting that there may be a visual deficit, a maze test can be performed. Maze testing can be difficult in the equine patient as horses can pick up cues from the person with the lead rope. Vision in each eye can be assessed independently with a blackout mask over the contralateral eye. Once blindness has been confirmed, it must be localized to a preretinal, retinal, optic nerve, or cortical deficiency. The easiest way to rule out preretinal causes of blindness (eg, anterior uveitis, corneal opacity, cataract, or vitreal opacity) is to determine whether a tapetal reflex is visible. This technique is known as retroillumination and is performed by shining a light at arm's length away into the eye. This technique is most successful if the clinician is positioned below the level of the eye so that the light reflects back from the tapetum (**Fig. 4**). An ocular opacity that is substantial enough to cause blindness should block this tapetal reflex. It is important for the clinician to keep in mind that the tapetal reflex

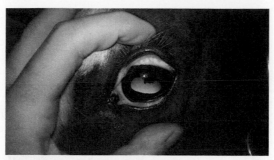

Fig. 4. A normal tapetal reflex in a horse using the clinical technique of retroillumination. Note the sharp pupillary margins and even orange color of the tapetal reflection.

may be blue, yellow, red, or green. A positive tapetal reflex should localize the lesion as posterior to the vitreous (retina, optic nerve, or visual cortex).

The PLR can then help to localize the lesion. The swinging flashlight test is critical to identifying a prechiasmal lesion. A Marcus-Gunn sign represents the scenario in which a light causes both eyes to constrict when the normal eye is illuminated, but when the light is moved to the abnormal contralateral side, the pupil dilates in the face of direct illumination. In this test, the light is held to one eye to activate the direct PLR and the consensual PLR to the contralateral eye. The flashlight is quickly moved to the other eye to assess the contralateral pupil's response. A positive swinging flashlight test indicates that there is an afferent defect in the blind eye located before the optic chiasm. To further localize the lesion, the retina and optic nerve head is then assessed. Retinal damage must be severe to result in blindness. Detachment is the most likely cause of a unilateral retinal blindness and should result in a dilated pupil that is nonresponsive to direct illumination in the eye.

Patients with optic neuritis may present with a swollen disc but if the disease is localized further down the pathway of the optic nerve, the optic papilla observed on fundic examination may appear normal. MRI is the best modality for evaluating a suspected optic nerve condition. Optic neuritis is typically associated with other intraocular changes such as uveitis and has been associated with several viral and other infectious agents. Treatment is focused on the underlying cause of the inflammation, and if infectious agents are ruled out, systemic immunosuppression can be attempted. Currently no studies give prognostic data on the success of treating optic neuritis in horses.

Tumors of the optic nerve are uncommon in the horse, with sporadic reports of optic nerve neoplasia in the literature. Advanced Imaging is necessary to show the presence of an optic nerve tumor. Depending on the location and extent of the lesion, exenteration of the globe and surrounding tissues may be advised with the caveat that some orbital tumors such as extra-adrenal paraganglimoas can result in expulsive and life-threatening hemorrhage.[9]

Damage to the optic nerve head as a result of hypoxia, compression, or traumatic stretching are also common conditions. Ischemic optic neuropathy is associated with a sudden loss of oxygenation such as severe blood loss or surgical occlusion of the external and internal carotid arteries.[10] In these cases, the patient becomes acutely blind with an absent or decreased direct PLR within 1 to 2 days of the hypoxic event. Initial fundic examination is often normal, but the optic nerve head will atrophy over time resulting in a poor prognosis for return of vision. Compressive optic neuropathy occurs from compression of the nerve within the orbit caused by inflammatory, neoplastic, or infectious causes.[11] Again, diagnosis is aided by advanced imaging,

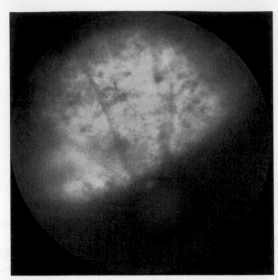

Fig. 5. Optic nerve hyperemia and edema associated with traumatic optic neuropathy. (*Courtesy of* Dr R. McMullen.)

and prognosis for return of vision is guarded. Traumatic optic neuropathy is the result of rapid pulling on the optic nerve as the result of head trauma. It is characterized by the presence of optic nerve edema and hemorrhage, acute vision loss, and a dilated pupil (**Fig. 5**). Treatment consists of systemic immunosuppression, and the prognosis for vision is grave.

Lesions further along the visual pathway including the optic tract, lateral geniculate nucleus, and visual cortex can be caused by myriad agents. These cases must be approached like any brain disease with evaluation for other neurologic lesions and advanced imaging. Postanesthetic cortical blindness has been reported in horses as has temporary blindness after seizure.[12,13]

Neuro-ophthalmic disease in the horse is uncommon and requires a thorough neuro-ophthalmic examination to localize lesions. A stepwise approach helps the practitioner identify and treat these lesions successfully.

REFERENCES

1. Schwarz BC, Sallmutter T, Nell B. Keratoconjunctivitis sicca attributable to parasympathetic facial nerve dysfunction associated with hypothyroidism in a horse. J Am Vet Med Assoc 2008;233(11):1761–6.

2. Matthews A. Nonulcerative keratopathies in the horse. Equine Veterinary Education 2000;12(5):271–8.

3. Dan Wolf E, Merideth R. Parotid duct transposition in the horse. J Equine Vet Sci 1981;1(4):143–5.

4. Rebhun WC, Loew ER, Riis RC, et al. Clinical manifestations of night blindness in the Appaloosa horse. Compend Contin Educ Pract Vet 1984;6:S103–6.

5. Baird JD, Mackenzie CD. Cerebellar hypoplasia and degeneration in part-arab horses. Aust Vet J 1974;50(1):25–8.

6. Green SL, Cochrane SM, Smith-Maxie L. Horner's syndrome in ten horses. Can Vet J 1992;33(5):330.

7. Mayhew IG. Horner's syndrome and lesions involving the sympathetic nervous system [Horses, eyes]. Equine Practice (USA) 1980;2:44–7.
8. Usenik EA. Sympathetic innervation of the head and neck of the horse: neuro-pharmacological studies of sweating in the horse: Thesis 1957. Univ Minnesota. pp. 1–125
9. Miesner T, Wilkie D, Gemensky-Metzler A, et al. Extra-adrenal paraganglioma of the equine orbit: six cases. Vet Ophthalmol 2009;12(4):263–8.
10. Hardy J, Robertson J, Wilkie D. Ischemic optic neuropathy and blindness after arterial occlusion for treatment of guttural pouch mycosis in two horses. J Am Vet Med Assoc 1990;196(10):1631–4.
11. Barnett K, Blunden A, Dyson S, et al. Blindness, optic atrophy and sinusitis in the horse. Vet Ophthalmol 2008;11(s1):20–6.
12. McKay J, Forest T, Senior M, et al. Postanaesthetic cerebral necrosis in five horses. Vet Rec 2002;150(3):70–4.
13. Tofflemire KL, David Whitley R, Wong DM, et al. Episodic blindness and ataxia in a horse with cholesterinic granulomas. Vet Ophthalmol 2013;16(2):149–52.

Periocular Neoplasia in the Horse

Krista Estell, DVM

KEYWORDS

- Sarcoid • Squamous cell carcinoma • Periocular • Neoplasia • Chemotherapy
- Radiation therapy • Immunotherapy

KEY POINTS

- Response to therapy is more likely to be achieved when the lesion is small.
- The "wait-and-see" approach is outdated and can be harmful.
- Benign does not mean that a tumor is not fatal.
- "Benign" tumors, such as sarcoids, can be locally aggressive and may compromise vision and quality of life. Squamous cell carcinoma and melanoma can be locally aggressive and may metastasize to distant organs.
- Treatments should be proven, effective, and safe.
- Controlled prospective studies and clinical trials are the next step in researching new developments in the treatment of neoplasia.

INTRODUCTION

Neoplasia of the eye, adnexa, and surrounding integument is a common occurrence in equine practice. Cutaneous neoplasia accounts for 30% of all equine dermatologic lesions, and neoplasia of the periorbital skin and adnexa occur frequently.[1] Squamous cell carcinoma (SCC) is the most frequently diagnosed neoplastic condition of the globe and orbit.[2] The most common equine skin tumors include sarcoid, squamous cell carcinoma, and lymphoma.[1] Melanomas are less commonly reported in the literature, although this likely represents the lack of referral of melanomas to a tertiary hospital for diagnosis rather than a lower incidence of disease. Various other neoplastic conditions have been reported to affect the eye, adnexa, and periorbital skin, including papilloma, hemangioma, mast cell tumor, basal cell carcinoma, fibrosarcoma, adenoma, adenocarcinoma, and myxosarcoma, among others.[2,3]

The author has no relevant financial interests or funding sources to disclose.
Department of Equine Internal Medicine, Marion duPont Scott Equine Medical Center, Virginia–Maryland College of Veterinary Medicine, 17690 Old Waterford Road, Leesburg, VA 20176, USA
E-mail address: Krista.estell@gmail.com

Vet Clin Equine 33 (2017) 551–562
http://dx.doi.org/10.1016/j.cveq.2017.08.004
0749-0739/17/© 2017 Elsevier Inc. All rights reserved.

DIAGNOSIS

The first step to developing an effective treatment strategy for periocular neoplastic conditions in the horse is obtaining a diagnosis. Careful evaluation of the globe and adnexal structures and digital palpation of the bony orbit should be performed to determine the extent of the tumor. Additionally, the local lymph nodes should be palpated for a change in size or texture that may indicate tumor metastasis. The treatment algorithm shown in **Fig. 1** can be applied to suspected cases of periocular neoplasia.

Biopsy is the recommended method of diagnosis for periocular neoplasia. The submission of a punch biopsy or other relatively large sample of tissue allows for accuracy in most cases. Non-neoplastic conditions including habronemiasis, pythiosis, and excessive granulation tissue are very similar in appearance to sarcoids and SCC, although treatment and prognosis differ wildly. Additionally, stromal invasive SCC may be mistakenly classified as keratitis unless a deep biopsy is performed.[4] Biopsy also should be performed on any enlarged local lymph nodes either with a punch biopsy instrument or via incisional wedge biopsy. Fine-needle aspirates are nearly always non-diagnostic in horses, with the exception of aspirates of melanocytic tumors, which often reveal a grossly black aspirate sample. Occasionally, a diagnosis can be made using an impression smear of the lesion, although there is increased risk of a non-diagnostic sample or a misdiagnosis when compared with tissue biopsy.

Excisional biopsy is ideal for lesions that are small or in a favorable location, whereas an incisional biopsy that includes normal tissue at the lesion margin is recommended for large masses that are in areas in which an incision with primary closure is not an option. If an excisional biopsy is performed, then the margins of the biopsy should be evaluated to determine if neoplastic cells extend to the edge of the submitted tissue. In general, confirmation of "clean margins" should be made only if there is at least 5 mm of normal tissue at all margins. In the case of sarcoids, however, which

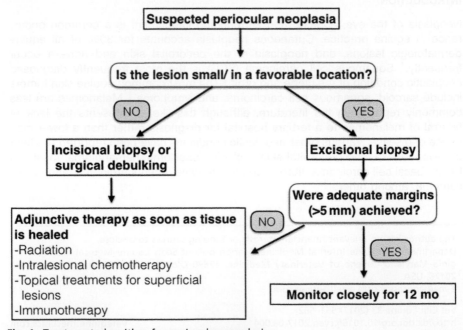

Fig. 1. Treatment algorithm for periocular neoplasia.

are quite locally aggressive, margins should not be considered clean unless 1.0 cm of normal tissue is present around all margins of the lesion.

It is a common misnomer that biopsy without complete excision results in malignant transformation of the tumor. Although biopsy does not cause malignancy, surgical excision or trauma of any kind may accelerate neoplastic growth. This has led to many veterinarians prescribing the "wait-and-see" approach to periocular neoplasia, which unfortunately often results in clients waiting until the neoplasia is too large to be easily treated. In all cases of neoplasia, but particularly when the globe, adnexa, or periorbital skin is involved, it is the author's conviction that there is no lesion too small to be treated. Excisional biopsies have the potential to be curative when masses are small, whereas larger lesions can be extremely challenging to treat due to the tissue tension of the periorbital skin and the general limits of accessibility of the conjunctiva and other adnexal structures.

SURGICAL OPTIONS

Surgical excision followed by the evaluation of surgical margins is the treatment of choice for all periorbital neoplasia. Although all gross tumor may be removed, microscopic tumor cells may extend into the surrounding normal-appearing tissue. Sarcoids can be particularly invasive, and often infiltrate skin 2 cm or more away from the visible tumor.[5] High tissue tension and limited ability to resect the periorbital skin curb the use of surgical excision in periorbital neoplasia, although if enucleation or exenteration is performed, then more extensive surgical margins can be taken with successful outcome.[6,7] Carbon dioxide laser ablation can be effective, although adequate margins must still be achieved.[8] Cryotherapy is less effective, particularly in larger lesions, and results in relatively more scar tissue that may complicate additional treatment.[5] For neoplasia of the sclera or cornea, surgical removal without follow-up adjunctive therapy can have a low success rate.[9] Other options for adjunctive therapy include topical treatments, intralesional chemotherapy, radiation therapy, and immunotherapy.

ADJUNCTIVE THERAPY

When lesions cannot be addressed surgically, or for tumors that have been debulked, but adequate surgical margins have not been achieved, adjunctive therapy needs to be considered. When considering an adjunctive treatment modality for periocular neoplasia, the veterinarian should apply 3 conditions before recommending treatment: (1) Is it proven? (2) Is it effective? (3) Is it safe?

To determine if a treatment has been proven to be effective and safe, the veterinarian should critically evaluate the available literature. Ideally, a prospective or good retrospective study evaluating the treatment should be published in a respected peer-reviewed journal. The study should include histopathologic diagnosis as part of the inclusion criteria, should have an adequate sample size, and have veterinary follow-up for at least 1 year after cessation of treatment.

Topical Agents

Topical therapies are commonly used to treat periocular neoplasia in horses due to ease of administration. In general, topical agents should be used only for superficial tumors, as topicals do not penetrate tissue well. It is often difficult to determine the appropriate time to discontinue the application of topical agents, as many are caustic, and application results in severe tissue inflammation that is indiscernible from neoplasia. Commonly used topical agents, their mechanisms of action, and documentation of effectiveness are listed in the following sections:

5-Fluorouracil

- Chemotherapeutic agent that inhibits DNA synthesis.
- Proven effective against penile/preputial SCC.[10]
- Less effective for the treatment of sarcoids.[6]
- Treatment course: for SCC, apply once a week for 5 weeks, then reassess.
- Local inflammation can cause considerable discomfort.

Mitomycin C

- Chemotherapeutic agent that inhibits RNA and alkylates DNA resulting in chromosomal breakage.
- Treatment course: If used for sole treatment, apply 0.04% mitomycin C topically 3 to 4 times a day for 7 days, followed by a break in treatment for 7 days. Repeat until the lesion has resolved.
- As sole therapy, response is good with success rates of 75% if a single ocular/adnexal structure is affected. Prognosis for response to therapy decreases if the conjunctiva or multiple areas are involved.[11]
- Side effects are minimal, and include epiphora.

Imiquimod (Aldara)

- Immune modulating agent that effects the innate and cell-mediated immune response resulting in increased production of multiple cytokines.
- Treatment course: Apply topically 3 times a week for up to 32 weeks or until the neoplasia is gone.
- Causes severe local inflammation that may make it difficult to continue to treat appropriately and determine when the neoplastic lesion is resolved.
- Reported to result in resolution in 60% of sarcoids, though follow-up time was very short in some cases.[12]

Acyclovir

- Antiviral purine analog that inhibits viral replication. Notably, acyclovir must be phosphorylated and activated by viral proteins. Bovine papilloma virus, which is likely involved in the etiology of sarcoids, lacks the ability to phosphorylate acyclovir.
- Treatment course: Apply once a day for 2 months or until tumor regression occurs.
- In a retrospective of clinically diagnosed sarcoids, application of acyclovir either after laser ablation or as a sole treatment, resulted in resolution of 68% of lesions. Increased thickness of lesions and diameter >5 cm were less likely to resolve. Follow-up time was as short as 1 month in some cases.[13]
- Application of acyclovir was significantly associated with treatment failure in a retrospective of 230 cases of sarcoids.[14]

Mistletoe extract (Viscum album)

- Alternative/complementary therapeutic occasionally used in the treatment of cancer in people.
- Shown to have immunomodulatory effects and display in vitro growth inhibition of some human tumor cell lines, although multiple meta-analyses have failed to prove its effectiveness.[15,16]

- In a prospective, randomized, blinded clinical trial, mistletoe extract was compared with a placebo for treatment of clinically diagnosed sarcoids (not histopathologically confirmed). Horses were injected subcutaneously 3 times a week for 15 weeks. In the treatment group, 41% of horses showed at least partial regression. Spontaneous regression of clinically diagnosed sarcoids were also seen in the placebo group.[17]

Intralesional Chemotherapeutics

Intralesional chemotherapy is recommended for the treatment of tumors that are smaller than 10 cm in diameter, or as an adjunctive treatment after surgery when clean margins are not achieved (**Fig. 2**). The pharmacologic advantage of intralesional drug administration includes increased concentration of the drug in the target site and low risk of systemic complications. This advantage is optimized by techniques that prolong dwelling time within a tumor. Cisplatin, a broad-spectrum chemotherapeutic agent that causes apoptosis of neoplastic cells by cross-linking DNA and interfering with cellular repair mechanisms, is the most effective and well-researched intralesional chemotherapeutic agent.[18] Two methods to retain cisplatin within the target tissue are to emulsify the cisplatin in sesame oil, which results in a slow release of cisplatin into the tissues, or to administer cisplatin in the form of a slowly biodegradable bead. In a retrospective analysis that included 573 tumors injected with cisplatin in sesame oil and a minimum of 2 years of follow-up, cisplatin was quite effective for the treatment of sarcoids and SCC, although success decreased as size of the tumor increased.[19] Cisplatin bead placement had a similar success rate for the treatment of sarcoids, and poses less risk of chemotherapy exposure to clients and personnel.[20] It is important to note that both cisplatin administration options require multiple treatments with precise techniques, and that results will not be as good as those described by the authors unless those techniques are followed exactly.[14]

Systemic Chemotherapeutics

The administration of systemic chemotherapeutic agents for periocular neoplasia in horses should be considered for cases in which there is evidence that the neoplasia has metastasized, or for cases in which it is necessary to shrink the tumor before surgical excision can be performed. Several chemotherapeutic regimens have been described; it is the recommendation of the author that a board-certified oncologist or large-animal internist with experience in the administration of chemotherapy be consulted to

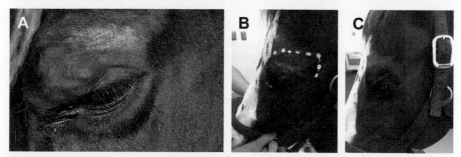

Fig. 2. (*A*) Mixed nodular/occult sarcoid in the superior lid. (*B*) The lid after surgical debulking of the nodular sarcoid. White dots are used for planning for intratumoral cisplatin in sesame oil injections. Note that the area of cisplatin treatment extends 2 cm away from grossly abnormal tissue and the surgical incision. (*C*) The lid 6 months after treatment with surgical debulking and 4 cisplatin in oil injections at 2-week intervals.

formulate a treatment plan. Clients are often interested in pursuing systemic chemotherapy provided a good quality of life can be maintained for their horses. In most horses, the severe adverse effects that are seen in people treated with chemotherapy, such as poor appetite, weight loss, and gastrointestinal upset, do not occur. A safety and efficacy study evaluating doxorubicin for the treatment of neoplasia in horses showed good response to treatment for SCC and lymphoma, although sarcoids and melanomas were poorly responsive to treatment.[21] Common side effects of doxorubicin include hyperthermia and transient colic signs, as well as immunosuppression. In the author's experience, horses are clinically normal between treatments and can be lightly ridden.

Radiation Therapy

The goal of radiation therapy is to cause neoplastic cell double-stranded DNA breaks that ultimately result in the destruction of tumor cells. Radiation therapy is relatively broad-spectrum, although different types of cutaneous tumor have varying sensitivity. Radiation has been used to successfully treat a variety of cutaneous periocular tumors, including sarcoids, myxosarcoma, and SCC. Unfortunately, melanocytic tumors are relatively radio-resistant; the doses of radiation that are needed may irreparably damage surrounding healthy tissue and organs. During treatment of the primary tumor, there is inevitable damage to the surrounding healthy tissue. Although healthy tissue is by nature less sensitive to radiation than neoplastic tissue, damage does occur. Adverse effects of radiation can be ameliorated by collimation, decreasing the dose of radiation administered (fractionation) and by shielding the nearby tissue with lead. Special concern needs to be applied to the ocular tissues (cornea, lens, retina, optic nerve), lacrimal gland, and to tissues that have fast cell cycles like the conjunctiva. Acute radiation damage occurs within 2 to 3 weeks of a course of radiation and results in erythema, swelling, ulceration, and epiphora. Chronic radiation effects include leukotrichia, dry eye due to lacrimal gland damage and bone necrosis.

External beam radiation, interstitial brachytherapy with radioactive beads or wires, and surface plesiotherapy with strontium have all been shown to be extremely effective in the treatment of periocular neoplasia, with success rates as high as 98%.[22–24] Unfortunately, due to anesthetic logistics as well as the availability and licensure of radioactive isotopes, there are few facilities that provide radiation therapy for horses.

Immunotherapy

Immunotherapy is one of the most interesting developing facets of veterinary and human oncology. The goal of immunotherapy is to activate and sensitize the host immune system to neoplastic cells. As tumor antigens are self-antigens, overcoming the immune system's innate self-tolerance has been the primary challenge in immunotherapy. There are 2 major pathways to accomplish this goal: (1) activate the cell-mediated immune system through administration of cytokines or bacterial antigens that cause the nonspecific activation of cytotoxic T cells, and (2) expose antigen-presenting cells to tumor antigens in hopes that this will overcome self-tolerance. Both mechanisms of immunotherapy have proven challenging in practice.

The most frequently used general immune stimulant for neoplasia in horses is the Bacillus Calmette-Guérin (BCG) vaccine. This is a live attenuated vaccine derived from *Mycoplasma bovis* that is used in human medicine for tuberculosis prevention as well as for primary therapy of bladder carcinoma in situ. Primarily used for the treatment of sarcoids in horses, the BCG vaccine has been shown in vitro to stimulate macrophages, dendritic cells, and T lymphocytes. When injected into clinically diagnosed periocular sarcoids, the injections resulted in a 59% to 69% resolution rate.[6] Response rate seemed to depend on type of sarcoid, as verrucous and occult sarcoids responded much less favorably to BCG injection in this study. Adverse effects of vaccination include local inflammation and granuloma formation in addition to fatal anaphylaxis. Several studies have detailed the administration of various inflammatory interleukin cytokines, either systemically or intratumorally, for the treatment of neoplasia in horses. Although most studies show a response to treatment, results have not been overwhelmingly positive, and these interleukins are currently not commercially available.[25,26]

Several different immunization options are available with the goal of exposing antigen-presenting cells to neoplastic antigens in the hope that the immune system will recognize these antigens as "non-self." There has been much anticipation of the application of the canine anti-melanoma vaccine Oncept (Merial Ltd, Athens, GA) to horses with severe melanoma. This vaccine is labeled for use in dogs with melanoma in which all gross melanoma tumor has been removed. It is a xenogeneic vaccine that codes for human tyrosinase. Tyrosinase, the enzyme that is responsible for melanin synthesis, is overexpressed in equine melanoma tissue as compared with non-neoplastic melanocytes and unpigmented tissue.[27] In a study in which Oncept was administered to normal horses, the vaccine was found to be safe, and to result in the production of anti-tyrosinase antibody.[28] Results of a clinical trial are needed to determine efficacy, and have not yet been published. Anecdotal results are mixed, with some reports of tumor resolution or stasis of growth, as well as reports of continued or even accelerated growth after vaccination.

Autologous vaccination, or inoculation of the host by injection of surgically excised tumor, has been used in an attempt to stimulate the immune system to attack neoplastic cells for decades. Although there are several studies documenting the results of autologous vaccination, many have had a relatively small sample size, with short follow-up time and variable histopathologic confirmation of diagnosis.[29] Autologous vaccination without modification of the tumor antigen would seem to have a similar problem of stimulating the immune system to recognize "self" proteins that allow neoplastic tumors to grow unchecked. The ImmuneFx vaccine (Veterinary Oncology Services, Tampa, FL) seeks to overcome this problem of self-tolerance by engineering autologous neoplastic cells to express a bacterial antigen on their surface. Although in vitro studies showing stimulation of both B cells and cytotoxic T cells, and in vivo studies in mice with glioblastoma are promising, a prospective clinical trial in horses has not been performed. A single case report describing treatment of a horse with metastatic melanoma stated that on average, melanoma lesions decreased in size by 40.3%.[30] As yet, no adverse reactions have been reported.

COMMON PERIOCULAR NEOPLASIA
Squamous Cell Carcinoma

SCC is the most common neoplasm of the globe and adnexa in the horse. Clinically, SCC typically presents as a fleshy pink growth on the nictitating membrane, conjunctiva, eyelid, or limbus. When identified early in the course of disease, SCC may present as a small, hyperemic, ulcerative lesion. Later in the progression of disease, a significant amount of bacterial infection may complicate SCC. Additionally, SCC may cause corneal ulceration from either abrading the cornea or by compromising eyelid function. There is a single case report of a pigmented ocular SCC and another case report in which both hemangiosarcoma and SCC were identified, which underscores the necessity of histopathologic confirmation of diagnosis.[31,32] In general, ocular SCC is locally invasive and slow to metastasize, although it is important to note that metastasis has been reported in up to 18.6% of ocular SCC cases.[33–36] Severe cases of ocular SCC may invade the calvarium and central nervous system via the optic nerve, or may spread to the central nervous system through metastasis.[34,35] In preputial and penile SCC, frequency of metastasis has been associated with more poorly differentiated SCC, although this correlation has not been investigated in periocular SCC.[37]

The etiology of SCC has not been completely elucidated and is likely multifactorial. Risk factors for the development of SCC include increasing age, ultraviolet radiation, and unpigmented skin.[38] Additionally, a genetic link with an autosomal recessive mode of inheritance has been suggested in Halflingers; genetics likely plays a role in other breeds as well.[39]

The prognosis for the treatment of SCC is good if lesions are identified and treated when they are small. Surgical excision is relatively unsuccessful if performed alone, but adjunctive treatment with radiation, cryotherapy, CO_2 laser ablation, photodynamic therapy, application of mitomycin C, or a combination of treatments significantly improves outcome (**Fig. 3**).[9,11,40–42] The exception seems to be SCC of the nictitating membrane, which has a good prognosis after surgical excision with a very low recurrence rate, although it is important to note that the study evaluating success of surgical excision of the nictitans included horses that were treated with adjunctive therapy if incomplete excision was noted on histopathology.[3] In addition to size of the lesion and type of treatment used, the location of SCC has an effect on prognosis. Recurrence rates after excision are higher in eyelid SCC as compared with other locations. As such, eyelid SCC and large tumors that invade the orbit have a poor long-term prognosis.[43]

Sarcoid

Sarcoids are a common neoplastic condition of the periocular skin in horses and account for most cutaneous neoplasia.[1] Clinically, sarcoids are characterized by appearance into 5 categories: occult, verrucous, nodular, fibroblastic, or mixed. Occult sarcoids are flat, alopecic areas that may be hyperkeratotic. Verrucous sarcoids are dry "warty" masses. Nodular sarcoids are firm ovoid masses that may be movable beneath the skin, although there is nearly always epidermal involvement with alopecia and hyperkeratosis. Fibroblastic sarcoids have a thick, fleshy appearance and an ulcerated surface. Most sarcoids are a combination of these 4 clinical types with a single type predominating. Fibroblastic sarcoids are typically the most aggressive type of sarcoid, but it is important to note that all sarcoids may grow rapidly, particularly if they are subjected to trauma, irritation, or ineffective treatment.

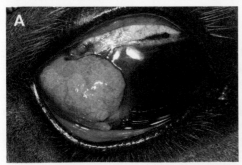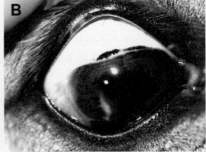

Fig. 3. (*A*) Classic appearance of an SCC at the lateral limbus. The mass is 2 × 1.5 cm, raised, cobblestoned, and pink to white. (*B*) The same eye after combination therapy with surgical keratoconjuntivectomy followed by strontium brachytherapy. The corneal fibrosis and neovascularization is consistent with mild postradiation keratopathy.

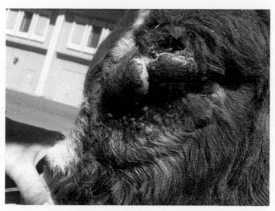

Fig. 4. Severe locally aggressive fibroblastic/nodular periocular sarcoid in a mini donkey that recurred following incomplete excision and topical application of a bloodroot-containing product.

Histologically, sarcoids are characterized by spindle-shaped fibroblastic cells that have poorly defined margins. Neoplastic cells will often extend up to 2 cm outside of the grossly abnormal area. Due to wide, poorly defined margins, recurrence rates after surgical excision of sarcoids are high, as high as 82% in the periocular area where there is limited tissue for resection. Although good results can still be achieved for periocular sarcoids, as treatment is most successful when lesions are small it is paramount to treat with the most effective therapies available early in the course of disease (**Fig. 4**).

The pathogenesis and etiology of equine sarcoids has not been fully described and is still a subject of debate. Sarcoids have been identified in horses as young as 2 years and have been reported in nearly all breeds. There have been reports of both genetic predisposition and epizootic outbreaks.[44] Several studies have associated the bovine papilloma virus (BPV) with equine sarcoids, and have found BPV DNA or protein in up to 100% of sarcoid tissue sampled.[45,46] Interestingly, BPV genetic material was occasionally identified in normal skin from horses with sarcoids, but was not present in skin from healthy horses or tissue from non-sarcoid neoplastic tumors.[45] It has been postulated that sarcoids develop due to inactivation of tumor suppressor gene p53 by BPV in addition to enhanced immunotolerance and upregulation of regulatory T cells.[47,48] It is likely that there are multiple factors at work in the pathogenesis of equine sarcoids, a combination of viral infection and immunologic genetic predisposition.

FUTURE INVESTIGATION

Additional research is needed to identify the underlying pathophysiology of periocular neoplastic conditions in the horse to determine the most effective treatment modality. Periocular neoplasia can be extremely challenging to treat, and even when the most effective therapies are applied early in the course of disease, treatment failures may occur. Currently there is no established "gold-standard" treatment for periocular neoplasia in the horse.

ACKNOWLEDGMENTS

The author thanks Alain Theon and Catherine Glines for their mentorship in equine oncology, support, and their compassion for all horses.

REFERENCES

1. Knowles EJ, Tremaine WH, Pearson GR, et al. A database survey of equine tumours in the United Kingdom. Equine Vet J 2016;48:280–4.
2. Giuliano EA. Equine periocular neoplasia: current concepts in aetiopathogenesis and emerging treatment modalities. Equine Vet J Suppl 2010;(37):9–18.
3. Labelle AL, Metzler AG, Wilkie DA. Nictitating membrane resection in the horse: a comparison of long-term outcomes using local vs. general anaesthesia. Equine Vet J Suppl 2011;(40):42–5.
4. Kafarnik C, Rawlings M, Dubielzig RR. Corneal stromal invasive squamous cell carcinoma: a retrospective morphological description in 10 horses. Vet Ophthalmol 2009;12:6–12.
5. Martens A, De Moor A, Vlaminck L, et al. Evaluation of excision, cryosurgery and local BCG vaccination for the treatment of equine sarcoids. Vet Rec 2001;149: 665–9.
6. Knottenbelt DC, Kelly DF. The diagnosis and treatment of periorbital sarcoid in the horse: 445 cases from 1974 to 1999. Vet Ophthalmol 2000;3:169–91.
7. Beard WL, Wilkie DA. Partial orbital rim resection, mesh skin expansion, and second intention healing combined with enucleation or exenteration for extensive periocular tumors in horses. Vet Ophthalmol 2002;5:23–8.
8. Carstanjen B, Jordan P, Lepage OM. Carbon dioxide laser as a surgical instrument for sarcoid therapy–a retrospective study on 60 cases. Can Vet J 1997; 38:773–6.
9. Mosunic CB, Moore PA, Carmicheal KP, et al. Effects of treatment with and without adjuvant radiation therapy on recurrence of ocular and adnexal squamous cell carcinoma in horses: 157 cases (1985-2002). J Am Vet Med Assoc 2004;225:1733–8.
10. Fortier LA, Mac Harg MA. Topical use of 5-fluorouracil for treatment of squamous cell carcinoma of the external genitalia of horses: 11 cases (1988-1992). J Am Vet Med Assoc 1994;205:1183–5.
11. Malalana F, Knottenbelt D, McKane S. Mitomycin C, with or without surgery, for the treatment of ocular squamous cell carcinoma in horses. Vet Rec 2010;167: 373–6.
12. Nogueira SA, Torres SM, Malone ED, et al. Efficacy of imiquimod 5% cream in the treatment of equine sarcoids: a pilot study. Vet Dermatol 2006;17:259–65.
13. Stadler S, Kainzbauer C, Haralambus R, et al. Successful treatment of equine sarcoids by topical aciclovir application. Vet Rec 2011;168:187.
14. Haspeslagh M, Vlaminck LE, Martens AM. Treatment of sarcoids in equids: 230 cases (2008-2013). J Am Vet Med Assoc 2016;249:311–8.
15. Evans M, Bryant S, Huntley AL, et al. Cancer patients' experiences of using mistletoe (Viscum album): a qualitative systematic review and synthesis. J Altern Complement Med 2016;22:134–44.
16. Horneber MA, Bueschel G, Huber R, et al. Mistletoe therapy in oncology. Cochrane Database Syst Rev 2008;(2):CD003297.
17. Christen-Clottu O, Klocke P, Burger D, et al. Treatment of clinically diagnosed equine sarcoid with a mistletoe extract (Viscum album austriacus). J Vet Intern Med 2010;24:1483–9.
18. Theon AP, Pascoe JR, Madigan JE, et al. Comparison of intratumoral administration of cisplatin versus bleomycin for treatment of periocular squamous cell carcinomas in horses. Am J Vet Res 1997;58:431–6.

19. Theon AP, Wilson WD, Magdesian KG, et al. Long-term outcome associated with intratumoral chemotherapy with cisplatin for cutaneous tumors in Equidae: 573 cases (1995-2004). J Am Vet Med Assoc 2007;230:1506–13.

20. Hewes CA, Sullins KE. Use of cisplatin-containing biodegradable beads for treatment of cutaneous neoplasia in Equidae: 59 cases (2000-2004). J Am Vet Med Assoc 2006;229:1617–22.

21. Theon AP, Pusterla N, Magdesian KG, et al. A pilot phase II study of the efficacy and biosafety of doxorubicin chemotherapy in tumor-bearing Equidae. J Vet Intern Med 2013;27:1581–8.

22. Byam-Cook KL, Henson FM, Slater JD. Treatment of periocular and non-ocular sarcoids in 18 horses by interstitial brachytherapy with iridium-192. Vet Rec 2006;159:337–41.

23. Theon AP, Pascoe JR. Iridium-192 interstitial brachytherapy for equine periocular tumours: treatment results and prognostic factors in 115 horses. Equine Vet J 1995;27:117–21.

24. Bradley WM, Schilpp D, Khatibzadeh SM. Electronic brachytherapy used for the successful treatment of three different types of equine tumours. Equine Vet Educ 2017;29:293–8.

25. Muller JM, Wissemann J, Meli ML, et al. In vivo induction of interferon gamma expression in grey horses with metastatic melanoma resulting from direct injection of plasmid DNA coding for equine interleukin 12. Schweiz Arch Tierheilkd 2011;153:509–13.

26. Heinzerling L, Burg G, Dummer R, et al. Intratumoral injection of DNA encoding human interleukin 12 into patients with metastatic melanoma: clinical efficacy. Hum Gene Ther 2005;16:35–48.

27. Phillips JC, Lembcke LM, Noltenius CE, et al. Evaluation of tyrosinase expression in canine and equine melanocytic tumors. Am J Vet Res 2012;73:272–8.

28. Lembcke LM, Kania SA, Blackford JT, et al. Development of immunologic assays to measure response in horses vaccinated with xenogeneic plasmid DNA encoding human tyrosinase. J Equine Vet Sci 2012;32:607–15.

29. Rothacker CC, Boyle AG, Levine DG. Autologous vaccination for the treatment of equine sarcoids: 18 cases (2009-2014). Can Vet J 2015;56:709–14.

30. Brown EL, Ramiya VK, Wright CA, et al. Treatment of metastatic equine melanoma with a plasmid DNA vaccine encoding Streptococcus pyogenes EMM55 protein. J Equine Vet Sci 2014;34:704–8.

31. McCowan C, Stanley RG. Pigmented squamous cell carcinoma of the conjunctiva of a horse. Vet Ophthalmol 2004;7:421–3.

32. Gearhart PM, Steficek BA, Peteresen-Jones SM. Hemangiosarcoma and squamous cell carcinoma in the third eyelid of a horse. Vet Ophthalmol 2007;10:121–6.

33. Gelatt KN, Myers VS Jr, Perman V, et al. Conjunctival squamous cell carcinoma in the horse. J Am Vet Med Assoc 1974;165(7):617–20.

34. Bacon CL, Davidson HJ, Yvorchuk K, et al. Bilateral Horner's syndrome secondary to metastatic squamous cell carcinoma in a horse. Equine Vet J 1996;28:500–3.

35. D'Angelo A, Bertuglia A, Capucchio MT, et al. Central vestibular syndrome due to a squamous cell carcinoma in a horse. Vet Rec 2007;161:314–6.

36. King TC, Priehs DR, Gum GG, et al. Therapeutic management of ocular squamous cell carcinoma in the horse: 43 cases (1979-1989). Equine Vet J 1991;23:449–52.

37. van den Top JG, de Heer N, Klein WR, et al. Penile and preputial squamous cell carcinoma in the horse: a retrospective study of treatment of 77 affected horses. Equine Vet J 2008;40:533–7.

38. Rebhun WC. Tumors of the eye and ocular adnexal tissues. Vet Clin North Am Equine Pract 1998;14:579–606, vii.

39. Lassaline M, Cranford TL, Latimer CA, et al. Limbal squamous cell carcinoma in Haflinger horses. Vet Ophthalmol 2015;18:404–8.

40. Michau TM, Davidson MG, Gilger BC. Carbon dioxide laser photoablation adjunctive therapy following superficial lamellar keratectomy and bulbar conjunctivectomy for the treatment of corneolimbal squamous cell carcinoma in horses: a review of 24 cases. Vet Ophthalmol 2012;15:245–53.

41. Bosch G, Klein WR. Superficial keratectomy and cryosurgery as therapy for limbal neoplasms in 13 horses. Vet Ophthalmol 2005;8:241–6.

42. Giuliano EA, Johnson PJ, Delgado C, et al. Local photodynamic therapy delays recurrence of equine periocular squamous cell carcinoma compared to cryotherapy. Vet Ophthalmol 2014;17(Suppl 1):37–45.

43. Dugan SJ, Roberts SM, Curtis CR, et al. Prognostic factors and survival of horses with ocular/adnexal squamous cell carcinoma: 147 cases (1978-1988). J Am Vet Med Assoc 1991;(198):298–303.

44. Abou Neel EA, Bozec L, Knowles JC, et al. Collagen–emerging collagen based therapies hit the patient. Adv Drug Deliv Rev 2013;65:429–56.

45. Carr EA, Theon AP, Madewell BR, et al. Bovine papillomavirus DNA in neoplastic and nonneoplastic tissues obtained from horses with and without sarcoids in the western United States. Am J Vet Res 2001;62:741–4.

46. Carr EA, Theon AP, Madewell BR, et al. Expression of a transforming gene (E5) of bovine papillomavirus in sarcoids obtained from horses. Am J Vet Res 2001;62: 1212–7.

47. Mahlmann K, Hamza E, Marti E, et al. Increased FOXP3 expression in tumour-associated tissues of horses affected with equine sarcoid disease. Vet J 2014; 202:516–21.

48. Bucher K, Szalai G, Marti E, et al. Tumour suppressor gene p53 in the horse: identification, cloning, sequencing and a possible role in the pathogenesis of equine sarcoid. Res Vet Sci 1996;61:114–9.

Ocular Manifestations of Systemic Disease in the Horse

Kathryn L. Wotman, DVM[a],*, Amy L. Johnson, DVM[b]

KEYWORDS

• Equine • Ophthalmology • Systemic • Ocular • Disease

KEY POINTS

• A thorough ophthalmic examination can aid in diagnosis of systemic abnormalities in horses and can easily be performed at the farm.
• The ophthalmic examination should be performed in a systematic sequence (eg, anterior structures to posterior), which allows for the periocular structures and globe to be fully examined.
• Ophthalmic findings should be used in conjunction with complete physical examination to elucidate accurate diagnosis and treatment plan.
• A variety of systemic diseases can cause ocular abnormalities, including bacterial, fungal, viral, and protozoal diseases, as well as parasites and endocrine abnormalities.

The diagnosis of systemic disease in horses can be elusive and the ophthalmic examination as part of a complete physical examination is often an underused tool for creating a differential diagnosis list. This article is organized for the equine practitioner as quick reference for systemic diseases causing ocular changes based on location around and in the eye. Many of these systemic diseases can cause multiple ocular ailments however the most common are presented here. Other exhaustive references for ocular manifestations of systemic disease include *Equine Ophthalmology*, 3rd edition, Dr Brian C. Gilger (2017) and *Veterinary Ophthalmology*, 5th Edition, Dr Kirk N. Gelatt, Dr Brian C. Gilger, and Dr Thomas J. Kern (2013).

[a] Comparative Ophthalmology, Department of Clinical Sciences, College of Veterinary Medicine and Biomedical Sciences, Colorado State University, 300 West Drake, Fort Collins, CO 80523-1678, USA; [b] Department of Clinical Sciences, Clinical Studies – New Bolton Center, University of Pennsylvania School of Veterinary Medicine, 382 West Street Road, Kennett Square, PA 19348, USA
* Corresponding author.
E-mail address: Kathryn.Wotman@colostate.edu

Vet Clin Equine 33 (2017) 563–582
http://dx.doi.org/10.1016/j.cveq.2017.08.002
0749-0739/17/© 2017 Elsevier Inc. All rights reserved.

vetequine.theclinics.com

GLOBE ABNORMALITIES

Any disease of the central or peripheral nervous system that affects CN function might result in globe and lid functional abnormalities, specifically in abnormalities of palpebral fissure size, eyelid function, and globe position or movement. Of the 12 cranial nerves (CN), 7 (CN II, III, IV, V, VI, VII, VIII) directly affect ocular structure or function. Sympathetic nerves also affect globe appearance. For excellent reviews of neuroophthalmology in horses, readers are referred to (See Kathern E. Myrna's article, "Neuro-ophthalmology in the Horse," in this issue for further details) and a previous issue of this journal.[1] In brief, palpebral fissure size and symmetry can be affected by deficits of CN III, CN VII, and sympathetic nerves. Eyelid function is affected by CN VII deficits. Globe position and movement are affected by CN III, IV, VI, and VIII deficits.

Many infectious and noninfectious nervous system diseases can affect CN function, either centrally (within the brainstem) or peripherally. In the authors' experience, the most common diseases to manifest with globe abnormalities include equine protozoal myeloencephalitis (EPM), viral encephalitides, bacterial meningoencephalitis, temporohyoid osteoarthropathy (THO), polyneuritis equi, and head trauma. If CN VII is involved, the predominant ocular finding might be corneal disease rather than globe or lid abnormalities. Brief descriptions of selected diseases are provided.

Parasitic

Tapeworm: Echinococcus granulosus

Exophthalmos may develop secondary to retrobulbar formation of hydatid cysts owing to *Echinococcus granulosus*. The definitive host for this tapeworm is the dog, and horses, as well as humans, serve as an intermediate host. Dogs and other canids, as the definitive hosts, harbor the intestinal stage of the tapeworm, which produces infective eggs.[2] The intermediate hosts and human are infected by ingesting the eggs in contaminated food or water.

After oral ingestion of *E granulosus* eggs, cysts may develop in many anatomic sites, including the liver.[3] Retrobulbar cyst formation may be detected via ultrasound imaging; however, definitive diagnosis is made by histopathologic identification of tissue taken after enucleation, which is often necessary for resolution of orbital disease.[3,4]

Bacterial

Tetanus

Rapid globe retraction and resulting "flashing" third eyelid elevation are 2 well-recognized ocular signs of tetanus in the horse.[5] Hyperesthesia is also a common finding.[6] The anaerobic, gram-positive, spore-forming bacterium *Clostridium tetani* produces the exotoxin tetanospasmin, which is responsible for the ocular clinical signs as well as systemic signs, which commonly include rigidity of the face and neck, and "sawhorse" stance followed by tonic muscle spasms and recumbency.[7,8] In the advanced stages of the disease, dilated pupil and ventrolateral strabismus may be present.[6] Horses are most commonly infected by the spores of *C tetani* contamination of a wound from inoculated soil, manure, metal objects, or contaminated surgical sites.

Treatment with supportive care, including muscle relaxation via phenothiazine sedative, barbiturate, benzodiazepines, or high doses of magnesium sulfate, are needed in addition to cleaning the contaminated wounds. Antibiotics will aid in elimination of infection. Penicillin has been commonly used; however, metronidazole is currently the preferred antimicrobial at a dosage of 20 to 30 mg/kg by mouth every 12 hours, or 40 to 60 mg/kg per rectum if the patient is not able to safely take oral medications for 3 to 5 days is the preferred antimicrobial.[7,8] Tetanus antitoxin can be infused around the wound to help neutralize any unbound toxin; however, owners should be warned of possible hepatic necrosis (Theiler's disease) several weeks after administration of the antitoxin. Vaccinating for tetanus provides safe, reliable protection against the bacterium.

Viral

Rabies

The rabies virus is a neurotropic enveloped virus belonging to the family *Rhabdoviridae*. Various types of wildlife such as bats, raccoons, foxes, and skunks serve as reservoirs for the RNA virus and transmit rabies to a "naïve" species via a bite wound and saliva.[7] Transmission by ingestion and inhalation of the virus has also been reported.[9] Once a horse is bitten by a rabies-infected animal, the incubation period can range from a few days to up to 6 months, depending on the area bitten in relation to distance from the brain. The longest incubation times occur in animals bitten on distal limbs because the virus has a longer path to the brain via peripheral nerves. Death typically occurs within 10 days of clinical signs.

Green reported the 5 most common clinical signs over the course of disease owing to rabies in horses as recumbency, hyperesthesia, tail and anal paralysis, ataxia and paraplegia, and fever.[10] Ocular signs are not the most prominent clinical sign in the rabid horse, but may include prolapse of the third eyelid gland and changes in globe position, including nystagmus and strabismus. Blindness owing to encephalopathy is often noted as the disease progresses.[10,11] A diagnosis of rabies is generally based on rapid deterioration of the animal with accompanying neurologic sings and no diagnostic test is available to definitively confirm the diagnosis antemortem; however, reverse transcriptase polymerase chain reaction (PCR) for viral detection in skin, saliva, or corneal impressions has been used.[12]

Euthanasia of afflicted animals is recommended because there is no treatment for rabies. Confirmation of the virus is made on postmortem examination via identification of intracytoplasmic Negri bodies on histologic examination of the brain and neurons, which is not 100% reliable, or via positive direct or indirect fluorescent antibodies on central nervous system tissue. Horses showed the strongest immunoreactivity in the cervical spinal cord, followed by the brainstem for the most accurate diagnosis.[13] Rabies can be prevented via preexposure vaccination, which has been shown to provide excellent protection against infection with the rhabdovirus for at least 1 year.[14]

Protozoal

Equine protozoal myeloencephalitis

EPM is the most frequently diagnosed infectious neurologic disease in the United States. It is most commonly caused by the protozoal parasite *Sarcocystis neurona*, although infection with other protozoa such as *Neospora hughesi* has also been reported.[15] Horses are infected with *S neurona* via consumption of food or water contaminated with opossum feces containing sporocysts. Depending on geography and environment, a high percentage of horses can be exposed to *S neurona*, but only a small percentage develop clinical signs of neurologic disease.

Clinical signs are highly variable and can manifest insidiously or suddenly, with subsequent slow or rapid progression. Any part of the central nervous system can be affected, although the most common clinical signs reflect damage to spinal cord white and gray matter. These signs include general proprioceptive ataxia with paresis and muscle atrophy, which is often asymmetric. Although spinal cord signs are probably most commonly observed by most general practitioners, a referral population of horses diagnosed with EPM most commonly showed signs localized to the brainstem

(7/19 horses; 37%).[16] EPM can cause very focal lesions as well as more extensive multifocal disease. If disease is restricted to CN nuclei essential for normal eye function, it is possible that only eye abnormalities would be observed.

Antemortem diagnosis of EPM is challenging owing to widespread equine exposure to the causative organisms, with positive serologic results in the absence of clinical disease. The best possible presumptive diagnosis requires 3 criteria: presence of neurologic disease, exclusion of other likely causes through appropriate diagnostic testing, and confirmation of *S neurona*-specific (or *N hughesi*-specific) antibodies in the cerebrospinal fluid (CSF), serum, or, ideally, both.[17] There are several commercially available tests that detect antibodies against *S neurona*, including Western blot, indirect fluorescent antibody test (IFAT), or enzyme-linked immunosorbent assay (ELISA). IFAT and ELISA are available to detect antibodies against *N hughesi*. Positive serum results do not confirm nervous system disease, regardless of the magnitude of the titer. With the exception of recently infected horses, negative serum results indicate a lack of exposure and hence a lack of disease. The most accurate method to diagnose clinical disease and active nervous system infection is to perform quantitative antibody testing on both serum and CSF, allowing detection of intrathecal antibody production.[18,19] This method improves overall diagnostic accuracy to 93% to 97%, as compared with serum alone, which has an overall accuracy of 54% to 56%.[19,20] The authors generally submit paired CSF and serum samples for an *S neurona* SAG2, 4/3 ELISA (or *Neospora* ELISA) serum:CSF titer ratio, which allows identification of intrathecal antibody production. IFAT can also be used for this purpose.

Currently, there are 3 EPM treatment products that have been approved by the US Food and Drug Administration and are commercially available.[17] Efficacy seems to be similar across products, with published treatment success rates of approximately 60% for all medications. Unfortunately, clinical trials directly comparing the medications and various treatment protocols have not been performed. There is a liquid combination product consisting of pyrimethamine (1 mg/kg by mouth daily) and sulfadiazine (20 mg/kg by mouth daily), generally administered for a minimum of 90 days. Ponazuril paste, a benzeneacetonitrile antiprotozoal drug, is labeled for a loading dose of 15 mg/kg by mouth followed by 5 mg/kg by mouth daily for 26 days. Pelleted diclazuril, a similar benzeneacetonitrile antiprotozoal drug, is labeled for use at 1 mg/kg by mouth daily for 28 days. Because there is no clearly superior treatment, drug choice is generally based on veterinarian and owner preference, preferred medication form (liquid vs paste vs pellet), financial considerations, or potential for adverse effects. Ponazuril and diclazuril are highly selective for apicomplexan parasites, and adverse effects are not expected. Pyrimethamine and sulfadiazine inhibit enzymes in the folic acid pathway and can cause bone marrow suppression with long-term use. Additional adverse effects include diarrhea, abortions, and congenital defects.[21]

Miscellaneous

Hyperkalemic periodic paralysis

Hyperkalemic periodic paralysis (HYPP) is an inherited myopathy of Quarter Horses, American Paint Horses, Appaloosas, and Quarter Horse crossbreds. It occurs as an autosomal-dominant trait in horses that are related to the Quarter Horse stallion Impressive.[22] Clinical manifestations include myotonia, muscle fasciculations and weakness, and/or paralysis resulting from failure of inactivation of sodium channels in skeletal muscles when serum potassium levels increase, resulting in persistent depolarization of muscle cells and fatigue.[23] Episodes of HYPP can occur during periods of increased serum potassium, including after change in feed to high potassium diets such as alfalfa or electrolyte supplementation, or with stressors, which may include transportation, general anesthesia, fasting, and other concurrent systemic diseases, including renal disease.

Ocular signs of HYPP include globe retraction owing to spasm of the retractor bulbi muscle with subsequent elevation of the third eyelid, which may present as one of the early clinical signs of an episode.[7] Owners educated to monitor for changes in third eyelid position as well as other initial signs of sweating and muscle fasciculations over the neck, shoulder, and flank may be able to prevent progression of the attack by feeding grain or corn syrup to help decrease serum potassium via facilitating movement across cell membranes.[7,24] More severe attacks should be addressed via intravenous supplementation of calcium gluconate, glucose, or sodium bicarbonate.

Owners should be educated on proper diet for afflicted horses, including keep dietary potassium low and maintaining renal loss of potassium to prevent HYPP attacks. Feeds supplemented with sugar or beet molasses should be avoided because it is high in potassium, as well as alfalfa, orchard grass, and brome hay. Meals should be fed in small and frequent quantities and regular exercise should be allowed. Horses that show recurrent episodes of muscle weakness and fasciculations can be managed with daily oral medications that promote renal potassium excretion, such as oral acetazolamide.[7,24] Genetic testing has been made available to help identify foals and horses with HYPP ancestry and horses positive for the genetic disease should not be bred.

Vestibular disease
Horses with vestibular disease typically show vestibular ataxia, characterized by balance loss, head/neck tilt or turn, and potentially abnormal nystagmus or strabismus. The vestibular system can be affected peripherally (outside the central nervous system) or centrally (within the central nervous system). Additional signs typical of central vestibular disease include an abnormal mental state (obtundation), multiple CN deficits (outside of CN VII and VIII), and general proprioceptive ataxia with weakness.

Ocular abnormalities with peripheral vestibular disease include ventral strabismus of the globe on the affected side, which is often positional (noted with head elevation), and horizontal nystagmus with the fast phase away from the affected side. Strabismus and nystagmus are more variable with central disease, occurring in any direction and potentially changing direction.

Causes of peripheral vestibular disease include those diseases that affect CN VIII as it leaves the brainstem and travels within the petrous temporal bone; these include THO, polyneuritis equi, otitis media interna, and head trauma resulting in petrous temporal bone fracture. The first 2 diseases are discussed in more detail under Corneal and Tear Film Abnormalities. The most common causes of central vestibular disease include EPM (discussed elsewhere in this article), head trauma resulting in basilar skull bone fracture, bacterial or viral meningoencephalitis, neoplasia, or aberrant parasite migration.

EYELID, NICTITANS, AND CONJUNCTIVAL ABNORMALITIES

Abnormalities in the eyelids or conjunctiva can result from a variety of infectious and noninfectious diseases. It is important to accurately evaluate the periocular tissues because they can be a good source of indication of systemic disease, as with icterus secondary to hemolysis. The surrounding ocular tissue can also be a good source for diagnostics including cytology, culture, and biopsy without disturbing the globe itself and can often be done in the field.

Parasitic

Onchocerciasis

Onchocerciasis is caused by *Onchocerca cervicalis* in the horse and commonly causes dermatitis as well as ocular changes, particularly in older horses. The larvae of *Onchocerca* are transmitted to the horse by biting midges, *Culicoides* spp, or black flies, *Simulium* spp. After inoculation, the larvae migrate to the nuchal ligament, where they develop into adult worms. The matured worms then produce microfilaria, which can migrate and cause clinical disease. Migrating microfilaria have shown a preference for the ventral midline and face of the horse where they can be ingested by *Culicoides* spp. to help complete the cycle.[25,26]

Dermal clinical signs and pruritis often result from inflammation as antigens are released as the microfilaria die. Preferential microfilaria localization associated with the ocular tissues includes the lower eyelid and lateral limbus of the eye. Depigmentation (vitiligo) of the conjunctiva around the temporal limbus is a distinguishing clinical sign. Other ocular clinical signs during the acute inflammatory stage include conjunctivitis with accompanying conjunctival hyperemia and chemosis as well as small white nodular formation at the limbus. Keratitis with focal subepithelial punctuate corneal opacities, vascularization, and corneal stromal inflammation and edema may also develop.[27,28] The microfilaria may migrate beyond the conjunctiva and cornea into the uveal tract. Subsequent death of the parasite incites inflammation of anterior segment, uveitis, with clinical signs that are nonspecific to *Onchocerca* spp. infection and include miosis, aqueous flare, white blood cells within the anterior chamber, and ocular hypotension. Posterior segment involvement may manifest as vitritis with inflammatory cells in the vitreous and/or chorioretinitis. Signs of chorioretinal edema and exudates are present and appear ophthalmoscopically as hyporeflective lesions when active, and classically seen as "butterfly" lesions in the peripapillary region in the chronic stages.[25,27]

Diagnosis of *Onchocerca* spp. as the cause of keratoconjunctivitis is often made by noting the common ocular clinical signs. A more definitive diagnosis can be reached by conjunctival or corneal biopsy. A keratectomy sample is generally obtained under general anesthesia; however, conjunctival biopsies can be taken standing with topical anesthesia. Samples are examined for the presence of the microfilaria and accompanying inflammatory cells including neutrophils, plasma cells, lymphocytes, and eosinophils.[29]

Treatment is aimed at controlling the inflammation associated with the die off the microfilaria and may include use of systemic corticosteroids (prednisolone 0.5 to mg/kg by mouth every 24 hours with a tapering dose) and nonsteroidal antiinflammatories (flunixin meglumine 0.5–1.1 mg/kg by mouth or intravenously every 12–24 hours, phenylbutazone 2.2–4.4 mg/kg by mouth every 12–24 hours) as well as topically applied steroids (0.1% dexamethasone sodium phosphate or 1% prednisolone acetate) if no corneal ulceration is present. Subconjunctival steroids can help to alleviate intraocular inflammation if safe to use, depending on the condition of the cornea.[7,30] Microfilaricide therapy with oral ivermectin or moxidectin is used to eliminate microfilaria; however, no treatment eliminates the adult worms from persistently infecting the nuchal ligament.[26,28,31] Therefore, regular deworming is recommended to routinely eliminate microfilaria.[32,33]

Habronemiasis

Harbronemiasis, also known as summer sores, is caused by the nematodes *Harbronema muscae, H microstoma*, and *Draschia megastoma*.[34] The larvae from these nematodes may be deposited on the skin, causing cutaneous harbronemiasis, or on the ocular tissue causing the ocular form. Larvae are transmitted to the horse by their intermediate hosts, the house fly and horse fly; as they feed on the skin and ocular surfaces, the larvae are subsequently deposited. The nematode larvae are typically found in the equine stomach. The aberrant migration of the larvae into the skin and ocular tissues creates a granulomatous hypersensitivity reaction.

Ocular signs of habronemiasis include nodule formation at the site of the hypersensitivity reaction and appear as yellow, raised, caseous lesions ("sulfur granules") most often at the medial canthus, but can also form in the conjunctiva and periocular region.[7] The horse may develop pruritis associated with the nodules, which can progress to fistulous tracts in the medial canthus. In some cases, keratitis and corneal ulceration develop if the eyelids become irregular from nodular formation.

The presence of the larvae within the granulomatous reaction is diagnostic. Conjunctival scrapings can also be performed and show an inflammatory reaction with neutrophils, eosinophils, mast cells, and macrophages, but generally lack evidence of the larvae.[34] Diagnosis can also be aided by other factors common to habronemiasis, including the prevalence of the disease in the warmer months owing to the active fly population. Some horses also seem to be predisposed to the condition, which may be owing in part to coat color because flies seem to prefer lighter colored skin and hair areas.[34]

Treatment of habronemiasis is aimed at controlling the intermediate host, the fly. Oral ivermectin (0.2 mg/kg) has been the treatment of choice because it provides effective kill of the adults and larvae in the equine stomach where they typically reside.[32,34] Refractory nodular lesions may necessitate debridement with additional treatment of topical or systemic corticosteroids for the inflammatory reaction.[35] Support for the cornea with topical steroids, if no ulceration is present, or topical antibiotics may be necessary to improve the horse's ocular comfort until the lesions subside.

Protozoal

Piroplasmosis

Blood protozoans that cause ocular signs in horses include *Theileria equi* (formerly *Babesia equi*) and *B caballi*. They are transmitted by ticks from the genera *Dermacentor, Hyalomma*, and *Rhipicephalus* and can also be transmitted iatrogenically via blood-contaminated equipment.[36] The United States and Canada are considered nonendemic areas for equine piroplasmosis and infected horses are quarantined under monitoring by the US Department of Agriculture.[36] Acute clinical signs after the 5- to 28-day incubation period include fever, lethargy, icterus, hemolytic anemia, hemoglobinuria, and possible death. Ocular signs include icterus and edema of the conjunctiva and sclera, with possible petechiation. Eyelid swelling and blood-tinged tears may also be present.[37]

Infected horses may become persistent carriers of the disease with or without apparent chronic clinical signs, including persistent lethargy, mild anemia, and general signs of poor health.[38] Diagnosis can be made by the finding the intraerythrocytic protozoa on Geimsa-stained blood smear in addition to common clinicopathologic changes of anemia and frequent thrombocytopenia and hemoglobinuria. The official testing method for importation into the United States is the competitive ELISA. Other testing with improved sensitivity to detect carriers of piroplasmosis without clinical signs include immunofluorescence assay, complement fixation test, and Western blot.[36]

Treatment in nonendemic areas such as the United States is aimed at prevention of transmission via clearance of the parasite. *T equi* is reportedly much more difficult to clear.[39] Generally, no specific treatment is required for the ophthalmic signs, which should resolve as the clinical signs improve. Imidocarb dipropionate is considered the treatment of choice to aid in improving clinical signs and support clearance of either parasite. Imidocarb given at a dosing range of 2.2 to 4.4 mg/kg intramuscularly at the initial dose followed by 2.2 mg/kg intramuscularly every 24 to 72 hours will aid in clearance of the protozoa.[36,40] During treatment with imidocarb, horses should be closely monitored for signs of colic owing to the drug's anticholinesterase activity and local injection site reactions are common. Infected horses must be registered in the US Department of Agriculture treatment program and undergo appropriate quarantine and testing, including serial negative PCR results before release.[36]

Rickettsial

Equine granulocytic ehrlichiosis

Equine granulocytic ehrlichiosis is caused by *Anaplasma phagocytophila* (previously named *Ehrlichia equi*) and is transmitted to horses by ticks in the genus *Ioxdes*.[41] The rickettsial organism has a tropism for the cytoplasm of neutrophils and eosinophils, where it replicates within morulae. Subsequent cell sequestration and destruction causes the clinical pathologic changes and illness.[42]

General clinical signs in the horse include fever, lethargy, inappetance, petechia, peripheral limb edema, icterus, weakness, and possible ataxia. Ophthalmic abnormalities associated with ehrlichia include icterus of the conjunctiva and sclera, petechiation of the conjunctiva, as well as uveitis.[43] Laboratory abnormalities include anemia, leukopenia (granuloycytopenia and lymphopenia), and thrombocytopenia. Diagnosis can be made by finding the morulae within the cytoplasm of neutrophils and eosinophils during the acute febrile phase of infection as well as a positive PCR assay for *A phagocytophila* in the buffy coat, and a greater than 4-fold increase in the immunofluorescence assay titer from of paired samples.[44–46]

Intravenous oxytetracycline (7 mg/kg) or oral doxycycline (10 mg/kg by mouth 2 times a day) are effective at resolving the fever within 24 hours, and clinical signs generally resolve within 1 week of treatment.[47] Specific treatment for the ocular signs is generally not necessary because they resolve once treatment is started. Prevention is directed at control of tick exposure.

Fungal

Dermatophytosis (ringworm)

Ringworm in the horse is caused by dermatophytes of the *Microsporum* or *Trichophyton* genera and results in skin disease on any part of the body.[48,49] The fungal infection is more common in the summer and/or in areas that have high humidity and heat, and younger horses seem to be more susceptible to infection. It is spread by direct contact or via fomites such as shared grooming and riding equipment.

Dermatophytosis causes alopecia on the eyelids with possible scaling and crusting of the periocular skin. Horses may be pruritic, which can cause secondary self-trauma around the eye. Positive fungal culture from hair, biopsy, or skin scraping of the causative species is diagnostic.

Treatment often is not necessary because the skin disease is commonly self-limiting; however, topical antifungal or chlorhexidine shampoos may be effective and are safer than systemic treatments.[35,48] Prevention of ringworm is through proper hygiene by using single use equipment or thorough cleaning of brushes and riding equipment.

Bacterial

Streptococcus equi subspecies equi (strangles)

Strangles is caused by the gram-positive coccoid bacteria, S equi subsp. equi, and is well-recognized by the classic clinical signs of fever, nasal discharge, and swollen abscessed retropharyngeal and submandibular lymph nodes. The highly contagious disease is spread via direct contact with infected horses or with fomites containing infected secretions, such as feed buckets and water troughs.

The bacteria colonize the lymph nodes within a few hours of transmission, which incites a migration of polymorphonuclear neutrophils to the area, resulting in abscessation of the nodes within days of infection. Draining of the lymph nodes into the guttural pouch may result in guttural empyema and can be a source of subclinical carriers of S equi. Bastard strangles occurs with metastasis to other regions, including the abdominal and thoracic lymph nodes. A more severe complication of S equi is an immune-mediated type III hypersensitivity reaction referred to as purpura hemorrhagica, resulting in vasculitis and pitting edema primarily in the distal limbs. However, the head and trunk are frequently involved. Other organ systems may be affected by the antigen–antibody immune complexes including kidneys, gastrointestinal tract, muscles, lungs, and myocardium, which require aggressive treatment with systemic corticosteroids.[35]

Ocular signs of strangles most commonly include serous to mucopurulent ocular discharge. Periorbital abscesses have also been reported and cause severe swelling of the eyelids and S equi–laden ocular discharge.[7,50] Other less common ocular changes include panophthalmitis, chorioretinitis,[51] and blindness secondary to brain abscess formation.[52]

Early diagnosis of strangles in the horse is important for containment of the disease. Daily measuring of rectal temperature will help with monitoring of infected horses as fever occurs 24 to 48 hours before mucosal inhabitation by S equi.[7,53] Bacterial culture of abscess aspirates, nasopharyngeal swabs, and nasopharyngeal and guttural pouch washes had been the gold standard diagnostic for strangles. However, direct PCR of nasopharyngeal swab, nasopharyngeal or guttural pouch wash are more sensitive than cultures and most often the two are performed together.[7,53–58]

Treatment of strangles often depends on the clinical stage of the disease and veterinarian preference and experience. The signs of ocular discharge are self-limiting as the disease progresses. Nonsteroidal antiinflammatory drugs are useful in the early course of the disease when fever causes the horse to be lethargic with a poor appetite and water intake. Encouraging drainage from the peripheral lymph nodes abscesses via hot packing is useful and may hasten the course of disease.

Prevention via vaccination is somewhat controversial and we refer the reader to more complete reviews on S equi, including the American College of Internal Medicine consensus statement[53] and the American Association of Equine Practitioners Infectious Disease Committee recommendations.

Viral

Equine herpes virus and equine influenza

Eyelid and conjunctival manifestations of viral disease in the horse tend to be mild and indistinguishable from each other. Both equine herpesvirus 1 (EHV-1) and equine influenza can present with upper respiratory signs, most commonly in younger horses with a more active routine, including frequent travel and exposure to other horses. Generally, signs of these viral infections include mild to moderate nasal discharge, fever, and lethargy. EHV-1 is also a cause of abortion and neurologic disease. Outward ocular signs of EHV-1, EHV-4, and influenza include serous to mucopurulent ocular discharge, chemosis, and conjunctival hyperemia.[59] Other ocular signs of EHV are discussed in elsewhere in this article. Treatment for the viral respiratory diseases is generally symptomatic and the ocular signs resolve once the animal recovers from the respiratory signs. Vaccine for both herpesvirus and influenza are generally recommended twice yearly to decrease the severity and duration of clinical signs of respiratory disease.[7]

Immune-Mediated Dermatoses

Pemphigus foliaceus

Pemphigus foliaceus is the most common autoimmune skin disorder recognized in the horse and is characterized by lesions on the head and distal limbs, which can progress to any part of the body. Autoantibodies to keratinocytes prevent normal intercellular connections leading to vesicle, bullae, and pustule formation, which progress to areas of alopecia, crusting, and scaling.[60] Ocular lesions include crusting and ulceration of the eyelids, conjunctival, and/or corneal ulcerations, as well as mucoid ocular discharge.

A diagnosis of pemphigus foliacueus is based on cytologic findings of skin biopsies, including acantholytic keratinocytes, intraepidermal pustules, and neutrophilic inflammation.[61] Oral corticosteroids, prednisolone, 1 to 2 mg/kg daily or dexamethasone 0.05 to 0.1 mg/kg daily at tapering doses, is the most common treatment used for horses with pemphigus. Other therapies including injectable gold salts or oral azathioprine can also be used in conjunction with oral corticosteroid therapy, although they carry risks of systemic side effects.[60,61] Long-term therapy is often necessary for control of the disease and can carry a poor prognosis both owing to the disease course and treatment complications in adult horses.

Acquired Hematologic Disease

Neonatal isoerythrolysis

Neonatal isoerythrolysis is a condition characterized by destruction of the foals antigenically different red blood cells (RBCs), inherited from the sire, to alloantibodies from the mare. The mare becomes sensitized to RBC antigens, most commonly Aa or Qa, during previous pregnancies, via blood transfusion, or through transplacental exposure to the fetus' RBC antigen in utero.[62] The foal is generally healthy at birth and develops clinical signs after ingesting colostrum with the mare's alloantibodies. Clinical signs develop 24 to 36 hours after birth and include icterus, pallor of mucous membranes, and progressive lethargy, tachycardia, and tachypnea from the developing anemia.[62] Ocular signs of neonatal isoerythrolysis include pale conjunctiva with marked icterus and possible sclera and conjunctival hemorrhages.

A diagnosis of neonatal isoerythrolysis is made the progressive clinical signs after ingestion of colostrums as well as decreased indicators of RBC concentration (packed cell volume, hemoglobin, and RBC count), increased total bilirubin levels, and hemolytic crossmatch between the mare's colostrum or serum and the effected foal's RBCs.[63] Treatment includes supportive care, including intravenous fluids to dilute the large hemoglobin load, minimization stress, and strict restriction of activity owing to anemia and exercise intolerance. Use of blood transfusions if the packed cell volume decrease becomes severe (packed cell volume <15%) may be necessary if compatible blood is available.[62] The ocular hemorrhages and icterus resolve as the hematologic abnormalities improve and the overall prognosis is generally good with adequate care.

CORNEAL AND TEAR FILM ABNORMALITIES

Diseases that affect facial nerve function can manifest as ocular problems owing to effects on ability to blink or tear production. Loss of eyelid tone and function can lead to exposure keratitis, frequently resulting in complicated corneal ulcers. Likewise, neurogenic keratoconjunctivitis sicca can result in severe corneal disease. One of the most common diseases to affect facial nerve function in horses is THO, described elsewhere in this article. Additionally, diseases that affect the brainstem or CN VII peripherally can cause a similar clinical picture; these diseases include EPM, polyneuritis equi, and head trauma.

Viral

Equine herpesvirus-2

EHV-2 has been associated with upper respiratory tract and ocular disease and can also be isolated from healthy horses of all ages brining to question its causative role in equine infections.[64,65] Outbreaks of EHV-2–associated keratoconjunctivitis have been reported and horses present with epiphora, conjunctival hyperemia with mucopurulent discharge, corneal vascularization, cornea edema, and linear or punctate dendritic keratopathy. Recurrence of the ocular clinical signs, as with most herpesviruses, is not uncommon.

A definitive diagnosis of EHV-2 as the cause of keratoconjunctivitis is made difficult owing to the virus' ubiquitous nature in normal eyes of horses. Conjunctival swabs seem to be the preferred method of isolating viral DNA via PCR when compared with conjunctival biopsies.[66] Resolving conjunctival inflammation and corneal disease in response to topical antiviral therapy (0.1% idoxuridine 4–12 times daily, 0.5% cidofovir twice daily) may provide the most evidence for EHV-2 as the causative agent of equine keratoconjunctivitis in many cases.[64,67]

Metabolic

Pituitary pars intermedia dysfunction: Equine Cushing's disease

Pituitary pars intermedia dysfunction (PPID) is one of the most common diseases diagnosed in geriatric horses and ponies. Hypertrophy or hyperplasia of the pars intermedia results from loss of dopaminergic innervation. The increasing size of the pars intermedia leads to greater secretion of pro-opiomelanocortin–derived peptides including corticotropin, α-melanocyte–stimulating hormone, and, endorphin which all signal the adrenal cortex to increase production of plasma glucocorticoids. The hyperplastic pars intermedia also decreases the function of the adjacent neuroendocrine tissues.[68,69]

The most commonly recognized clinical signs of PPID include hypertrichosis (hirsutism), laminitis, abnormal fat deposits including in the supraorbital fossa, weight loss with muscle atrophy, polyuria, polydipsia, lethargy, and abnormal sweat patterns.[68] Beech and colleagues[70] evaluated the corneal sensitivity in older horses with PPID (age >15 years) when compared with aged horses without PPID (age >15 years) and normal control horses (age ≤10 years). Corneal sensitivity was measured by Cochet-Bonnet aesthesiometer and showed that aged horses with PPID had a significant decrease in corneal sensitivity compared with the 2 other groups.[70] Decreased corneal sensitivity may predispose horses with PPID to an increased incidence of abnormal healing patterns of corneal wounds including nonhealing ulcers. A recent study showed increased levels of cortisol in tears of aged horses with PPID when compared with normal young and aged horses without PPID. Glucocorticoids are known to decrease healing times both systemically and in the cornea; therefore, increased exposure to higher tear cortisol concentrations in horses with PPID may contribute to delayed corneal wound healing times.[71] Abnormal vision in horses with PPID attributed to compression at the level of the optic chiasm owing to hyperplasia of the pituitary pars intermedia, and retinal degeneration in the form of senile retinopathy with alterations of pigment in the nontapetum have been described.[72,73]

The treatment of horses with PPID includes good general management practices to boost overall health as well as administration of the dopamine agonist, pergolide (0.002 mg/kg initial oral dose per day). Cyproheptidine may need to be used in addition in horses resistant to pergolide therapy alone.[68]

Genetic

Hereditary equine regional dermal asthenia (hyperelastosis cutis)

Hereditary equine regional dermal asthenia (HERDA) is a genetic condition that has been recognized in Quarter Horses most commonly and can be traced back to a single sire origin. It has also been noted in Paint horses, Appaloosas with Quarter Horse lineage, and crossbred Arabian horses.[74] HERDA follows an autosomal-recessive mode of inheritance and the condition is likely present at birth; however, clinical signs are often not recognized until the horse begins preparation for riding.[75,76] The causative mutation involves equine cyclophilin B, which leads to defects in collagen organization in the middle to deep dermis. Common clinical signs in affected horses include decreased tensile strength of skin, particularly over the back and sides of neck with spontaneous wound and laceration formation, seroma, and hematoma development, leading to unsightly scarring.[77]

Ocular signs of HERDA include an increased incidence of corneal ulcers in affected horses. The corneal thickness is decreased in multiples areas in horses with HERDA, and increased corneal curvature as well as increased frequency of corneal opacity has been described.[78] Scanning electron microscopy–confirmed abnormal collagen arrangement within the cornea.[79] Affected horses were also shown to have high increased Schirmer tear test I values.[79]

There is no specific treatment for HERDA. Horses can be maintained with proper management, including decreased exposure to ultraviolet radiation and heat, and fastidious wound management, including close monitoring for the development of corneal ulcers. DNA testing is available to determine carrier or affected status (The Veterinary Genetics Laboratory at the University of California—Davis) and horses that are carriers or affected with HERDA should be removed from breeding programs.

Miscellaneous

Temporohyoid osteoarthropathy

THO is a unique equine disease caused by pathologic fusion of the temporohyoid articulation that can cause fractures of the petrous temporal bone, in which the peripheral components of CN VII and VIII are located. Clinical signs generally reflect discomfort from the abnormal articulation and pathologic fractures or damage to the peripheral components of CN VII and VIII. Discomfort is frequently manifested as abnormal chewing, reluctance to eat or drink, or sensitivity around the head.

Damage to CN VII results in typical signs of facial nerve paresis or paralysis: ear droop with decreased movement, decreased eyelid tone and loss of ability to blink, decreased lip tone with deviation of the nose to the unaffected side, and lower lip droop. Damage to CN VIII causes signs of peripheral vestibular disease, including head tilt, loss of balance with vestibular ataxia, and abnormal eye position or movements such as ventral strabismus or nystagmus (generally horizontal with fast phase away from the affected side). When CN VII is affected, ocular signs include keratitis and possibly ulceration, which typically occurs in the ventrotemporal third of the corneal and might be extensive.[1] If parasympathetic fibers that supply the lacrimal gland are affected by the pathologic fracture, neurogenic keratoconjunctivitis sicca develops, and abnormal Schirmer tear test results (<10) are observed.

A diagnosis of THO is generally confirmed by visualization of the abnormal temporohyoid articulation via guttural pouch endoscopy, skull radiography, or skull computed tomography. Depending on imaging modality and fracture location, fractures may not be specifically identified.

Treatment of the underlying condition can be conservative or surgical. Conservative treatment generally entails antiinflammatory drugs (nonsteroidal antiinflammatory drugs or corticosteroids) to decrease pain and inflammation, as well as provision of easily masticated feedstuffs to encourage consumption. Antibiotic treatment is recommended regardless of whether conservative or surgical management is chosen, because a small number of horses with THO have or subsequently develop otitis media interna. Additionally, fractures of the petrous temporal bone that penetrate through the calvarium can result in an ascending bacterial meningoencephalitis, with devastating consequences. Surgical treatment generally leads to immediate improvement in comfort and potentially to faster and more complete resolution of neurologic abnormalities. Another benefit of surgical treatment is a decreased chance of additional pathologic fractures developing in the future. Surgical options include partial stylohyoidectomy and ceratohyoidectomy; the authors prefer the latter procedure when possible owing to complications associated with the former.[80]

THO-induced ocular disease should be addressed immediately. Corneal ulceration develops rapidly and often becomes vision or globe threatening. Treatment involves frequent lubrication, appropriate ulcer treatment, and temporary or reversible tarsorrhaphy.[1]

Polyneuritis equi
Polyneuritis equi, previously known as neuritis of the cauda equina, is a poorly understood disease that likely has an immune-mediated basis. The disease results in progressive granulomatous inflammation of nerve roots and nerves; the cauda equina and CNs are affected most commonly. Initial clinical signs might include hyperesthesia of the head or perineal region, which is generally followed by loss of sensation. Progressive paralysis of the tail, bladder, rectum, and anus frequently develops. One or several CNs might also be involved, and sometimes CN deficits are noted before the hind end signs.

This disease should be considered if CN abnormalities are recognized without convincing evidence of central nervous system disease. Depending on CN involvement, ocular signs might be the only initial abnormalities. If the facial nerve is involved, corneal disease frequently develops, as described with THO.

Antemortem diagnosis is challenging. CSF cytology often shows an increased white cell count with a mixed mononuclear or neutrophilic pleocytosis and variably increased protein concentration. One report describes diagnosis via transrectal sonography of the extradural sacral nerve roots as well as histology of a sacrocaudalis dorsalis lateralis muscle biopsy.[81]

Treatment is generally unrewarding; immunosuppressive treatment with steroids or other immunosuppressant drugs is most common. Some horses can survive for extended periods if supportive care for fecal and urinary incontinence is provided.

UVEAL TRACT AND ANTERIOR CHAMBER ABNORMALITIES, INCLUDING UVEITIS

Many infectious organisms that cause systemic disease can also directly infect the anterior chamber. Some are known for triggering an immune-mediated response that leads to uveitis in the absence of local infection. The most common types of infections that cause uveitis directly or indirectly include generalized bacterial sepsis or bacterial meningoencephalitis (foals more so than adults), *Rhodococcus equi* infections, leptospirosis, and borreliosis. Less commonly, parasites such as *Sertaria*, *Dirofilaria*, or *Parelaphostrongylus tenuis* can infest the anterior chamber. Please refer to the article by for a more thorough explanation regarding commonly encountered uveitic diseases in the horse including equine recurrent uveitis. Borreliosis is covered more specifically in this section.

Bacterial

Borrelliosis

Horses living in endemic regions are frequently infected with *Borrelia burgdorferi*, the gram-negative spirochete bacterium that causes Lyme disease. Infection occurs when the horse is bitten by an *Ixodes* spp. tick carrying *B burgdorferi*, and the organism is transmitted to the horse in tick saliva. Most horses seem to be infected subclinically and either eliminate the organism without specific treatment or remain persistently infected without clinical ramifications.

However, *B burgdorferi* infection has been associated with several syndromes in horses, including neurologic disease (neuroborreliosis), uveitis (ocular borreliosis), and dermal masses at the sites of tick bites (pseudolymphoma).[82–84] Additional clinical signs that historically have been attributed to *B burgdorferi* infection but are less well-described include chronic weight loss, sporadic lameness, stiffness, arthritis, joint effusion, muscle soreness, hepatitis, laminitis, and abortion.

Signs of ocular disease attributed to *B burgdorferi* are typical of severe, often end-stage uveitis. These include blepharospasm, epiphora, aqueous flare, fibrin or hypopyon within the anterior chamber, miosis, decreased intraocular pressure, synechiae, dyscoria, retinal detachment, visual loss, and phthisis bulbi. Ocular borreliosis can occur without other systemic signs of disease, but more commonly occurs concurrently with neurologic disease. In some cases, ocular signs precede the development of neurologic signs.

Diagnosis of ocular borreliosis can be challenging. Suggested diagnostic criteria in humans include occurrence in patients living in an endemic area, lack of evidence for other diseases, nonophthalmic clinical findings consistent with Lyme disease, positive serology, and response to treatment.[85] Likewise, diagnostic criteria for horses should include potential exposure to *Borrelia* via residence in or travel to an endemic area, exclusion of other causes of uveitis, and potentially other systemic signs that could be attributed to *Borrelia*. Unfortunately, affected horses are not consistently seropositive for antibodies against *B burgdorferi*, so negative Lyme serologic results do not rule out the condition. Conversely, horses in endemic areas are frequently seropositive in the absence of ocular disease. Currently, available serologic tests for horses include IFAT, ELISA whole cell, Western blot, bead-based multiple antigen ELISA assay (Multiplex), and point-of-care ELISA kits (C6 SNAP).

Because noninfectious (traumatic or immune-mediated) uveitis is a far more common entity in horses than uveitis owing to infectious agents, positive Lyme serology in a horse with uveitis is more likely to be an incidental finding than to reflect the cause of ocular disease. However, if additional systemic signs are present, particularly neurologic signs or marked muscle atrophy or fever, ocular borreliosis should be considered more strongly. Additional testing that may lend support to a diagnosis includes ocular fluid cytology, PCR testing, or immunologic testing. Affected horses might have spirochetes visible on cytology, positive PCR results on aqueous or vitreous humor, or detectable antibody levels in ocular fluids, despite potentially negative serologic results.[83] Histopathology on affected eyes can confirm the diagnosis; lesions typically consist of lymphoplasmacytic and suppurative uveitis and endophthalmitis with intralesional argyrophilic spirochetes consistent with *Borrelia*.

The optimal treatment for borreliosis is unknown and might depend on the extent of infection. A small experimental infection study indicated that intravenous tetracycline was more effective than oral doxycycline or intramuscular ceftiofur.[86] However, these drugs do not reliably obtain effective concentrations in cerebrospinal or ocular fluids. Minocycline, which has better bioavailability than doxycycline and obtains adequate CSF levels when dosed at 4 mg/kg bodyweight every 12 hours, was not shown to reach adequate aqueous humor levels in normal or mildly inflamed eyes at that dose.[87] Whether standard dosing would obtain adequate levels in severely inflamed eyes or whether higher doses are required is unknown. High-dose, parenteral penicillin or third-generation cephalosporins with good blood–brain barrier and blood–aqueous barrier penetration (cefotaxime, ceftazidime) might also be appropriate choices. In addition to systemic antimicrobials with activity against *Borrelia*, standard uveitis treatment with antiinflammatory drugs (nonsteroidal or steroidal as appropriate) and atropine is warranted.

RETINAL AND CHOROIDAL ABNORMALITIES

As noted in this article, many systemic diseases can manifest as inflammation resulting in damage to the choroid and/or retina of the horse. In many cases, other signs of infection and neurologic abnormality my prompt the fundic examination. The fundus changes that often accompany disease such as equine motor neuron disease (EMND) can be very useful in identifying a cause of the systemic abnormalities. A more comprehensive review of retinal diseases and their diagnosis can be found elsewhere in this issue.

Equine Motor Neuron Disease

Horses with EMND are unlikely to be presented owing to ocular complaints. However, if an ophthalmic examination is performed for another reason, subclinical (or mildly clinical) cases of EMND might be detected. EMND is a neurodegenerative disorder that most commonly develops in adult horses deficient in vitamin E.[88] The disease is characterized histologically by degeneration of motor neurons in the ventral horn of the spinal cord and specific brain stem nuclei. Consequently, denervation atrophy of skeletal muscle occurs. Highly oxidative type I postural muscles are predominantly affected.

Clinical signs include marked weight loss, owing to profound muscle atrophy, despite an excellent appetite. Generalized weakness causes horses to adapt a short-strided gait and base narrow posture, with low head carriage, frequent limb shifting, and increased recumbency. Horses show muscle tremors, particularly after exertion, and sweat excessively.

Ocular findings can be very helpful in diagnosis. EMND causes a distinctive retinopathy, and fundic examination reveals a mosaic pattern of dark brown–black to yellow–brown pigment deposited in the tapetal zone coupled with a horizontal band of pigment at the tapetal–nontapetal junction.[89] This pigment has been shown to be ceroid lipofuscin. Although not present in every case of EMND, when this retinopathy is observed the disease should be highly suspected and critical evaluation of the horse's vitamin E status, body condition, and neuromuscular function performed.

Helpful diagnostic tests include serum or plasma vitamin E level, sacrocaudalis dorsalis medialis muscle biopsy, or spinal accessory nerve biopsy. Vitamin E supplementation (10–20 IU/kg by mouth daily) may halt progression of the disease, but rarely leads to substantial improvement in moderately or severely affected horses.

OPTIC NERVE ABNORMALITIES AND BLINDNESS OWING TO CENTRAL DISEASE

Any brain disease that causes disruption in the central visual pathways from the lateral geniculate nuclei to the visual cortex causes blindness with normal pupillary light reflexes. Depending on the severity of other neurologic signs, blindness might be the most obvious abnormality and reason for seeking veterinary attention. When ophthalmic examination does not reveal an ocular cause of blindness, and pupillary light responses are normal, brain diseases should be considered.

Metabolic encephalopathies (hepatic, uremic, intestinal) are the most common cause of central blindness in horses in the authors' practices. Hepatic and uremic encephalopathy usually can be diagnosed based on other clinical signs of liver or kidney disease in conjunction with biochemistry results. Intestinal encephalopathy, also known as intestinal hyperammonemia, is a unique disease of horses thought to result most commonly from intestinal tract disease that leads to excessive ammonia absorption, overwhelming the hepatic capacity for metabolism.[90] Biochemistry does not typically show evidence for hepatic dysfunction, but blood ammonia levels are markedly elevated.

Less common causes of central blindness in horses include postictal change; head trauma; encephalitis owing to viral, protozoal, fungal (*Aspergillosis* spp. associated with guttural pouch mycosis), or bacterial infection; leukoencephalomalacia ("moldy corn poisoning" owing to the mold *Fusarium moniliforme* and its mycotoxin fumonisin); space-occupying masses such as tumors, abscesses, granulomas; thiamine deficiency; and complications from anesthesia or inadvertent intracarotid injection.

REFERENCES

1. Irby NL. Neuro-ophthalmology in horses. Vet Clin North Am 2011;27(3):455–79.
2. Zhang W, Li J, McManus DP. Concepts in immunology and diagnosis of hydatid disease. Clin Microbiol Rev 2003;16(1):18–36.
3. Rezabek GB, Giles RC, Lyons ET. Echinococcus granulosus hydatid cysts in the livers of two horses. J Vet Diagn Invest 1993;5(1):122–5.
4. Barnett KC, Cottrell BD, Rest JR. Retrobulbar hydatid cyst in the horse. Equine Vet J 1988;20(2):136–8.
5. Scagliotti RH. Comparative neuro-ophthalmology. In: Gelatt KN, editor. Veterinary ophthalmology. 3rd edition. Philadelphia: Lippincott, Williams & Wilkins; 1999.
6. Green SL, Little CB, Baird JD, et al. Tetanus in the horse: a review of 20 cases (1970 to 1990). J Vet Intern Med 1994;8(2):128–32.
7. Cullen CJ, Webb AA. Ocular manifestations of systemic disease. In: Gelatt KN, Gilger BC, Kern TJ, editors. Part 3: The Horse, in Veterinary Ophthalmology. 5th edition. Ames (IA): Wiley-Blackwell; 2015.
8. Mackay RJ. Disease of the nervous system-tetanus. In: Smith BP, editor. Llarge animal internal medicine. 5th edition. St. Louis (MO): Elsevier; 2015.
9. Gibbons RV. Cryptogenic rabies, bats, and the question of aerosol transmission. Ann Emerg Med 2002;39(5):528–36.

10. Green SL, Smith LL, Vernau W, et al. Rabies in horses: 21 cases (1970-1990). J Am Vet Med Assoc 1992;200(8):1133–7.
11. Hudson LC, Weinstock D, Jordan T, et al. Clinical presentation of experimentally induced rabies in horses. Zentralbl Veterinarmed B 1996;43(5):277–85.
12. Woldehiwet Z. Rabies: recent developments. Res Vet Sci 2002;73(1):17–25.
13. Stein LTL. Immunohistochemical study of rabies virus within the central nervous system of domestic and wildlife species. Vet Pathol 2007;47(4):630–3.
14. Harvey AM, Watson JL, Brault SA, et al. Duration of serum antibody response to rabies vaccination in horses. J Am Vet Med Assoc 2016;249(4):411–8.
15. Marsh AE, Barr BC, Madigan J, et al. Neosporosis as a cause of equine protozoal myeloencephalitis. J Am Vet Med Assoc 1996;209(11):1907–13.
16. Johnson AL, Burton AJ, Sweeney RW. Utility of 2 immunological tests for ante-mortem diagnosis of equine protozoal myeloencephalitis (Sarcocystis neurona infection) in naturally occurring cases. J Vet Intern Med 2010;24(5):1184–9.
17. Reed SM, Furr M, Howe DK, et al. Equine protozoal myeloencephalitis: an updated consensus statement with a focus on parasite biology, diagnosis, treatment, and prevention. J Vet Intern Med 2016;30(2):491–502.
18. Furr M, Howe D, Reed S, et al. Antibody coefficients for the diagnosis of equine protozoal myeloencephalitis. J Vet Intern Med 2011;25(1):138–42.
19. Reed SM, Howe DK, Morrow JK, et al. Accurate antemortem diagnosis of equine protozoal myeloencephalitis (EPM) based on detecting intrathecal antibodies against Sarcocystis neurona using the SnSAG2 and SnSAG4/3 ELISAs. J Vet Intern Med 2013;27(5):1193–200.
20. Johnson AL, Morrow JK, Sweeney RW. Indirect fluorescent antibody test and surface antigen ELISAs for antemortem diagnosis of equine protozoal myeloencephalitis. J Vet Intern Med 2013;27(3):596–9.
21. Johnson AL. Update on infectious diseases affecting the equine nervous system. Vet Clin North Am 2011;27(3):573–87.
22. Bowling AT, Byrns G, Spier S. Evidence for a single pedigree source of the hyperkalemic periodic paralysis susceptibility gene in Quarter Horses. Anim Genet 1996;27(4):279–81.
23. Rudolph JA, Spier SJ, Byrns G, et al. Periodic paralysis in quarter horses: a sodium channel mutation disseminated by selective breeding. Nat Genet 1992;2(2):144–7.
24. Spier SJ. Diseases of Muscle-Hyperkalemic Periodic Paralysis (HYPP) in Large Animal Internal Medicine (5th edition) Smith BP ed. Elsevier Mosby, St. Louis, 2015.
25. Cello RM. Ocular onchocerciasis in the horse. Equine Vet J 1971;3(4):148–54.
26. Lloyd S, Soulsby EJ. Survey for infection with Onchocerca cervicalis in horses in eastern United States. Am J Vet Res 1978;39(12):1962–3.
27. Moran CT, James ER. Equine ocular pathology ascribed to Onchocerca cervicalis infection: a re-examination. Trop Med Parasitol 1987;38(4):287–8.
28. Schmidt GM, Krehbiel JD, Coley SC, et al. Equine onchocerciasis: lesions in the nuchal ligament of midwestern U.S. horses. Vet Pathol 1982;19(1):16–22.
29. Schmidt GM, Krehbiel JD, Coley SC, et al. Equine ocular onchocerciasis: histo-pathologic study. Am J Vet Res 1982;43(8):1371–5.
30. Gemensky Metzler AJ. Diseases of the Eye-Ocular Onchocerciasis in Large Animal Internal Medicine (5th edition) Smith BP ed. Elsevier Mosby, St. Louis, 2015.
31. Lyons ET, Swerczek TW, Tolliver SC, et al. Prevalence of selected species of internal parasites in equids at necropsy in central Kentucky (1995-1999). Vet Parasitol 2000;92(1):51–62.

32. Herd RP, Donham JC. Efficacy of ivermectin against Onchocerca cervicalis microfilarial dermatitis in horses. Am J Vet Res 1983;44(6):1102–5.

33. Mancebo OA, Verdi JH, Bulman GM. Comparative efficacy of moxidectin 2% equine oral gel and ivermectin 2% equine oral paste against Onchocerca cervicalis (Railliet and Henry, 1910) microfilariae in horses with naturally acquired infections in Formosa (Argentina). Vet Parasitol 1997;73(3):243–8.

34. Pusterla N, Watson JL, Wilson WD, et al. Cutaneous and ocular habronemiasis in horses: 63 cases (1988-2002). J Am Vet Med Assoc 2003;222(7):978–82.

35. Oldenkamp EP. Treatment of ringworm in horses with natamycin. Equine Vet J 1979;11(1):36–8.

36. Wise LN, Pelzel-McCluskey AM, Mealey RH, et al. Equine piroplasmosis. Vet Clin North Am Equine Pract 2014;30(3):677–93.

37. Sippel WL, Cooperrider DE, Gainer JH, et al. Equine piroplasmosis in the United States. J Am Vet Med Assoc 1962;141:694–8.

38. Wise LN, Kappmeyer LS, Mealey RH, et al. Review of equine piroplasmosis. J Vet Intern Med 2013;27(6):1334–46.

39. Kuttler KL, Zaugg JL, Gipson CA. Imidocarb and parvaquone in the treatment of piroplasmosis (Babesia equi) in equids. Am J Vet Res 1987;48(11):1613–6.

40. de Waal DT. Equine piroplasmosis: a review. Br Vet J 1992;148(1):6–14.

41. Reubel GH, Kimsey RB, Barlough JE, et al. Experimental transmission of ehrlichia equi to horses through naturally infected ticks (Ixodes pacificus) from Northern California. J Clin Microbiol 1998;36(7):2131–4.

42. Dziegiel B, Adaszek L, Kalinowski M, et al. Equine granulocytic anaplasmosis. Res Vet Sci 2013;95(2):316–20.

43. Ziemer EL, Keenan DP, Madigan JE. Ehrlichia equi infection in a foal. J Am Vet Med Assoc 1987;190(2):199–200.

44. Ristic M, Holland CJ, Dawson JE, et al. Diagnosis of equine monocytic ehrlichiosis (Potomac horse fever) by indirect immunofluorescence. J Am Vet Med Assoc 1986;189(1):39–46.

45. Madigan JE, Rikihisa Y, Palmer JE, et al. Evidence for a high rate of false-positive results with the indirect fluorescent antibody test for Ehrlichia risticii antibody in horses. J Am Vet Med Assoc 1995;207(11):1448–53.

46. Mott J, Rikihisa Y, Zhang Y, et al. Comparison of PCR and culture to the indirect fluorescent-antibody test for diagnosis of Potomac horse fever. J Clin Microbiol 1997;35(9):2215–9.

47. Madigan JE, Pusterla N. Ehrlichial diseases. Vet Clin North Am Equine Pract 2000;16(3):487–99, ix.

48. Weese JS, Yu AA. Infectious folliculitis and dermatophytosis. Vet Clin North Am Equine Pract 2013;29(3):559–75.

49. Cafarchia C, Figueredo LA, Otranto D. Fungal diseases of horses. Vet Microbiol 2013;167(1–2):215–34.

50. Boyle AG. Diseases of the Respiratory System-Streptococcus Equi Infection (Strangles) in Large Animal Internal Medicine (5th edition) Smith BP ed. Elsevier Mosby, St. Louis, 2015.

51. Roberts SR. Chorioretinitis in a band of horses. J Am Vet Med Assoc 1971;158(12):2043–6.

52. Spoormakers TJ, Ensink JM, Goehring LS, et al. Brain abscesses as a metastatic manifestation of strangles: symptomatology and the use of magnetic resonance imaging as a diagnostic aid. Equine Vet J 2003;35(2):146–51.

53. Sweeney CR, Timoney JF, Newton JR, et al. Streptococcus equi infections in horses: guidelines for treatment, control, and prevention of strangles. J Vet Intern Med 2005;19(1):123–34.
54. Boyle AG. Streptococcus equi detection polymerase chain reaction assay for equine nasopharyngeal and guttural pouch wash samples. J Vet Intern Med 2001;30(1):276–81.
55. Cordoni G, Williams A, Durham A, et al. Rapid diagnosis of strangles (Streptococcus equi subspecies equi) using PCR. Res Vet Sci 2015;102:162–6.
56. Lindahl S, Baverud V, Egenvall A, et al. Comparison of sampling sites and laboratory diagnostic tests for S. equi subsp. equi in horses from confirmed strangles outbreaks. J Vet Intern Med 2013;27(3):542–7.
57. North SE, Wakeley PR, Mayo N, et al. Development of a real-time PCR to detect Streptococcus equi subspecies equi. Equine Vet J 2014;46(1):56–9.
58. Newton JR, Verheyen K, Talbot NC, et al. Control of strangles outbreaks by isolation of guttural pouch carriers identified using PCR and culture of Streptococcus equi. Equine Vet J 2000;32(6):515–26.
59. Gilkerson JR, Bailey KE, Diaz-Méndez A, et al. Update on viral diseases of the equine respiratory tract. Vet Clin North Am Equine Pract 2015;31(1):91–104.
60. Rosenkrantz W. Immune-mediated dermatoses. Vet Clin North Am Equine Pract 2013;29(3):607–13.
61. Vandenaboole SIJ, White SD, Affolter VK, et al. Pemphigus foliaceus in the horse: a retrospective study of 20 cases. Vet Dermatol 2004;15(6):381–8.
62. Boyle AG, Magdesian KG, Ruby RE. Neonatal isoerythrolysis in horse foals and a mule foal: 18 cases (1988-2003). J Am Vet Med Assoc 2005;227(8):1276–83.
63. Becht JL, Semrad SD. Hematology, blood typing, and immunology of the neonatal foal. Vet Clin North Am 1985;1(1):91–116.
64. Kershaw O, von Oppen T, Glitz F, et al. Detection of equine herpesvirus type 2 (EHV-2) in horses with keratoconjunctivitis. Virus Res 2001;80(1–2):93–9.
65. Borchers K, Ebert M, Fetsch A, et al. Prevalence of equine herpesvirus type 2 (EHV-2) DNA in ocular swabs and its cell tropism in equine conjunctiva. Vet Microbiol 2006;118(3–4):260–6.
66. Hollingsworth SR, Pusterla N, Kass PH, et al. Detection of equine herpesvirus in horses with idiopathic keratoconjunctivitis and comparison of three sampling techniques. Vet Ophthalmol 2015;18(5):416–21.
67. Collinson PN, O'Rielly JL, Ficorilli N, et al. Isolation of equine herpesvirus type 2 (equine gammaherpesvirus 2) from foals with keratoconjunctivitis. J Am Vet Med Assoc 1994;205(2):329–31.
68. McFarlane D. Equine pituitary pars intermedia dysfunction. Vet Clin North Am Equine Pract 2011;27(1):93–113.
69. Schott HC 2nd. Pituitary pars intermedia dysfunction: equine Cushing's disease. Vet Clin North Am Equine Pract 2002;18(2):237–70.
70. Miller C, Utter ML, Beech J. Evaluation of the effects of age and pituitary pars intermedia dysfunction on corneal sensitivity in horses. Am J Vet Res 2013;74(7):1030–5.
71. Hart KA, Kitchings KM, Kimura S, et al. Measurement of cortisol concentration in the tears of horses and ponies with pituitary pars intermedia dysfunction. Am J Vet Res 2016;77(11):1236–44.
72. Brosnahan MM, Paradis MR. Assessment of clinical characteristics, management practices, and activities of geriatric horses. J Am Vet Med Assoc 2003;223(1):99–103.

73. Chandler KJ, Billson FM, Mellor DJ. Ophthalmic lesions in 83 geriatric horses and ponies. Vet Rec 2003;153(11):319–22.
74. White SD, Affolter VK, Bannasch DL, et al. Hereditary equine regional dermal asthenia ("hyperelastosis cutis") in 50 horses: clinical, histological, immunohistological and ultrastructural findings. Vet Dermatol 2004;15(4):207–17.
75. Tryon RC, White SD, Famula TR, et al. Inheritance of hereditary equine regional dermal asthenia in Quarter Horses. Am J Vet Res 2005;66(3):437–42.
76. Tryon RC, Penedo MC, McCue ME, et al. Evaluation of allele frequencies of inherited disease genes in subgroups of American Quarter Horses. J Am Vet Med Assoc 2009;234(1):120–5.
77. Rashmir-Raven A. Heritable equine regional dermal asthenia. Vet Clin North Am Equine Pract 2013;29(3):689–702.
78. Badial PR, Cisneros-Alvarez LE, Brandao CV, et al. Ocular dimensions, corneal thickness, and corneal curvature in quarter horses with hereditary equine regional dermal asthenia. Vet Ophthalmol 2015;18(5):385–92.
79. Mochal CA, Miller WW, Cooley AJ, et al. Ocular findings in Quarter Horses with hereditary equine regional dermal asthenia. J Am Vet Med Assoc 2010;237(3):304–10.
80. Pease AP, van Biervliet J, Dykes NL, et al. Complication of partial stylohyoidectomy for treatment of temporohyoid osteoarthropathy and an alternative surgical technique in three cases. Equine Vet J 2004;36(6):546–50.
81. Aleman M, Katzman SA, Vaughan B, et al. Antemortem diagnosis of polyneuritis equi. J Vet Intern Med 2009;23(3):665–8.
82. Johnstone LK, Engiles JB, Aceto H, et al. Retrospective evaluation of horses diagnosed with neuroborreliosis on postmortem examination: 16 cases (2004-2015). J Vet Intern Med 2016;30(4):1305–12.
83. Priest HL, Irby NL, Schlafer DH, et al. Diagnosis of Borrelia-associated uveitis in two horses. Vet Ophthalmol 2012;15(6):398–405.
84. Sears KP, Divers TJ, Neff RT, et al. A case of Borrelia-associated cutaneous pseudolymphoma in a horse. Vet Dermatol 2012;23(2):153–6.
85. Lesser RL. Ocular manifestations of Lyme disease. Am J Med 1995;98(4):60S–2S.
86. Chang Y, Ku Y, Chang C, et al. Antibiotic treatment of experimentally Borrelia burgdorferi-infected ponies. Vet Microbiol 2005;107(3–4):285–94.
87. Schnabel LV, Papich MG, Divers TJ, et al. Pharmacokinetics and distribution of minocycline in mature horses after oral administration of multiple doses and comparison with minimum inhibitory concentrations. Equine Vet J 2012;44(4):453–8.
88. Divers TJ, Mohammed HO, Cummings JF, et al. Equine motor neuron disease: findings in 28 horses and proposal of a pathophysiological mechanism for the disease. Equine Vet J 1994;26(5):409–15.
89. Riis RC, Jackson C, Rebhun W, et al. Ocular manifestations of equine motor neuron disease. Equine Vet J 1999;31(2):99–110.
90. Dunkel B, Chaney KP, Dallap-Schaer B, et al. Putative intestinal hyperammonaemia in horses: 36 cases. Equine Vet J 2011;43(2):133–40.

Antifungal Therapy in Equine Ocular Mycotic Infections

Eric C. Ledbetter, DVM

KEYWORDS

- Antifungal • Horse • Equine • Keratomycosis • Fungal keratitis • Mycotic infection

KEY POINTS

- Keratomycosis is the most common ocular fungal infection treated in equine medicine; however, a diverse range of mycotic infections, affecting numerous other ocular tissues, may also be encountered in clinical practice.
- A comprehensive knowledge of the relative characteristics and properties of the antifungal medications used in equine ophthalmology is essential to selecting an optimal treatment strategy for a particular case.
- Clinicians must select both an appropriate antifungal medication and an effective medication administration route to achieve the best outcome.
- Many newer medication delivery methods and devices are now available for the treatment of ocular fungal infections in horses and can contribute to an improved outcome in select situations.

INTRODUCTION

Fungi are frequent and clinically important causes of ocular infections in the horse. Keratomycosis is the most common ocular fungal infection treated in equine medicine; however, a diverse range of mycotic infections affecting numerous other ocular tissues may also be encountered in clinical practice. Many equine mycoses are diagnostic and therapeutic challenges for the clinician. Prompt and appropriate treatment is essential to minimize morbidity and reduce the likelihood of vision loss associated with ocular fungal infections.

The antifungal pharmaceutical treatment options available to veterinarians are more limited when compared with the range of antimicrobials used as therapy for equine bacterial infections. A thorough knowledge of the relative characteristics and properties of the antifungal medications used in equine ophthalmology is essential to

Disclosure Statement: The author has nothing to disclose.
Department of Clinical Sciences, Cornell University College of Veterinary Medicine, Cornell University Hospital for Animals, CVM Box 34, Ithaca, NY 14853, USA
E-mail address: ecl32@cornell.edu

Vet Clin Equine 33 (2017) 583–605
http://dx.doi.org/10.1016/j.cveq.2017.08.001
0749-0739/17/© 2017 Elsevier Inc. All rights reserved.

vetequine.theclinics.com

selecting an optimal treatment strategy for a particular case. This includes selection of both an appropriate antifungal medication and an effective medication administration route. In addition, newer medication delivery methods and devices are now available for the treatment of ocular fungal infections in horses and can contribute to an improved outcome in select situations.

TYPES OF EQUINE OCULAR FUNGAL INFECTIONS
Keratomycosis

Keratomycosis is a relatively common ocular disease in horses compared with most other domestic animal species, and it is the most clinically important equine ocular fungal infection.[1–3] The high prevalence of fungal keratitis in horses is believed to result from host and environmental factors that increase exposure and susceptibility of the equine cornea to fungi.[4] Risk factors identified for development of fungal keratitis in the horse include prior treatment with topical ocular antimicrobials, prior treatment with topical ocular corticosteroids, vegetative corneal foreign bodies, and external corneal trauma.[1–3,5] Keratomycosis is a vision and globe-threatening infection that must be aggressively managed to achieve an optimal functional outcome. The clinical features, progression, and response to treatment can vary greatly among individual equine cases and the therapeutic plan must be tailored to the individual horse.[1–7]

The clinical presentation and appearance of keratomycosis can differ dramatically between horses. Fungal infections of the cornea may be ulcerative or nonulcerative and can affect superficial or deep tissue layers of the cornea. General clinical forms of fungal keratitis that occur in the horse include epithelial keratopathies, subepithelial infiltrates, superficial corneal ulcers, deep corneal ulcers (that can progress to descemetoceles or corneal perforations), and stromal abscesses.[8–11] Specific clinical findings during ophthalmic examination that suggest a diagnosis of fungal keratitis in the horse include white, yellow, green, brown, or black corneal plaques, often with a feathery or fluffy appearance; corneal satellite lesions; corneal furrowing; and deep stromal abscessation (**Fig. 1**).[1,4,6] These examination findings should increase the suspicion of fungal infection, but clinical features alone should not be relied on to suggest a diagnosis of fungal keratitis in horses. Diagnostic evaluation for fungal involvement should be pursued for all cases of ulcerative and nonulcerative keratitis in horses when the cause is not readily apparent from historical information or clinical ophthalmic examination findings.

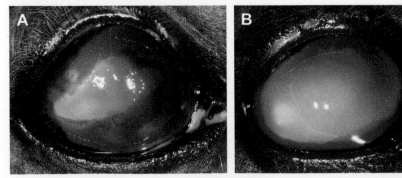

Fig. 1. Clinical photographs of equine keratomycosis in 2 horses. Fungal corneal ulcer (*A*) associated with a white corneal fungal plaque and mild hypopyon. Fungal stromal abscess (*B*) associated with marked keratitis and anterior uveitis.

Aspergillus and Fusarium spp are the most frequently isolated infectious organisms in equine keratomycosis; however, a variety of other filamentous fungi (eg, Absidia, Acremonium, Alternaria, Chrysosporium, Cladosporium, Cunninghamella, Curvularia, Cylindrocarpon, Cystodendron, Drechslera, Epidermophyton, Gliocladium, Graphium, Microsporum, Mortierella, Mucor, Paecilomyces, Papulaspora, Penicillium, Phycomyces, Pseudallescheria, Rhizoctonia, Rhizopus, Scedosporium, Scopulariopsis, Scytalidium, Stemphylium, Trichoderma, and Verticillium spp) and yeasts (eg, Candida, Cryptococcus, Histoplasma, Pichia, Rhodotorula, Saccharomyces, and Trichosporon spp) are also reported.[1–23] Most of these fungi are normal inhabitants of the equine extraocular microflora and environment.[24–30] Fungi are capable of invading the cornea only after circumvention of normal ocular anatomic, physiologic, and immunologic protective barriers.[31] Following penetration into the corneal epithelium and stroma, fungi multiply and induce an inflammatory response with subsequent tissue destruction.[32]

Blepharitis

The equine eyelids are basically composed of modified skin and are, therefore, potentially susceptible to any etiologic agent of cutaneous mycosis in horses. Fungal blepharitis may occur with cutaneous infection by numerous fungal organisms, including Alternaria spp, Aspergillus spp, Bipolaris spp, Candida spp, Cladosporium spp, Curvularia spp, Cryptococcus spp, Exserohilum rostratum, Geotrichum candidum, Histoplasma spp, Madurella mycetomatis, Microsporum spp, Rhinosporidium spp, Scedosporium apiospermum, Penicillium spp, Pseudallescheria boydii, Sporothrix schenckii, and Trichophyton spp[33–36] Basidiobolus spp are also specifically reported to cause eyelid granulomas in horses.[37] Alopecia, erythema, desquamation, hyperkeratosis, pruritus, and ulceration of the eyelids are common clinical lesions. Fungal blepharitis is associated with nodular granulomas or the development of chronic draining tracts in some cases.[35] Mycotic infections of the equine eyelids are believed to most commonly result from penetrating plant material cutaneous trauma, secondary infections of damaged skin, or regional spread of a generalized dermatosis.[38]

Epizootic lymphangitis is a chronic, contagious disease of equids associated with infection by Histoplasma farciminosum.[39] Infection is characterized by lymphangitis and lymphadenitis. Clinically, the disease has cutaneous, respiratory, and ocular forms. The ocular form of this disease includes the formation of granulomatous nodules of the eyelids, conjunctiva, nictitans membrane, and nasolacrimal system.[40,41] These nodules are frequently ulcerated. Epizootic lymphangitis is endemic in specific geographic regions, including parts of Africa, Asia, and the Middle East, but is not known to occur in North America.[39]

Conjunctivitis

Reported conjunctival fungal infections in the horse include granulomatous conjunctivitis resulting from Scedosporium apiospermum infection.[42] This mycotic infection represents a subconjunctival form of eumycetoma and appears clinically as solitary or multiple firm masses in the subconjunctival tissues.[43] Histopathologically, the subconjunctival mycetomas are characterized by phaeohyphomycosis with pyogranulomatous inflammation. This uncommon equine infection is suspected to occur following penetrating conjunctival trauma that introduces fungal spores into a conjunctival wound or the subconjunctival space.[42,43] Additional fungal causes of conjunctivitis frequently mentioned to affect horses, but without detailed published descriptions, include species of *Aspergillus*, *Blastomyces*, *Rhinosporidium*, and *Sporothrix*.[33]

Intraocular Mycotic Infections

Intraocular fungal infections described in the horse include iris abscesses, intralenticular infection, and endophthalmitis.[44] Fungal abscesses of the iris appear as focal, yellow-white, masses or accumulations of flocculent material adherent to the iridal surface or corpora nigra (**Fig. 2**).[44] Mycotic iris abscesses are typically associated with severe anterior uveitis, often characterized as anterior chamber fibrin and hyphema. Deep corneal stromal abscess are concurrently present with iris abscesses in some horses. In rare cases, fungi may also penetrate within the anterior lens capsule and lens cortex.[44] The introduction of fungi into the interior of the eye by corneal micropuncture trauma or hematogenous fungal dissemination to uvea tissues are proposed pathophysiologies that may produce this clinical syndrome in the horse.

Optic Neuritis

Fungal optic neuritis can develop in the horse in association with gutturomycosis or *Cryptococcus neoformans* meningitis.[45,46] Inflammation of the optic nerve may include papillitis (inflammation of the intraocular section of the optic nerve that is visible by ophthalmoscopy) or be restricted to the retrobulbar section of the optic nerve (which is not visible by ophthalmoscopy). Clinically, unilateral or bilateral blindness and mydriasis are observed.[45,47] Anisocoria and reduced or absent pupillary light reflexes may also be present. Vision or pupillary abnormalities may also develop in horses with cryptococcal meningitis as a result of lesions of the central nervous system. Equine central nervous system and optic nerve cryptococcosis are believed to result from hematogenous or lymphatic dissemination of fungal organisms from a primary site of infection (eg, gastrointestinal or pulmonary infection) or direct invasion across the cribriform plate from an infection of the nasal region.[48] Extension of an *Aspergillus* granuloma from the guttural pouch to the intracranial optic nerve is also described in a horse, and multiple ischemic infarcts were presented histologically in the optic nerve.[46]

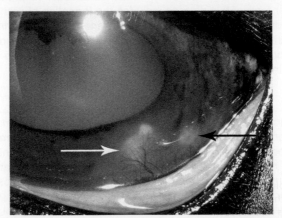

Fig. 2. Deep stromal fungal abscess (*white arrow*) and an associated iris abscess (*black arrow*) in a horse.

Orbital Disease

Fungal orbital disease is uncommon in the horse, but orbital abscesses and cellulitis can occur with *Scedosporium apiospermum* or *Cryptococcus neoformans* infection.[49–51] Exophthalmos, strabismus, resistance to globe retropulsion, periorbital swelling, and exposure keratitis are noted clinically. An orbital eumycetoma was described in a horse that occurred after severe trauma resulting from a horse kick injury to the orbit.[49] In the reported horse, the orbital infection and osteomyelitis spread extensively to the adjacent sinuses and the nasal cavity.[49]

DIAGNOSIS OF EQUINE OCULAR FUNGAL INFECTIONS

A variety of diagnostic modalities for the detection of fungi in equine ocular infections are available to the clinician. The selection of any tests should be tailored to each specific clinical scenario. Factors that affect this decision include the ocular lesions present and their rate of progression, the ocular tissues involved and their accessibility for sampling, availability of specimen collection and imaging equipment, and the accessibility of diagnostic laboratory support.

General diagnostic assays available for the detection of fungi in equine ocular lesions include cytology, histopathology, culture, polymerase chain reaction (PCR) assays, and in vivo confocal microscopy. Cytologic evaluation of tissue swabs or scrapings provides a comparatively rapid result, is relatively atraumatic to perform, samples can typically be collected in awake or sedated horses, and does not require specialized equipment.[52] Cytology is less sensitive than some other diagnostic techniques and deep tissue infections may be inaccessible for adequate sampling.[53] Histopathology is more sensitive for the detection of fungal elements than cytology but requires more traumatic sampling techniques and, in some instances, deep sedation or general anesthesia to safely collect adequate samples from diseased and fragile ocular tissues (**Fig. 3**A).[54]

Fungal culture is highly sensitive for most fungi and permits antifungal susceptibility testing to be performed on isolates.[53,54] Culture often requires lengthy periods for

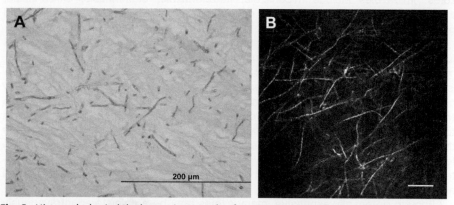

Fig. 3. Histopathologic (*A*) photomicrograph of an anterior lamellar keratectomy specimen from a horse with keratomycosis. The specimen is stained with hematoxylin-eosin stain (H&E) and displays numerous filamentous fungi. Confocal microscopic (*B*) photomicrograph of the cornea of a horse with keratomycosis displaying numerous filamentous fungal elements. Bar = 50 μm.

assay completion and some fastidious fungal organisms may be difficult to grown in vitro (particularly when antifungal medications are already being administered to the horse before culture sample collection). PCR assays are available for the detection of fungal DNA in equine ocular infections.[55] These PCR assays are highly sensitive and can identify many common fungal genera associated with equine infections. The frequent presence of potentially pathogenic fungi in the equine periocular microfloras and immediate external environment can make result interpretation difficult in some instances. Great care must be taken to avoid contamination of samples during collection and transportation to the diagnostic laboratory.

In vivo confocal microscopy is a relatively new imaging technology that permits noninvasive, real-time examination of tissues at the cellular level. The high resolution and magnification images produced by confocal microscopy allows for the detection of fungal elements within tissues (see **Fig. 3**B).[56,57] This technique requires clear tissue media, so its use in equine ocular infections is restricted to the cornea and superficial conjunctival epithelium. In vivo confocal microscopy of the cornea can be used for ulcerative and nonulcerative lesions and can detect fungal structures in both superficial and deep corneal layers. Although confocal microscopy is an excellent technique for the diagnosis of equine keratomycosis, current availability of this imaging equipment in equine ophthalmology is limited.

PHARMACOLOGIC ANTIFUNGAL TREATMENT OPTIONS

Classes of antifungals that are used most frequently for equine ocular infections include the azoles, polyenes, pyrimidines, echinocandins, allylamines, chitin synthesis inhibitors, silver sulfadiazine, and iodophors.

Azoles

The azole class of antifungals includes many of the most common antifungal agents used in equine ophthalmology. Azoles bind to the fungal enzyme cytochrome P450 and inhibit the biosynthesis of ergosterol in the plasma membrane.[58] The result is increased membrane permeability and growth inhibition. Azoles are considered fungistatic agents and are divided into 2 main classes: the imidazoles and the triazoles. Imidazoles include miconazole, ketoconazole, clotrimazole, enilconazole, and econazole. Triazoles include itraconazole, fluconazole, voriconazole, and posaconazole.

Azoles have a broad spectrum of activity against many yeasts and filamentous fungi. Miconazole, itraconazole, fluconazole, enilconazole, and voriconazole are common compounded topical ophthalmic medications and dermatologic creams administered to horses with fungal infections (**Table 1**). Itraconazole is frequently combined with dimethyl sulfoxide to improve solubility and is reported as an effective topical treatment of equine keratomycosis.[59] Ophthalmic voriconazole administered topically to horses penetrates the intact corneal epithelium and can be detected in the aqueous humor in concentrations exceeding the minimum inhibitory concentration for many common fungal pathogens of horses.[60] Miconazole may also be administered to horses by the subconjunctival route and voriconazole by both subconjunctival and intracorneal routes.

Although potentially expensive, many azoles may be administered intravenously or orally to horses. Fluconazole administered long-term intravenously or orally resulted in detectable aqueous humor concentrations in horses.[61] Following intravenous or oral administration to horses, voriconazole is detected in the preocular tear film and aqueous humor in concentrations exceeding the therapeutic

Table 1
Common topical ophthalmic antifungal agents used in horses: medication concentrations, formulations, and administration frequencies

Antifungal	Drug Class	Concentration or Formulation	Administration Frequency
Fluconazole	Triazole	0.2% solution	q2h–q6h
Itraconazole	Triazole	1% ointment (with 30% DMSO)	q2h–q6h
Ketoconazole	Imidazole	1% solution	q2h–q6h
Miconazole	Imidazole	1% solution	q2h–q6h
Voriconazole	Triazole	1% solution	q2h–q6h
Amphotericin B	Polyene	0.075% to 0.5% solution	q2h–q6h
Natamycin	Polyene	5% suspension	q2h–q6h
Flucytosine	Pyrimidine	1% solution	q2h–q6h
Terbinafine	Allylamine	0.2% solution	q2h–q6h
Silver sulfadiazine	Metal ion	1% ointment/cream	q6h–q24 h
Povidone-iodine	Iodophor	0.1% to 5% solution	q24 h

target for many pathogenic fungi.[62,63] Itraconazole administered to horses orally or intravenously achieves plasma concentrations inhibitory to many pathogenic fungi but is not detectable in the aqueous humor.[64] Ketoconazole demonstrated poor gastrointestinal absorption in horses after intragastric gavage.[65]

Polyenes

The polyenes include amphotericin B, natamycin, and nystatin. These fungicidal agents directly bind with ergosterol in the fungal cell membrane, resulting in loss of membrane integrity, oxidative damage, altered metabolic function, and ultimately cell death.[66]

Polyenes are the broadest-spectrum antifungal agents available, exhibiting activity against most yeasts, filamentous fungi, and dimorphic fungi associated with equine ocular infections. Natamycin is currently the only drug approved by the US Food and Drug Administration for the treatment of fungal keratitis in humans and is the only topical ophthalmic drug commercially available for this purpose (Natacyn, natamycin 5% ophthalmic solution, Alcon Laboratories, Fort Worth, TX, USA). Natacyn is a thick white suspension of natamycin that tends to accumulate within corneal ulcers, potentially increasing contact time. Natamycin is a commonly used topical ophthalmic medication for equine ocular fungal infections and is demonstrated in vitro to be fungicidal against many filamentous fungi isolated from horses with keratomycosis.[67] Natamycin is generally regarded as the treatment of choice for *Fusarium* keratomycosis in most animal species, but it is poorly water soluble and penetrates intact corneal epithelium poorly.

Nystatin and amphotericin may be compounded for topical ophthalmic use in the horse (see **Table 1**). Colloidal suspensions of nonliposomal amphotericin should be used and reconstituted with sterile water because saline decreases amphotericin stability. Amphotericin concentrations of 0.15% to 0.2% are most commonly used for topical ophthalmic applications. Subconjunctival and intracorneal injections of amphotericin can also be performed in the horse. Amphotericin can be administered intravenously to horses for systemic fungal infections, but ocular tissue distribution is unknown.[68]

Pyrimidines

Flucytosine is a pyrimidine with an intracellular mode of action that is unique among the available antifungal agents. After absorption into fungal cells, flucytosine is converted to 5-fluorouracil by the enzyme cytosine deaminase.[66] The compound 5-fluorouracil is a toxic antimetabolite and inhibits fungal DNA synthesis. Flucytosine exhibits both fungistatic and fungicidal properties. Flucytosine is currently used infrequently for equine ocular infections because it has a relatively narrow antifungal spectrum, poor penetration into ocular tissues, and fungal resistance develops rapidly when it is used as a sole therapeutic agent. It is particularly effective against yeasts such as Candida spp.

Echinocandins

Echinocandins are semisynthetic lipopeptides that inhibit glucan synthesis in the fungal cell wall, resulting in structural damage, osmotic imbalances, and cell lysis.[66] Caspofungin, micafungin, and anidulafungin are included in this drug class. Echinocandins are fungicidal against Candida spp, but are fungistatic or ineffective against filamentous fungi. Currently, echinocandins are not widely used in equine medicine and information regarding their clinical applications is limited.[69]

Allylamines

Terbinafine is an allylamine that inhibits the fungal enzyme squalene epoxidase. This prevents ergosterol synthesis, disrupts cell membrane synthesis, and results in the intracellular accumulation of cytotoxic squalene.[66] Terbinafine has fungicidal properties and exhibits broad-spectrum activity against many yeast and filamentous fungi.

Topical application of terbinafine 0.2% solution every 4 hours for 7 doses did not result in detectable aqueous humor concentrations in normal horse eyes, suggesting it may be ineffective for use in deep corneal or intraocular fungal infections.[70] Preliminary pharmacokinetic studies indicated that terbinafine bioavailability after oral administration in horses is limited by first-pass metabolism (ie, its concentration is greatly reduced before it reaches the systemic circulation) and may be associated with minor oral irritation, fever, and colic.[71,72]

Chitin Synthesis Inhibitors

Lufenuron is a benzoylphenyl urea-derived insecticide that inhibits chitin synthesis, polymerization, and deposition. Because it may disrupt chitin synthesis in fungal cell walls, it has been suggested as a potential topical or systemic therapeutic for equine fungal infections.[73] When evaluated in vitro, lufenuron had no effect on the growth of Aspergillus and Fusarium isolates obtained from infected equine corneas.[74] During an in vivo equine study, oral administration of lufenuron produced detectable blood concentrations in most evaluated horses without adverse effects, but the maximum blood lufenuron concentrations detected were below the concentrations demonstrated to be ineffective in vitro.[74] Further research is required to determine if lufenuron has any applications for equine ocular fungal infections, but current evidence does not support its clinical use.

Silver Sulfadiazine

Silver sulfadiazine reacts with fungal DNA and prevents unzipping of the double helix with inhibition of replication.[73] An in vitro study evaluating the antifungal properties of silver sulfadiazine against filamentous fungi isolated from horses with keratomycosis (eg, Aspergillus, Fusarium, Curvularia, Scopulariopsis, Penicillium, and Chrysosporium spp) determined it was fungicidal in its mechanism of action.[67] Silver sulfadiazine is inexpensive and anecdotally described to be safe and effective for topical use in horses with ocular fungal infections.[75]

Iodophors

The iodophor povidone-iodine is a stable chemical complex of polyvinylpyrrolidone and elemental iodine. It is a broad-spectrum microbicide with a nonspecific mode of action that is not completely understood but involves the disruption of microorganism cell walls and membranes. The use of dilute concentrations of povidone-iodine is anecdotally described as a topical therapy for equine keratomycosis (see **Table 1**).[75] Although inexpensive and readily available, povidone-iodine must be used with caution because it may cause ocular irrigation and local toxicity. To minimize irritation, povidone-iodine is generally applied no more frequently than once daily and is thoroughly flushed from the ocular surface within 5 minutes of application.

ANTIFUNGAL SUSCEPTIBILITY TESTING

Antifungal susceptibility testing is performed less commonly in equine medicine than antibacterial susceptibility testing. Currently, interpretation of results for individual cases may be complicated by the relative unavailability of reliable and reproducible antifungal susceptibility testing methods in many veterinary diagnostic laboratories, the lack of established susceptibility breakpoints for many fungi associated with equine infections (especially filamentous fungi), and the absence of published studies describing the clinical use of antifungal susceptibility information in equine patient care.[76] The length of time required for assay completion can also render the results of limited clinical value to individual cases. Despite these limitations, published descriptions of antifungal susceptibility patterns for equine ocular fungal isolates can assist with the empirical selection of antifungal medications for horses with ocular mycotic infections while susceptibility results are pending or in situations in which these tests cannot be performed.

In vitro antifungal susceptibility testing uses laboratory standards to attempt to predict the in vivo efficacy of antifungal medications. These standards are based on the anticipated serum concentrations safely achievable with a given medication and are influenced by each drug's pharmacokinetic, pharmacodynamic, and toxicity properties; the inherent susceptibility of a particular fungi to a drug; and the tissue site of infection. Currently, there are no separate standards for ocular tissue concentrations available for topically administered ophthalmic antifungals. The serum standards are used to estimate susceptibility for topical ocular treatment; however, tissue concentrations of antifungals administered topically are likely equal to or greater than serum concentrations in many clinical situations. Consequently, in vitro resistance may be overcome by high in vivo antifungal concentrations in some clinical situations, such as topical treatment of eyelid, conjunctival, or corneal infections.

The correlation between in vitro antifungal susceptibility testing and in vivo clinical effectiveness is not always predictable because clinical outcome is also influenced by host and fungal factors that cannot be quantitated in vitro. As a result, it has been suggested that the greatest clinical value of antifungal susceptibility testing may be in the identification of general trends.[77] This necessitates that the treatment of equine ocular mycotic infections with any antifungal agent always be combined with diligent clinical monitoring of treatment response.

There are 2 basic classifications of antifungal susceptibility testing that are commonly used: qualitative and quantitative.[78] Qualitative testing includes assays, such as the disk diffusion or Kirby-Bauer methods in which disks impregnated with an antifungal are placed on agar plates inoculated with the fungi to be tested. The antifungal drug diffuses into the plate in a descending concentration gradient away from the disk. The diameter of the zone of growth inhibition surrounding the disk is measured and cross-referenced to established ranges that correlate with susceptibility or resistance for that specific fungus to that particular drug. Minimal inhibitory concentration values are not provided by these tests.

Quantitative antifungal susceptibility testing methods include broth microdilution, broth macrodilution, and agar-based methods.[78,79] The broth microdilution method uses a plate with varying concentrations of antifungals in each well. Broth macrodilution testing is similar, but uses larger tubes and volumes of antifungals. In these methods, a standardized fungal inoculum and incubation period are used. Agar-based quantitative methods consist of plastic strips with predefined concentration gradients on an antifungal drug. The strips are applied to an agar surface inoculated with the fungus, which transfers the antifungal to the agar matrix. Quantitative testing methods provide specific minimum inhibitory concentrations (the lowest antifungal concentration that inhibits visible growth of a fungus), which correspond with a specific breakpoint for susceptibly interpretation. The breakpoints are provided by various sources, including the Clinical Laboratory Standards Institute and the European Committee on Antimicrobial Susceptibility Testing.

EQUINE ANTIFUNGAL SUSCEPTIBILITY STUDIES

There are relatively few published studies investigating the antifungal susceptibility patterns of equine ocular fungal isolates. To date, the available reports have primarily focused on keratomycosis. These published studies suggest that there is substantial geographic variation in both the frequency of particular fungal isolates and the isolates' antifungal susceptibility patterns. It is, therefore, expected that regional differences in the efficacy of antifungal medications will be encountered when treating ocular fungal infections horses.

In general, direct comparison of the results of studies evaluating antifungal susceptibility patterns in equine ophthalmology is not possible. Differences in testing methodologies and inconsistent study breakpoints for determination of susceptibility and resistance contribute to these difficulties. In addition, variation in how results are communicated makes comparisons problematic. Some studies report results as susceptible versus resistant. In other studies, absolute values for minimum inhibitory concentrations or minimal fungicidal concentrations are provided. Other publications only describe relative susceptibility of fungi to different antifungal drugs that are compared with each other. Finally, some studies report susceptibility patterns for grouped fungal isolates, whereas others describe results for individual fungal genera or species.

Studies evaluating equine corneal fungal isolates from California, Florida, and the northeastern United States (which included horses from New York, Pennsylvania, Connecticut, New Jersey, Maine, and Massachusetts) exemplify the geographic differences in fungal isolates and antifungal susceptibility patterns that are observed (**Tables 2–5**).[80–82] In California, *Aspergillus*, *Fusarium*, and *Rhizopus* spp were the most frequent fungi isolated.[80] Grouped fungal isolates from horses in California had the highest percentage of in vitro susceptibility by broth microdilution testing to (in declining order) voriconazole, posaconazole, natamycin, and amphotericin. In Florida, *Aspergillus, Fusarium,* and *Penicillium* spp were cultured most commonly and

Table 2
Antifungal susceptibility determinations for grouped fungi isolated from horses with keratomycosis

	California (Reed et al,[80] 2013)	Florida (Brooks et al,[81] 1998)	Northeastern United States (Ledbetter et al,[82] 2007)
Caspofungin	50% (2)	NA	NA
Clotrimazole	NA	NA	81% (72)
Ketoconazole	50% (2)	50% (22)	59% (74)
Miconazole	NA	77% (22)	28% (69)
Amphotericin	67% (3)	NA	59% (69)
Natamycin	67% (6)	77% (22)	88% (64)
Nystatin	NA	NA	89% (73)
Itraconazole	43% (7)	64% (22)	67% (49)
Fluconazole	25% (8)	4% (22)	16% (38)
Fluorocytosine	50% (2)	NA	59% (59)
Posaconazole	86% (7)	NA	NA
Voriconazole	89% (9)	NA	NA

Results are from 3 studies evaluating horses from California, Florida, and the northeastern United States. Results presented as percent susceptible (total number of isolates tested).
Abbreviation: NA, not applicable.
Data from Refs.[80–82]

natamycin, miconazole, itraconazole, and ketoconazole were the most effective antifungal medications evaluated using a broth microdilution testing method.[81] The most frequent fungi detected from horses with keratomycosis in the northeastern United States were *Aspergillus*, *Candida*, and *Fusarium* spp. Northeastern fungal isolates

Table 3
Antifungal susceptibility determinations for *Aspergillus* spp isolated from horses with keratomycosis

	California (Reed et al,[80] 2013)	Florida (Brooks et al,[81] 1998)	Northeastern USA (Ledbetter et al,[82] 2007)
Caspofungin	NA	NA	NA
Clotrimazole	NA	NA	91% (46)
Ketoconazole	100% (1)	78% (9)	57% (47)
Miconazole	NA	100% (9)	30% (43)
Amphotericin	NA	NA	65% (40)
Natamycin	50% (4)	100% (9)	82% (44)
Nystatin	NA	NA	96% (47)
Itraconazole	25% (4)	100% (9)	86% (28)
Fluconazole	0% (5)	0% (9)	8% (24)
Fluorocytosine	NA	NA	73% (41)
Posaconazole	100% (4)	NA	NA
Voriconazole	100% (5)	NA	NA

Results are from 3 studies evaluating horses from California, Florida, and the northeastern United States. Results presented as percent susceptible (total number of isolates tested).
Data from Refs.[80–82]

Table 4
Antifungal susceptibility determinations for *Fusarium* spp isolated from horses with keratomycosis

	California (Reed et al,[80] 2013)	Florida (Brooks et al,[81] 1998)	Northeastern USA (Ledbetter et al,[82] 2007)
Caspofungin	NA	NA	NA
Clotrimazole	NA	NA	43% (7)
Ketoconazole	NA	14% (7)	43% (7)
Miconazole	NA	43% (7)	0% (7)
Amphotericin	NA	NA	43% (7)
Natamycin	NA	71% (7)	100% (6)
Nystatin	NA	NA	43% (7)
Itraconazole	NA	0% (7)	0% (6)
Fluconazole	NA	0% (7)	0% (3)
Fluorocytosine	NA	NA	0% (5)
Posaconazole	NA	NA	NA
Voriconazole	NA	NA	NA

Results are from 3 studies evaluating horses from California, Florida, and the northeastern United States. Results presented as percent susceptible (total number of isolates tested).
Data from Refs.[80–82]

had the highest percentage of susceptibility to nystatin, natamycin, and clotrimazole using a disk diffusion antifungal susceptibility testing method.[82] In should also be noted that the antifungal medications evaluated in these studies were not always consistent.[80–82]

Table 5
Antifungal susceptibility determinations for *Candida* spp isolated from horses with keratomycosis

	California (Reed et al,[80] 2013)	Florida (Brooks et al,[81] 1998)	Northeastern USA (Ledbetter et al,[82] 2007)
Caspofungin	0% (1)	NA	NA
Clotrimazole	NA	NA	88% (8)
Ketoconazole	NA	NA	100% (8)
Miconazole	NA	NA	38% (8)
Amphotericin	0% (1)	NA	86% (7)
Natamycin	NA	NA	100% (4)
Nystatin	NA	NA	100% (8)
Itraconazole	0% (1)	NA	83% (6)
Fluconazole	0% (1)	NA	50% (4)
Fluorocytosine	0% (1)	NA	57% (7)
Posaconazole	0% (1)	NA	NA
Voriconazole	0% (1)	NA	NA

Results are from 3 studies evaluating horses from California, Florida, and the northeastern United States. Results presented as percent susceptible (total number of isolates tested).
Data from Refs.[80–82]

An in vitro study evaluated minimum inhibitory concentrations and antifungal susceptibility patterns of 8 *Aspergillus* and 6 *Fusarium* isolates obtained from horses with keratomycosis in the midwestern and southern United States.[83] Broth dilution antifungal susceptibility testing was used. In that study, grouped fungi were significantly more susceptible to voriconazole than natamycin, itraconazole, fluconazole, and kerataconzole.[83] Miconazole susceptibility was similar to voriconazole for the grouped isolates. When evaluating *Aspergillus* isolates separately, they were most susceptible to voriconazole, miconazole, and intraconazole.[83] *Fusarium* isolates susceptibility was greatest to natamycin and voriconazole. Fluconazole displayed consistently poor activity against the fungi included in the study.[83]

A study using a broth dilution method evaluated minimal inhibitory concentrations and minimal fungicidal concentrations for 16 equine cornea fungal isolates from Texas.[84] Tested isolates included *Aspergillus*, *Fusarium*, *Mucor*, *Paecilomyces*, *Penicillium*, and *Rhizoctonia* spp. That study determined that the imidazoles (eg, miconazole, ketoconazole, clotrimazole, and econazole) consistently displayed the lowest mean inhibitory titers for the tested filamentous fungi.[84] The polyene antifungals tested, including natamycin and amphotericin, displayed more variable in vitro activity against the isolates. Flucytosine was relatively less active than the other evaluated antifungals, with the exception of the *Paecilomyces* isolates in which it had excellent in vitro efficacy.[84]

The in vitro fungistatic and fungicidal activities of silver sulfadiazine and natamycin were evaluated with broth macrodilution testing methods for 17 fungi isolated from horses with keratomycosis.[67] Evaluated fungal organisms included various species of *Aspergillus*, *Fusarium*, *Curvularia*, *Scopulariopsis*, *Penicillium*, and *Chrysosporium*. The fungi were isolated from horses residing in Alabama, Florida, Georgia, Indiana, and Missouri. For all 17 fungi grouped together, minimum inhibitory concentration distribution ranged from less than or equal to 1 to greater than 64 µg/mL for silver sulfadiazine and 256 to greater than 1000 µg/mL for natamycin.[67] Minimum fungicidal concentration ranged from less than or equal to 1 to greater than 64 µg/mL for silver sulfadiazine and 512 to greater than 1000 µg/mL for natamycin.[67] The study concluded that silver sulfadiazine was fungicidal against all isolates tested in vitro and natamycin was fungicidal against some of the tested fungi at the evaluated drug concentrations.

A small and relatively specific study evaluated 10 *Aspergillus* isolates from horse with keratomycosis in Pennsylvania using a broth microdilution method.[85] Based on the calculated minimum inhibitory concentrations, it was determined 100% of isolates were susceptible to itraconazole and voriconazole at 24 hours. At 48 hours, 80% of isolates were susceptible to itraconazole and 40% to voriconazole. Two (20%) of the isolates were susceptible to miconazole at 24 and 48 hours. None of the tested *Aspergillus* isolates were susceptible to natamycin (minimum inhibitory concentrations ranged from 4 to 32 µg/mL).

In vitro antifungal susceptibility testing was performed for 5 *Aspergillus fumigatus* and 7 *Eurotium amstelodami* isolates from the conjunctival flora of horses in Switzerland without ocular disease.[86] Both agar-based and broth dilution antifungal susceptibility testing were used. *Aspergillus fumigatus* isolates had the lowest minimal inhibitory concentrations to voriconazole. *Eurotium amstelodami* isolates had the lowest minimal inhibitory concentrations to voriconazole and itraconazole. High minimal inhibitory concentrations were consistently detected for fluconazole. Amphotericin and miconazole in vitro activity was highly variable for the tested fungi from the Swiss horses.

Thirty-five filamentous fungi isolated form the conjunctival microflora of horses without ocular disease in Wisconsin were evaluated for antifungal susceptibility patterns with a diffusion testing method.[87] The study reported culturing a wide-variety of fungal genera from the horses, but which fungi were actually tested in vitro for antifungal susceptibility was not provided. Natamycin had the highest in vitro efficacy against the grouped isolates with 97% determined to be susceptible.[87] Nystatin (74% of isolates susceptible), miconazole (69% of isolates susceptible), amphotericin (51% of isolates susceptible), and fluorocytosine (49% of isolates susceptible) had intermediate activity. It was noted in the study that *Aspergillus* and *Fusarium* isolates were 100% susceptible to miconazole. Susceptibility percentages were lowest for ketoconazole (31%) and griseofulvin (3%).[87]

Minimum inhibitory concentrations for miconazole, ketoconazole, itraconazole, and natamycin were determined for 11 filamentous fungal isolates obtained from horses with fungal keratitis in Alabama, Florida, and Georgia.[88] Evaluated fungi included *Aspergillus*, *Fusarium*, *Penicillium*, *Cladosporium*, and *Curvularia* isolates. Based on relative minimum inhibitory concentrations determined with a broth microdilution assay, it was reported that the order of susceptibility to the antifungal medications was, from greatest to least: *Penicillium*, *Curvularia*, *Cladosporium*, *Aspergillus*, and *Fusarium*.[88] When a novel third-generation chelating agent (8 mm disodium EDTA dehydrate and 20 mm 2-amino-2-hydroxymethyl-1, 3-propanediol) was combined with the antifungal drugs, the minimum inhibitory concentrations were decreased by 50% to 100%.[88]

ANTIFUNGAL ADMINISTRATION ROUTES, TECHNIQUES, AND DEVICES IN EQUINE KERATOMYCOSIS

Topical ophthalmic application of antifungal medications remains the primary route for treatment of horses with fungal keratitis. This method of therapy provides the most direct administration route to the tissue site of infection, is simple to perform in most horses, will frequently produce much higher tissue concentrations of antifungals than other therapeutic routes, and permits treatment with some antifungal medications that may otherwise not be possible (eg, due to systemic toxicity, poor gastrointestinal absorption, or prohibitive cost of systemic therapy). Antifungal drugs for topical ophthalmic administration may be formulated as solutions, suspensions, gels, and ointments. The decision to use a specific drug formulation is based on numerous factors, including availability, drug characteristics, the ocular lesion to be treated, desired administration frequency, client preference, and horse temperament.

Subpalpebral lavage systems are commonly used for horses with ocular mycotic infections.[89,90] These are specialized catheters that permit medication solution administration through the lumen of a long tube (the injection port is typically placed around the withers) that runs through the eyelid to a footplate in the superior or inferior conjunctival fornix. Subpalpebral lavage systems facilitate simple, safe, and efficient topical ophthalmic drug delivery while minimizing horse discomfort, handling, and stress. These systems are especially useful for horses that are difficult to treat (due to temperament or painful ocular conditions) and horses with fragile globes (eg, deep corneal ulcers) that may be damaged by excessive manipulation during attempted medication administration. Indwelling nasolacrimal catheters are also described for use in horses but are more difficult to place and can become dislodged by horse rubbing or sneezing.[91] Antifungal solutions commonly administered to horses through subpalpebral lavage systems include voriconazole, natamycin, and miconazole. The commercially available formulation of natamycin is a thick white suspension that may clog lavage systems if not correctly used and flushed.

Topical ophthalmic antifungal solutions can also be administered as continuous infusions using specifically designed pump systems.[92] Implantation of nonbiodegradable subconjunctival pumps in horses is described but not currently in routine use in equine ophthalmology.[93] Subpalpebral lavage-based pump systems, however, are commonly used in horses to provide continuous delivery of ophthalmic medications with minimal labor. Both battery-powered pumps and commercially available latex reservoirs may be attached to subpalpebral lavage systems to achieve this purpose.[92]

Care should be exercised when using unfamiliar ophthalmic medications through pump systems. For example, voriconazole 1% solution was demonstrated to be incompatible for use in constant-rate infusion pump systems.[94] In the evaluated pump system, the voriconazole remained sterile but precipitated crystallized drug blocked the lavage system tubing. Unfortunately, the effects of the prolonged retention times within infusion pumps and the associated tubing on medication sterility and stability have not been determined for most ophthalmic antifungals. This raises concerns about the use of these systems with newer antifungal medications when possible interactions are unknown. The uncertainty of this situation is similar to the practice of mixing ophthalmic medications for the treatment of horses with fungal keratitis. Anecdotally, many clinicians combine ophthalmic drugs for administration through constant-rate infusion pumps. Some medication combinations (eg, natamycin, tobramycin, cefazolin, and serum) have been studied and demonstrated to be effective in vitro; however, most medication combinations have unknown efficacy and stability when used in this manner.[95] Even the studied combination of natamycin, tobramycin, cefazolin, and serum was noted to rapidly settle out of suspension, which could adversely affect delivery by an infusion pump.[95]

Adjunctive therapy with an oral antifungal, in particular fluconazole (14.0 mg/kg oral loading dose given once, then 5.0 mg/kg every 24 hours), is frequently described in horses with keratomycosis.[96] Fluconazole has excellent bioavailability in horses after oral administration and is relatively cost-effective antifungal medication. Although safe and well-tolerated in most horses, this route of therapy is currently of unproven clinical benefit. Antifungal susceptibility studies suggest that resistance to fluconazole is common among equine corneal isolates. Fluconazole administration can also produce prolonged anesthetic recovery times when anesthesia is induced with ketamine and midazolam.[97] The prolongation of recovery from anesthesia is likely mediated through fluconazole's effects on the CYP3A4 enzyme that is responsible for the metabolism of many anesthetic drugs. This possible drug interaction should be considered in potential surgical candidates.

Oral itraconazole therapy is also possible in horses with fungal keratitis, but there is unpredictable and poor gastrointestinal absorption among some of the drug formulations available (particularly the capsules).[64] The low drug bioavailability requires high oral dosages to help achieve therapeutic concentrations, which is not always feasible in some horses due to cost and administration volume limitations. When itraconazole is used, the oral solution that is complexed with cyclodextrins to improve solubility is recommended (5.0 mg/kg orally every 24 hours) due to its superior absorption relative to other formulations.

A potential alternative systemic antifungal for use in horses with ocular mycotic infections is voriconazole (3.0–4.0 mg/kg orally every 24 hours). Voriconazole displays excellent tissue distribution characteristics and possess a broad spectrum of action against common mycotic pathogens of the equine cornea.[62,63] Although oral voriconazole therapy is a promising adjunctive therapy for keratomycosis, current drug prices render this approach impractical for most clinical situations.

In addition to topical and oral antifungal administration routes, subconjunctival and intracorneal injections are now being used more frequently in horses with mycotic infections. These represent newer administration routes that seem very promising as therapy for select cases not responding to more conventional therapies.

Subconjunctival injections of antifungal medications are described for horses with keratomycosis.[96,98] Depending on the drug formulation injected, this route of antifungal administration may provide extended durations of high therapeutic drug levels in the cornea, and potentially the anterior segment, with less frequent administration than standard topical therapy. High corneal drug concentrations are facilitated by slow and continuous drug leakage from the subconjunctival space back into the tears. In addition, the lipid layers of the bulbar conjunctiva are bypassed, which may increase penetration of water-soluble medications across the sclera and into the interior of the globe or the cornea. Hematogenous dissemination of the drug through conjunctival vessels may further serve to improve medication penetration after injection. Subconjunctival injections are generally considered as an adjunctive therapy to topical medications; however, they may be considered as the sole treatment in select cases were topical medications cannot be administered (eg, due to horse temperament or client limitations). The primary disadvantages of subconjunctival injections are local irritation, potential toxicity, inability to remove the injected drug once administered, and the potential difficulties encountered with performance of the injections in horses with fragile globes.

Subconjunctival injections are volume-limited and ophthalmic formulations of medications should not be used for injections. Injections must be given in the bulbar subconjunctival space and the superior conjunctiva is the preferred site in the horse because it is the most accessible and observable. A 25-gauge or 27-gauge needle attached to a 1.0 to 3.0 mL syringe is used for the injection. One specific subconjunctival injection protocol is described[99] as follows: sedate the horse and then perform auriculopalpebral and supraorbital nerve blocks. Apply 0.5 mL of the topical anesthetic (eg, 5% proparacaine) to the superior bulbar conjunctiva. Irrigate the conjunctival fornix and ocular surface with 1% povidone iodine in sterile water. Thoroughly flush the ocular surface with 3.0 to 6.0 mL of sterile eye wash. Reapply topical anesthetic and then apply 0.5 mL of 2.5% phenylephrine to the superior bulbar conjunctiva. Insert an eyelid retractor and stabilize the conjunctiva with Colibri forceps (if required). The needle is held bevel-up and inserted into the subconjunctival space. The medication is then slowly injected to create a fluid bleb (**Fig. 4**A).

The subconjunctival injection of amphotericin and voriconazole is described in detail for horses with keratomycosis.[96,98,99] Anecdotal descriptions of subconjunctival injection of miconazole in horses also exist (0.5–1.0 mL of the 10 mg/mL intravenous solution every 24 hours for up to 5 days). The reported dosage for amphotericin is 0.2 to 0.3 mL of the 5 mg/mL amphotericin intravenous solution administered every other day for a total of 3 doses.[96,99] In a recent report, adverse effects of this regimen were most commonly limited to local irritation at the injection site (ie, conjunctival hyperemia, chemosis, and hemorrhage) and mild-to-moderate ocular pain (manifested as blepharospasm and epiphora).[99] Because amphotericin may burn when injected, a reaction from the horse should be anticipated. It is recommended that conjunctival injection sites be rotated to reduce compounding the local irritation that may develop. Voriconazole can be administered as a single 0.4 to 0.5 mL dose of 1% voriconazole intravenous solution.[98] Immediate postinjection complications described include conjunctival hyperemia, chemosis, and mild conjunctival hemorrhage. There

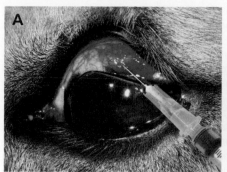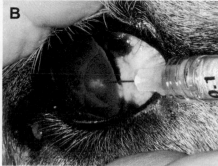

Fig. 4. Performance of subconjunctival (*A*) and intracorneal (*B*) voriconazole injections in a horse with a deep corneal stromal fungal abscess.

are no reports of multiple voriconazole injections being administered to an individual horse.

The newest method of delivering antifungal agents to horses with keratomycosis is by intrastromal corneal injection.[100] Intracorneal injections of both amphotericin and voriconazole are described in horses for the treatment of stromal abscesses.[98,100,101] Intrastromal injections are performed with the horse heavily sedated, or under general anesthesia, and with the aid of magnification such as a head loupe. Performance of these injection procedures requires advanced training because serious complications are possible, including corneal lamellar fracture, anterior stromal laceration, intracameral injection, intraocular contamination with microorganisms, and needle trauma to intraocular structures such as the uvea or lens.

The intracorneal injection of 100 to 150 μL of amphotericin solution was briefly reported in a horse but without a detailed description.[100] More detailed case descriptions are available for the use of intracorneal voriconazole injections in horses with deep stromal corneal abscesses.[98,101] The voriconazole injections were administered in the described horses after unsatisfactory response to more routine medical therapy and resulted in resolution of clinical ocular disease.

Both 1% and 5% voriconazole have been used in horses and are prepared by aseptically reconstituting injectable voriconazole lyophilized powder with sterile water.[98,101] Aliquots of approximately 0.1 to 0.2 mL voriconazole solution are prepared in advance in separate 1.0 to 3.0 mL Luer-lock syringes with 27-gauge or 30-gauge needles. The needles can be bent to a 30° to 45° angle near the hub, depending on the injection technique to be used.[101] If not under general anesthesia, horses are then sedated and auriculopalpebral and supraorbital nerve blocks performed. Retrobulbar blocks may also be used. The ocular surface is prepared routinely with dilute betadine solution and several rounds of topical anesthetic (eg, proparacaine or lidocaine) are applied. An eyelid speculum can be placed to increase exposure of the corneal surface.

Two different techniques are described for performance of the injections: linear injection or circumferential injection.[98,101] In the linear injection technique, prebent needles are used and inserted almost parallel to the corneal surface beginning at an anatomic point 2 to 3 mm abaxial to the near border of the lesion.[101] The needle travels horizontally along corneal stromal lamellar planes anterior to the corneal lesion and should stop just beyond the opposite border of the lesion. The voriconazole solution in then injected slowly as the needle is withdrawn. Additional injections are administered as needed to cover the bulk of the visible abscess. In

1 report, 3 injections of 5% voriconazole were used (dorsal, central, and ventral) per cornea and a total voriconazole dose of 22.5 mg was injected into each cornea.[101]

If performing the circumferential injection technique, straight needles are used and inserted into the cornea at an angle of 30° to 45°.[98] The tip of the needle is positioned adjacent to the border of the legion and the voriconazole solution slowly injected as the needle is withdrawn (see **Fig. 4**B). Four separate sites are injected around the abscess (3, 6, 9, and 12 o'clock positions) to create a drug deposit around the periphery of the corneal lesion. In 1 report, 4 injections were used per cornea and a total voriconazole dose of 150 to 400 µL of 1% voriconazole was injected into each cornea.[98]

Clinically successful intracorneal injections of both 1% and 5% voriconazole are described in horses.[98,100,101] In a recent study, the relative effects of 1% and 5% voriconazole were evaluated on clinically normal equine corneas and cultured equine keratocytes.[102] Injection of both 1% and 5% voriconazole produced similar structural alterations in the equine cornea (ie, stromal delamination). Higher aqueous humor concentrations of voriconazole were detected with injection of the 1% solution. Both 1% and 5% voriconazole exceeding the drug concentration demonstrated to be toxic to equine keratocytes in vitro after several hours of continuous exposure.[102]

FUTURE ANTIFUNGAL TREATMENT MODALITIES AND CONCLUSIONS

The continued development of more effective antifungal medications for use in equine ophthalmology is critical to achieving better outcomes for horses with mycotic infections. Research evaluating antifungal combinations and correlating ocular isolate antifungal susceptibly patterns and in vivo clinical outcome is also required to assist clinicians in making appropriate treatment choices. Additional administration routes and mechanisms are needed to facilitate the delivery of antifungal medications to horses, which can represent a major obstacle to adequate therapy in many cases. Biodegradable ocular implants, such as the scleral fluconazole implants designed for use in human patients, might provide an alternative method of treating horses.[103] Transcorneal and trans-scleral iontophoresis (the active noninvasive drug delivery method that transports charged and neutral drug particles across biological membranes) might also be adapted for the delivery of antifungal medications, or for riboflavin for corneal cross-linking therapy, in horses with keratomycosis or intraocular mycotic infection. Corneal cross-linking therapy is described in horses with keratomycosis and requires additional investigation and optimization.[104]

REFERENCES

1. Gaarder JE, Rebhun WC, Ball MA, et al. Clinical appearances, healing patterns, risk factors, and outcomes of horses with fungal keratitis: 53 cases (1978-1996). J Am Vet Med Assoc 1998;213(1):105–12.

2. Andrew SE, Brooks DE, Smith PJ, et al. Equine ulcerative keratomycosis: visual outcome and ocular survival in 39 cases (1987-1996). Equine Vet J 1998;30(2):109–16.

3. Grahn B, Wolfer J, Keller C, et al. Equine keratomycosis: clinical and laboratory findings in 23 cases. Prog Vet Comp Ophthalmol 1993;3:2–7.

4. Barton MH. Equine keratomycosis. Comp Cont Educ Pract 1992;14:936–44.

5. Galan A, Martin-Suarez EM, Gallardo JM, et al. Clinical findings and progression of 10 cases of equine ulcerative keratomycosis. Equine Vet Educ 2009;21:236–42.

6. Sansom J, Featherstone H, Barnett KC. Keratomycosis in six horses in the United Kingdom. Vet Rec 2005;156(1):13-7.

7. Bistner SI, Riis RC. Clinical aspects of mycotic keratitis in the horse. Cornell Vet 1979;69(4):364-74.

8. Hendrix DV, Brooks DE, Smith PJ, et al. Corneal stromal abscesses in the horse: a review of 24 cases. Equine Vet J 1995;27(6):440-7.

9. Brooks DE, Andrew SE, Denis H, et al. Rose bengal positive epithelial microerosions as a manifestation of equine keratomycosis. Vet Ophthalmol 2000;3(2-3): 83-6.

10. Brooks DE, Plummer CE, Mangan BG, et al. Equine subepithelial keratomycosis. Vet Ophthalmol 2013;16(2):93-6.

11. Galera PD, Brooks DE. Optimal management of equine keratomycosis. Vet Med Res Rep 2012;3:7-17.

12. Aho R, Tala M, Kivalo M. Mycotic keratitis in a horse caused by *Aspergillus fumigatus*. The first reported case in Finland. Acta Vet Scand 1991;32(3):373-6.

13. Beech J, Sweeney CR, Irby N. Keratomycosis in 11 horses. Equine Vet J 1983; 2(Supplement 2):39-44.

14. Hodgson DR, Jacobs KA. Two cases of *Fusarium* keratomycosis in the horse. Vet Rec 1982;110(22):520-2.

15. Richter M, Hauser B, Kaps S, et al. Keratitis due to *Histoplasma* spp. in a horse. Vet Ophthalmol 2003;6(2):99-103.

16. Friedman DS, Schoster JV, Pickett JP, et al. *Pseudallescheria boydii* keratomycosis in a horse. J Am Vet Med Assoc 1989;195(5):616-8.

17. Shadomy HJ, Dixon DM. A new Papulaspora species from the infected eye of a horse: Papulaspora equi sp. nov. Mycopathologia 1989;106(1):35-9.

18. Moore CP, Fales WH, Whittington P, et al. Bacterial and fungal isolates from equidae with ulcerative keratitis. J Am Vet Med Assoc 1983;182(6):600-3.

19. McLaughlin SA, Brightman AH, Helper LC, et al. Pathogenic bacteria and fungi associated with extraocular disease in the horse. J Am Vet Med Assoc 1983; 182(3):241-2.

20. Moore CP, Collins BK, Fales WH. Antibacterial susceptibility patterns for microbial isolates associated with infectious keratitis in horses: 63 cases (1986-1994). J Am Vet Med Assoc 1995;207(7):928-33.

21. Wada S, Hobo S, Ode H, et al. Equine keratomycosis in Japan. Vet Ophthalmol 2013;16(1):1-9.

22. Wada S, Ode H, Hobo S, et al. *Mortierella wolfii* keratomycosis in a horse. Vet Ophthalmol 2011;14(4):267-70.

23. Voelter-Ratson K, Pot SA, Florin M, et al. Equine keratomycosis in Switzerland: a retrospective evaluation of 35 horses (January 2000-August 2011). Equine Vet J 2013;45(5):608-12.

24. Andrew SE, Nguyen A, Jones GL, et al. Seasonal effects on the aerobic bacterial and fungal conjunctival flora of normal thoroughbred brood mares in Florida. Vet Ophthalmol 2003;6(1):45-50.

25. Samuelson DA, Andresen TL, Gwin RM. Conjunctival fungal flora in horses, cattle, dogs, and cats. J Am Vet Med Assoc 1984;184(10):1240-2.

26. Gemensky-Metzler AJ, Wilkie DA, Kowalski JJ, et al. Changes in bacterial and fungal ocular flora of clinically normal horses following experimental application of topical antimicrobial or antimicrobial-corticosteroid ophthalmic preparations. Am J Vet Res 2005;66(5):800-11.

27. Rosa M, Cardozo LM, da Silva Pereira J, et al. Fungal flora of normal eyes of healthy horses from the State of Rio de Janeiro, Brazil. Vet Ophthalmol 2003; 6(1):51–5.

28. Barsotti G, Sgorbini M, Nardoni S, et al. Occurrence of fungi from conjunctiva of healthy horses in Tuscany, Italy. Vet Res Commun 2006;30(8):903–6.

29. Johns IC, Baxter K, Booler H, et al. Conjunctival bacterial and fungal flora in healthy horses in the UK. Vet Ophthalmol 2011;14(3):195–9.

30. Khosravi AR, Nikaein D, Sharifzadeh A, et al. Ocular fungal flora from healthy horses in Iran. J Mycol Med 2014;24(1):29–33.

31. Thomas PA. Current perspectives on ophthalmic mycoses. Clin Microbiol Rev 2003;16(4):730–97.

32. Vemuganti GK, Garg P, Gopinathan U, et al. Evaluation of agent and host factors in progression of mycotic keratitis: a histologic and microbiologic study of 167 corneal buttons. Ophthalmology 2002;109(8):1538–46.

33. Lavach JD. Large animal ophthalmology. St Louis (MO): C.V. Mosby Company; 1990.

34. Figueredo LA, Cafarchia C, Otranto D. *Geotrichum candidum* as etiological agent of horse dermatomycosis. Vet Microbiol 2011;148(2–4):368–71.

35. Valentine BA, Taylor GH, Stone JK, et al. Equine cutaneous fungal granuloma: a study of 44 lesions from 34 horses. Vet Dermatol 2006;17(4):266–72.

36. Etana D. Isolates of fungi from symptomatic carthorses in Awassa, Ethiopia. Zentralbl Veterinarmed B 1999;46(7):443–51.

37. Connole MD. Equine phycomycosis. Aust Vet J 1973;49(4):214–5.

38. Blackford J. Superficial and deep mycoses in horses. Vet Clin North Am Large Anim Pract 1984;6(1):47–58.

39. al-Ani FK. Epizootic lymphangitis in horses: a review of the literature. Rev Sci Tech 1999;18(3):691–9.

40. Soliman R, Ebeid M, Essa M, et al. Ocular histoplasmosis due to *Histoplasma farciminosum* in Egyptian donkeys. Mycoses 1991;34(5–6):261–6.

41. Fouad K, Saleh MS, Sokkar S, et al. Studies on lachrymal histoplasmosis in donkeys in Egypt. Zentralbl Veterinarmed B 1973;20(8):584–93.

42. Berzina I, Trumble NS, Novicki T, et al. Subconjunctival mycetoma caused by *Scedosporium apiospermum* infection in a horse. Vet Clin Pathol 2011;40(1): 84–8.

43. Cortez KJ, Roilides E, Quiroz-Telles F, et al. Infections caused by *Scedosporium* spp. Clin Microbiol Rev 2008;21(1):157–97.

44. Brooks DE, Taylor DP, Plummer CE, et al. Iris abscesses with and without intralenticular fungal invasion in the horse. Vet Ophthalmol 2009;12(5):306–12.

45. Hart KA, Flaminio MJ, LeRoy BE, et al. Successful resolution of cryptococcal meningitis and optic neuritis in an adult horse with oral fluconazole. J Vet Intern Med 2008;22(6):1436–40.

46. Hatziolos BC, Sass B, Albert TF, et al. Ocular changes in a horse with gutturomycosis. J Am Vet Med Assoc 1975;167(1):51–4.

47. Welsh RD, Stair EL. Cryptococcal meningitis in a horse. J Equine Vet Sci 1995; 15:80–2.

48. Riley CB, Bolton JR, Mills JN, et al. Cryptococcosis in seven horses. Aust Vet J 1992;69(6):135–9.

49. Johnson GR, Schiefer B, Pantekoek JF. Maduromycosis in a horse in western Canada. Can Vet J 1975;16(11):341–4.

50. Scott EA, Duncan JR, McCormack JE. Cryptococcosis involving the postorbital area and frontal sinus in a horse. J Am Vet Med Assoc 1974;165(7):626–7.

51. Roberts MC, Sutton RH, Lovell DK. A protracted case of cryptococcal nasal granuloma in a stallion. Aust Vet J 1981;57(6):287–91.
52. Bradford KA, Allison RW, Love BC. What is your diagnosis? Corneal scraping from an ulcerative lesion in a Quarter horse. Vet Clin Pathol 2012;41(4):601–2.
53. Massa KL, Murphy CJ, Hartmann FA, et al. Usefulness of aerobic microbial culture and cytologic evaluation of corneal specimens in the diagnosis of infectious ulcerative keratitis in animals. J Am Vet Med Assoc 1999;215(11):1671–4.
54. Hamilton Hl, McLaughlin SA, Whitley EM, et al. Histological findings in corneal stromal abscesses of 11 horses: correlation with cultures and cytology. Equine Vet J 1994;26(6):448–53.
55. Zeiss C, Neaderland M, Yang FC, et al. Fungal polymerase chain reaction testing in equine ulcerative keratitis. Vet Ophthalmol 2013;16(5):341–51.
56. Ledbetter EC, Irby NL, Kim SG. In vivo confocal microscopy of equine fungal keratitis. Vet Ophthalmol 2011;14(1):1–9.
57. Ledbetter EC, Irby NL, Schaefer DM. In vivo confocal microscopy of corneal microscopic foreign bodies in horses. Vet Ophthalmol 2014;17(Suppl 1):69–75.
58. Peyton LR, Gallagher S, Hashemzadeh M. Triazole antifungals: a review. Drugs Today (Barc) 2015;51(12):705–18.
59. Ball MA, Rebhun WC, Gaarder JE, et al. Evaluation of itraconazole-dimethyl sulfoxide ointment for treatment of keratomycosis in nine horses. J Am Vet Med Assoc 1997;211(2):199–203.
60. Clode AB, Davis JL, Salmon J, et al. Evaluation of concentration of voriconazole in aqueous humor after topical and oral administration in horses. Am J Vet Res 2006;67(2):296–301.
61. Latimer FG, Colitz CM, Campbell NB, et al. Pharmacokinetics of fluconazole following intravenous and oral administration and body fluid concentrations of fluconazole following repeated oral dosing in horses. Am J Vet Res 2001; 62(10):1606–11.
62. Colitz CM, Latimer FG, Cheng H, et al. Pharmacokinetics of voriconazole following intravenous and oral administration and body fluid concentrations of voriconazole following repeated oral administration in horses. Am J Vet Res 2007;68(10):1115–21.
63. Passler NH, Chan HM, Stewart AJ, et al. Distribution of voriconazole in seven body fluids of adult horses after repeated oral dosing. J Vet Pharmacol Ther 2010;33(1):35–41.
64. Davis JL, Salmon JH, Papich MG. Pharmacokinetics and tissue distribution of itraconazole after oral and intravenous administration to horses. Am J Vet Res 2005;66(10):1694–701.
65. Prades M, Brown MP, Gronwall R, et al. Body fluid and endometrial concentrations of ketoconazole in mares after intravenous injection or repeated gavage. Equine Vet J 1989;21(3):211–4.
66. Prasad R, Shah AH, Rawal MK. Antifungals: mechanism of action and drug resistance. Adv Exp Med Biol 2016;892:327–49.
67. Betbeze CM, Wu CC, Krohne SG, et al. In vitro fungistatic and fungicidal activities of silver sulfadiazine and natamycin on pathogenic fungi isolated from horses with keratomycosis. Am J Vet Res 2006;67(10):1788–93.
68. Begg LM, Hughes KJ, Kessell A, et al. Successful treatment of cryptococcal pneumonia in a pony mare. Aust Vet J 2004;82(11):686–92.
69. Ben-Shlomo G. The use of 0.5% caspofungin, a member of a new class of antifungals, against aggressive ulcerative keratomycosis, refractory to

conventional therapy. Proceedings of the International Equine Ophthalmology Consortium Symposium. Stresa (Italy). June 5–7, 2014.

70. Clode A, Davis J, Davidson G, et al. Aqueous humor and plasma concentrations of a compounded 0.2% solution of terbinafine following topical ocular administration to normal equine eyes. Vet Ophthalmol 2011;14(1):41–7.

71. Williams MM, Davis EG, KuKanich B. Pharmacokinetics of oral terbinafine in horses and Greyhound dogs. J Vet Pharmacol Ther 2011;34(3):232–7.

72. Younkin TJ, Davis EG, Kukanich B. Pharmacokinetics of oral terbinafine in adult horses. J Vet Pharmacol Ther 2017;40(4):342–7.

73. Ford MM. Antifungals and their use in veterinary ophthalmology. Vet Clin North Am Small Anim Pract 2004;34(3):669–91.

74. Scotty NC, Evans TJ, Giuliano E, et al. In vitro efficacy of lufenuron against filamentous fungi and blood concentrations after PO administration in horses. J Vet Intern Med 2005;19(6):878–82.

75. Moore CP, Collins BK, Fales WH, et al. Antimicrobial agents for treatment of infectious keratitis in horses. J Am Vet Med Assoc 1995;207(7):855–62.

76. Eschenauer GA, Carver PL. The evolving role of antifungal susceptibility testing. Pharmacotherapy 2013;33(5):465–75.

77. Odds FC. Should resistance to azole antifungals in vitro be interpreted as predicting clinical non-response? Drug Resist Updat 1998;1(1):11–5.

78. Kuper KM, Coyle EA, Wanger A. Antifungal susceptibility testing: a primer for clinicians. Pharmacotherapy 2012;32(12):1112–22.

79. Alastruey-Izquierdo A, Melhem MS, Bonfietti LX, et al. Susceptibility test for fungi: clinical and laboratorial correlations in medical mycology. Rev Inst Med Trop Sao Paulo 2015;57(Suppl 19):57–64.

80. Reed Z, Thomasy SM, Good KL, et al. Equine keratomycoses in California from 1987 to 2010 (47 cases). Equine Vet J 2013;45(3):361–6.

81. Brooks DE, Andrew SE, Dillavou CL, et al. Antimicrobial susceptibility patterns of fungi isolated from horses with ulcerative keratomycosis. Am J Vet Res 1998; 59(2):138–42.

82. Ledbetter EC, Patten VH, Scarlett JM, et al. In vitro susceptibility patterns of fungi associated with keratomycosis in horses of the northeastern United States: 68 cases (1987-2006). J Am Vet Med Assoc 2007;231(7):1086–91.

83. Pearce JW, Giuliano EA, Moore CP. In vitro susceptibility patterns of *Aspergillus* and *Fusarium* species isolated from equine ulcerative keratomycosis cases in the midwestern and southern United States with inclusion of the new antifungal agent voriconazole. Vet Ophthalmol 2009;12(5):318–24.

84. Coad CT, Robinson NM, Wilhelmus KR. Antifungal sensitivity testing for equine keratomycosis. Am J Vet Res 1985;46(3):676–8.

85. Wotman KL, Utter ME, Rankin SC. Antifungal susceptibility testing of *Aspergillus* species isolates from horses with keratomycosis in Southeast Pennsylvania: 10 cases (2006 – 2007). Vet Ophthalmol 2008;11:413–29 [abstract: 56].

86. Voelter-Ratson K, Monod M, Unger L, et al. Evaluation of the conjunctival fungal flora and its susceptibility to antifungal agents in healthy horses in Switzerland. Vet Ophthalmol 2014;17(Suppl 1):31–6.

87. Moore CP, Heller N, Majors LJ, et al. Prevalence of ocular microorganisms in hospitalized and stabled horses. Am J Vet Res 1988;49(6):773–7.

88. Weinstein WL, Moore PA, Sanchez S, et al. In vitro efficacy of a buffered chelating solution as an antimicrobial potentiator for antifungal drugs against fungal pathogens obtained from horses with mycotic keratitis. Am J Vet Res 2006;67(4):562–8.

89. Sweeney CR, Russell GE. Complications associated with use of a one-hole sub-palpebral lavage system in horses: 150 cases (1977-1996). J Am Vet Med Assoc 1997;211(10):1271–4.

90. Giuliano EA, Maggs DJ, Moore CP, et al. Inferomedial placement of a single-entry subpalpebral lavage tube for treatment of equine eye disease. Vet Ophthalmol 2000;3(2–3):153–6.

91. Brooks D. Use of an indwelling nasal lacrimal cannula for the administration of medication to the eye. Equine Vet J Suppl 1983;11:135–7.

92. Myrna KE, Herring IP. Constant rate infusion for topical ocular delivery in horses: a pilot study. Vet Ophthalmol 2006;9(1):1–5.

93. Blair MJ, Gionfriddo JR, Polazzi LM, et al. Subconjunctivally implanted micro-osmotic pumps for continuous ocular treatment in horses. Am J Vet Res 1999; 60(9):1102–5.

94. Smith KM, Maxwell L, Gull T, et al. Stability of 1% voriconazole solution in a constant-rate infusion pump for topical ocular delivery to horses. Vet Ophthalmol 2014;17(Suppl 1):82–9.

95. Scotty NC, Brooks DE, Schuman Rose CD. In vitro efficacy of an ophthalmic drug combination against corneal pathogens of horses. Am J Vet Res 2008; 69(1):101–7.

96. Sherman AB, Clode AB, Gilger BC. Impact of fungal species cultured on outcome in horses with fungal keratitis. Vet Ophthalmol 2017;20(2):140–6.

97. Krein SR, Lindsey JC, Blaze CA, et al. Evaluation of risk factors, including fluconazole administration, for prolonged anesthetic recovery times in horses undergoing general anesthesia for ocular surgery: 81 cases (2006-2013). J Am Vet Med Assoc 2014;244(5):577–81.

98. Tsujita H, Plummer CE. Corneal stromal abscessation in two horses treated with intracorneal and subconjunctival injection of 1% voriconazole solution. Vet Ophthalmol 2013;16(6):451–8.

99. Telford CR, Gilger BC. Subconjunctival amphotericin B injection adjunctive therapy for refractory equine keratomycosis. Vet Ophthalmol 2016;19:E21–43 [abstract: 022].

100. Cutler TJ. Intracorneal administration of antifungal drugs in 4 horses. Vet Ophthalmol 2010;13:407–23 [abstract: 072].

101. Smith KM, Pucket JD, Gilmour MA. Treatment of six cases of equine corneal stromal abscessation with intracorneal injection of 5% voriconazole solution. Vet Ophthalmol 2014;17(Suppl 1):179–85.

102. Smith KM, Breshears MA, Maxwell LK, et al. In vitro and in vivo effect of voriconazole exposure on the equine cornea: a pilot study. Vet Ophthalmol 2015;18: E17–24 [abstract: 093].

103. Miyamoto H, Ogura Y, Hashizoe M, et al. Biodegradable scleral implant for intra-vitreal controlled release of fluconazole. Curr Eye Res 1997;16(9):930–5.

104. Hellander-Edman A, Makdoumi K, Mortensen J, et al. Corneal cross-linking in 9 horses with ulcerative keratitis. BMC Vet Res 2013;9:128.

Advanced Imaging of the Equine Eye

Brian C. Gilger, DVM, MS

KEYWORDS

- Equine • Eye • Imaging • Ultrasound • Computed tomography • MRI
- Optical coherence tomography • Confocal microscopy

KEY POINTS

- Advanced imaging is becoming more important and feasible for use in the diagnosis of equine ocular disease.
- Ultrasound imaging of the eye and periocular structures is the most common modality used and is indicated whenever there are cloudy ocular structures preventing direct examination of ocular structures.
- Optical coherence tomography and in vivo confocal microscopy are very promising techniques, especially for detailed examination of the cornea.
- Computed tomography with or without use of MRI are the most useful imaging modalities to thoroughly evaluate the equine orbit and periorbital structures.

INTRODUCTION

Advanced ocular imaging has revolutionized human ophthalmology with new technologies such as optical coherence tomography (OCT), which has developed into the primary method for the diagnosis of retinal diseases such as macular degeneration in humans.[1,2] Although there is a considerable need for better imaging techniques beyond ophthalmoscopy in equine ophthalmology, the routine use of advanced imaging has been relatively slow in acceptance. This is most likely due to several factors, including the high cost and lack of portability of the instruments and the inability to image the equine eye using human-designed equipment given the differences in anatomy and ocular size of the horse eye compared with the human eye. Furthermore, the need for general anesthesia to conduct many imaging techniques, such as computed tomography (CT) or MRI, limit their routine use in equine practice. However, improved instruments and advanced techniques such as the standing CT scanner have made these technologies more readily available, more feasible, and in some cases, such as ultrasound, quite practical to image the equine eye.

Disclosure Statement: The author has nothing to disclose.
Department of Clinical Sciences, NC State University College of Veterinary Medicine, 1060 William Moore Drive, Raleigh, NC 27607, USA
E-mail address: bgilger@ncsu.edu

Vet Clin Equine 33 (2017) 607–626
http://dx.doi.org/10.1016/j.cveq.2017.07.006
0749-0739/17/© 2017 Elsevier Inc. All rights reserved.

This article is organized by anatomic structure of the eye and diseases associated with each structure. Indications for imaging, suitable modalities, techniques, and interpretation of images of specific areas of the eye, such as the adnexa, cornea, anterior chamber, lens, vitreous, retina, and orbit, are reviewed. With this organization, the reader will be able to easily identify ways to image a specific disease entity or anatomic location, making this article a valuable reference source. Furthermore, although there are many advanced imaging modalities described for the eye in the human and research literature, this article concentrates on those techniques that have been reported in normal or diseased equine eyes. At first mention of the imaging modality, a brief description of the procedural steps for the modality is included in an adjacent text box. This article does not describe routine clinical imaging and examination techniques of the equine eye, such as slit lamp biomicroscopy, tonometry, color surface and retinal photography, and electroretinography, which have been described well recently.[3]

This article reviews the literature for studies describing advanced imaging of the equine eye to serve as a reference for practitioners to assist in choosing image modalities, be a reference for the procedural technique, and to help with interpretation of the image results. For the ocular adnexa (eyelids), we review studies describing the use of ultrasound imaging. For corneal imaging, we will review ultrasound imaging, high-frequency ultrasound imaging (ultrasound biomicroscopy [UBM]), OCT, and in vivo confocal microscopy. For nasolacrimal duct (NLD) assessment, we review studies using CT and endoscopy. For the anterior segment and lens, we review ultrasound imaging, infrared (IR) photography, and anterior segment angiography. For the vitreous, retina, and optic nerve, we review ultrasound imaging, posterior segment angiography, and OCT. For the orbit, periocular structures, and to assess blindness, we review studies using CT and MRI. Finally, we describe several other diagnostic methods using advanced imaging, such as ultrasound-guided aspirations and injections.

IMAGING OF THE OCULAR ADNEXA
Indications for Imaging

The most common reason that imaging, other than routine ocular examination, is needed for eyelids or periocular tissue is when trauma has occurred and the eyelids are very swollen or when there is a suspected abscess or foreign body in the eyelid (ie, draining tract).

Advanced Imaging Modalities Described

In nearly all cases, ultrasound is used to image the eyelid or anterior orbit. Ultrasonography is a safe and painless method to examine intraocular and retrobulbar structures in awake animals (**Box 1**). Depth of sound beam penetration is proportional to wave length of the ultrasound probe. A low-frequency transducer (5 MHz) gives greater tissue penetration but poor near-field axial resolution and a high-frequency transducer (10 MHz) gives lower tissue penetration, but high near-field axial resolution. Therefore, for the eye, the higher frequency transducer gives better resolution and is preferred. Ideally, a 10- to 20-MHz frequency transducer is used for ocular ultrasound. See this recent publication for more information on ultrasound imaging of the equine eye.[3]

Ultrasonic imaging of the lacrimal gland (either abscess or adenitis) was described in horses presenting with acute onset severe upper eyelid swellings.[4,5] On ultrasound imaging, approximately one-half of the eyelids with acute swelling had an enlarged lacrimal

---

Box 1
Technique for performing an ocular ultrasound examination

To perform a complete ultrasound examination of the globe and orbit, topical anesthesia of the cornea (proparacaine 0.5%) is always applied. Ultrasound coupling gel can be irritating to the cornea; therefore, a sterile methocellulose gel is placed on the transducer tip, eyelid, or corneal surface. The transducer is then placed directly on the cornea, upper eyelid, or area of swelling. If there is a corneal ulcer or perforation, then the scan must be performed through closed eyelids. The globe is imaged in both the horizontal and vertical planes through the visual axis. At the completion of the examination, the coupling gel should be irrigated from the eye and conjunctiva using sterile eyewash.

---

gland that seemed to be slightly heterogeneous in appearance with an extension of the gland from beneath the superior orbital rim (**Fig. 1**).[5] Therefore, the sonographic appearance of a painful and swollen eyelid of a horse can help to differentiate between an eyelid abscess, lacrimal gland dacryoadenitis, and the presence of foreign body (**Fig. 2**). This valuable information can help to determine therapeutic next steps, such as draining of an abscess, removal of a foreign body, or medical therapy for lacrimal gland adenitis.[4,5]

IMAGING OF THE NASOLACRIMAL DUCT
Indications for Imaging

The NLD is imaged when it is obstructed, which results in chronic epiphora and ocular discharge. Imaging of the NLD is done to determine the cause and location of the obstruction and to determine if the NLD obstruction can be repaired.

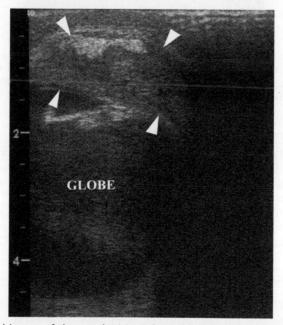

Fig. 1. Ultrasound image of dacryoadenitis. Enlarged lacrimal gland (*arrowheads*) appear slightly heterogeneous in appearance and extend beneath the superior orbital rim. (*Modified from* Reimer JM, Latimer CS. Ultrasound findings in horses with severe eyelid swelling, and recognition of acute dacryoadenitis: 10 cases (2004-2010). Vet Ophthalmol 2011;14:86–92; with permission.)

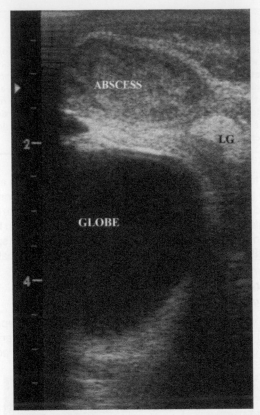

Fig. 2. Ultrasound image of an abscess of the upper eyelid. A well-circumscribed lesion (abscess) superior to the globe is visualized. LG, lacrimal gland. (*Modified from* Reimer JM, Latimer CS. Ultrasound findings in horses with severe eyelid swelling, and recognition of acute dacryoadenitis: 10 cases (2004-2010). Vet Ophthalmol 2011;14:86–92; with permission.)

Advanced Imaging Modalities Described

Although several methods have been described to image the NLD, including endoscopy, radiology, CT, and MRI, the most effective imaging modalities are those that also image the periocular sinuses and other structures of the head, with and without contrast injection of the NLD (ie, dacryocystorhinography; **Box 2**).[6–10] This imaging is important to evaluate the tissues surrounding the NLD that, when diseased, commonly impinge on the NLD causing obstruction. By injecting radiopaque dye, such as radiopaque iodine (Iohexol, Omnipaque, GE Healthcare, Chicago, IL), the

---

Box 2
Technique for performing dacryocystorhinography

Dacryocystorhinography has been described using both conventional radiography and computed tomography (CT). After imaging without injection of contrast (survey images), the nasal puncta is catheterized with an open-ended tomcat catheter and 5 mL of iodinated contrast medium is injected into one or both puncta. Immediately after injection, lateral and dorsoventral skull radiographs or CT scans are performed.

entire course of the NLD can be imaged. The location of narrowing or site of obstruction can, in most cases, be easily determined.

Dacryocystorhinography has been described using both conventional radiography and CT.[6,8–11] After imaging without injection of contrast (survey images), the nasal puncta is catheterized and 5 mL of iodinated contrast medium is injected into one or both NLD through the proximal or distal puncta, to compare diseased and normal NLDs, if available. Lateral and dorsoventral skull radiographs or CT scans are performed as soon as practical after the injection of the contrast medium.[9] Depending on available instruments, imaging can be performed either standing or under anesthesia; however, general anesthesia is generally preferred to provide excellent, high-contrast images. Advantages of CT scan dacryocystorhinography over conventional radiology include that CT provides superior resolution of the nasolacrimal apparatus and the ability to reconstruct in 3 dimensions for better visualization of the lesions **(Fig. 3)**.[6,9]

IMAGING OF THE CORNEA
Indications for Imaging

Imaging of the cornea is most commonly used to determine the cause and depth (extent) of an injury (eg, laceration), defect (eg, descemetocele), and/or infiltrate (cellular, infectious, or neoplastic). When the cornea is opaque, ocular ultrasound imaging, especially high-frequency ultrasound imaging, can be used to locate lesions and determine their depth. Despite the usefulness of this imaging modality, it has not been extensively described in the horse, only small animals. Other advanced imaging techniques include OCT **(Box 3)** and in vivo confocal microscopy.

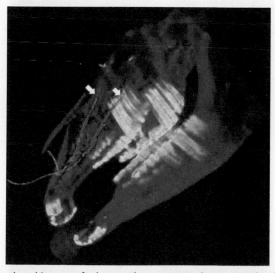

Fig. 3. Three-dimensional image of a horse after computed tomography dacryocystorhinography. The postprocessed image was constructed from sagittal and dorsal plane computed tomography sequences. The nasolacrimal contrast is colored red in this image. Other than proximal nasolacrimal fistulas (*arrows*), no additional nasolacrimal abnormalities were observed. (*Data from* Gilger BC, Histed J, Pate DO, et al. Anomalous nasolacrimal openings in a 2-year-old Morgan filly. Vet Ophthalmol 2010;13:339–42; with permission.)

> **Box 3**
> **Technique for performing ocular optical coherence tomography**
>
> The handheld probe of the optical coherence tomography (OCT) device is fitted with a 12-mm telecentric lens and regions of the cornea are scanned at with parameters such as 1000 A-scans per B-scan, and 100 B-scans in total, to generate a radial volume of 8 mm in diameter. Proper positioning of the handheld probe is confirmed using the horizontal and vertical B-scan aiming images on the OCT unit per manufacturer instructions. At the time of imaging, the upper eyelid is held manually against the upper bony orbit, avoiding pressure against the globe.

Advanced Imaging Modalities Described

Despite the availability of UBM for several years, it has only been described in a horse with an opaque corneal mass.[12] UBM revealed a hyperechoic mass that involved approximately one-third of the corneal depth and ultimately was determined to be a hemangioma (**Fig. 4**).[12] It would be particularly interesting to evaluate equine corneal stromal abscesses and other common equine corneal disease with UBM, but to date this has not been reported.

OCT obtains high-resolution cross-sectional images using interferometry, which correlates the light backscattered from tissue and light that has traveled a known distance to measure the magnitude and echo time delay of backscattered light.[13] Use of this noncontact, handheld device has been described for evaluating the normal horse cornea, providing excellent anatomic images (**Fig. 5**)[13] and corneal thickness

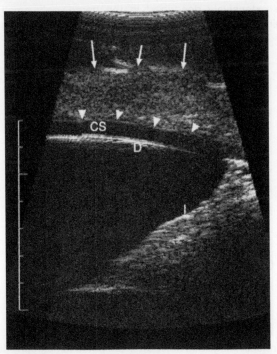

Fig. 4. High-resolution ultrasound image of a corneal mass in a horse. This hyperechoic mass (*arrows*), a hemangioma, involved approximately one-third of the corneal depth with normal cornea beneath the mass (*arrowheads*). CS, corneal stroma; D, Descemet's membrane; I, Iris. (*Modified from* Bentley E, Miller PE, Diehl KA. Diagnostic tool in veterinary ophthalmology. J Am Vet Med Assoc 2003;223:1617–22; with permission.)

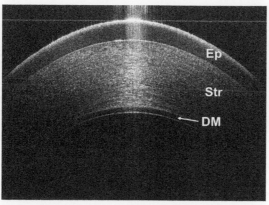

Fig. 5. Optical coherence tomography of a normal corneal of the horse. The corneal epithelium (Ep), stroma (Str), and Descemet's membrane (DM) are visualized.

measurements.[14] The advantage of OCT imaging is that it provides high resolution and magnification of ocular tissues that approaches the histopathologic level; however, OCT is limited by the need for clear media for penetration of light and limited patient and operator movement to minimize motion artifact. To date, few evaluations of equine corneal lesions with OCT have been reported. Although imaging of opaque structures may limit its use, it is possible with OCT to evaluate the depth of lesions and, in some cases, the extent of stromal fibrosis and infiltrate (**Fig. 6**). OCT evaluation of the cornea of horses with heterochromic iridocyclitis demonstrated areas of increases in light reflectivity associated with the characteristic pigmented keratic precipitates, with some aggregates projecting to the anterior chamber and other areas of thickened and detached Descemet's membrane and retrocorneal membrane (**Fig. 7**).[15]

In vivo confocal microscopy has been used to evaluate the normal equine corneal and limbal anatomy,[16] and for evaluation of a corneal foreign body[17] and fungal keratitis.[18] In normal horses, in vivo confocal microscopy, which required contact of the device with the cornea, was able to provide high-resolution and magnified imaging of the corneal epithelial layers, corneal innervation, endothelial

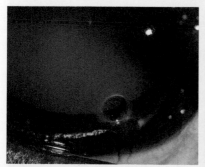
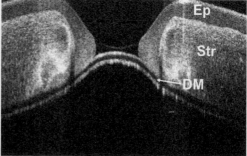

Fig. 6. Optical coherence tomography (OCT) image of a horse with a chronic Decemetocele. On the left is the clinical photograph and on the right is the OCT image. The epithelium (Ep) has grown down to cover the stroma (Str) and is in contact with the Descemet's membrane (DM). The tear film is seen as an arc above the DM.

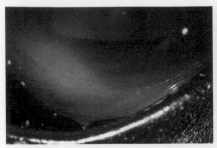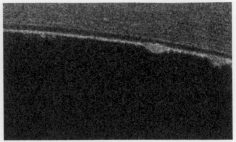

Fig. 7. Optical coherence tomography (OCT) image with heterochromic iridocyclitis (HIK). Horse diagnosed with HIK with characteristic clinical signs of corneal edema and pigmented keratitic precipitate (*left*) and endothelial deposits or keratitic precipitates visualized on OCT imaging (*right*).

cells and concentration, and corneal thickness measurements in normal horses (**Fig. 8**).[16] In another study, in vivo confocal microscopy was able to identify corneal foreign bodies, such as burdock bristles and other plant material, which appeared as hyperreflective linear, circular, or oval structures within the corneal tissue.[17] The diagnostic procedure was particularly helpful for surgical planning to determine the etiology of clinically idiopathic keratitis or to localize and identify corneal opacities.[17] Confocal microscopy was also demonstrated to be useful for identifying fungus, which appears as 200- to 400-μm long, linear, branching hyperreflective structures in ulcerative or nonulcerative keratitis, particularly in deep corneal stromal lesions.[18]

IMAGING OF THE ANTERIOR UVEA AND LENS
Indications for Imaging

The anterior uvea is most commonly imaged to evaluate anterior uveal masses (ie, differentiate between neoplastic and cystic structures), evaluate the state of the anterior chamber (eg, shallow or deep; clear or filled with hypopyon/fibrin), evaluate

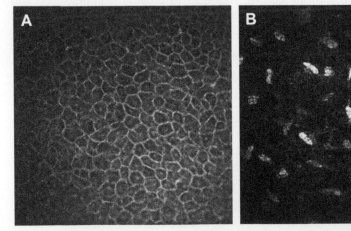

Fig. 8. In vivo confocal microscopy of the equine cornea. This imaging technique provides high resolution and magnified imaging of the cornea. (*A*) Superficial cornea and epithelium. (*B*) Corneal stroma. (*Courtesy of* Dr Eric Ledbetter, Ithaca, New York.)

for synechia, and to evaluate for lens abnormalities (luxation, rupture, cataract formation).

Advanced Imaging Modalities Described

The most common imaging modality for assessment of the anterior chamber, anterior uvea, and lens is b-mode ultrasound, although other modalities, such as OCT, anterior segment angiography, and IR photography may be helpful for the evaluation of disease when the cornea is not opaque, but has not yet reported in the horse.[19–22] Ultrasound imaging has the particular advantage to image through opaque cornea and anterior chambers (or miotic pupils), which may obstruct the view when using OCT and possibly angiography.

B-mode ultrasound imaging using probes of 10 to 35 mHz is a noninvasive diagnostic procedure that routinely can be performed in awake horses, even those with ocular pain.[23] Ocular ultrasound to image the anterior segment of the eye is typically performed with the ultrasound probe placed on the cornea (if the cornea is not ruptured or compromised [ulcerated]) or, alternatively, through the eyelids. In both approaches—transcorneal and transpalpebral—a sterile, water-soluble coupling gel such as methylcellulose gel should be used on the probe. After application of topical anesthetic, such as proparacaine, the probe is placed directly on the cornea with or without the use of a standoff pad. Without a standoff pad, depending on the type and megahertz of the probe, near field artifact may limit the image of the cornea. A standoff pad, such as a saline-filled latex glove finger or gel device will allow imaging of the cornea without artifact. Cross-sectional imaging of the globe should be performed in both the horizontal and vertical meridians. The iris and ciliary body appear as echogenic linear structures that extend from the periphery of the globe toward the lens with irregular echogenic structures at the end of the iris (ie, corpora nigra). Only the anterior and posterior lens capsules can be imaged in the normal lens, with the posterior lens capsule being a dense crescent-shaped hyperechoic structure (**Fig. 9**).[23,24] Loss of structural integrity of the corneal or sclera, lens luxation, solid or cystic masses, synechia, cellular infiltrate into the anterior chamber, lens rupture, and cataract can all be imaged with ultrasound (**Fig. 10**).[23–25] Identification of cataracts and posterior synechia are the most common anterior segment ocular abnormalities identified on equine ultrasound imaging.[26,27]

IR photography allows imaging of the anterior uveal tract in high resolution even if there is corneal opacity (**Fig. 11**). Because of IRs longer wavelengths, IR radiation is able to penetrate an opaque cornea, allowing better visualization of the anterior segment of the eye and cellular infiltrate in the cornea.[22] Standard cameras can be converted to IR or dedicated IR cameras can be purchased.

IMAGING OF THE OCULAR POSTERIOR SEGMENT
Indications for Imaging

The posterior segment is usually imaged to evaluate the integrity of the retina and optic nerve, especially when the ocular media in front of the retina is opaque (ie, with corneal disease, cataract, or vitreous opacity). Imaging can also be done to evaluate the state of the vitreous in posterior uveitis, for example, and for high detail retinal evaluation and to measure thickness of the retinal layers using modalities such as OCT. Finally, after anterior segment trauma, such as corneal perforations and lacerations, posterior segment imaging, primarily ultrasonography, is useful for

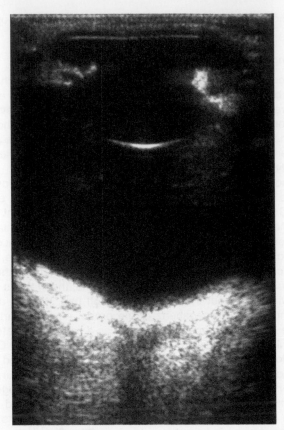

Fig. 9. B-mode ultrasound image of a normal equine eye. The anterior chamber, iris (with corpora nigra), posterior lens capsule crescent, hypoechoic vitreous, and posterior eye are all well-visualized in this image.

assessment of the extent of disease in the posterior segment to prognosis for return of vision.

Advanced Imaging Modalities Described

B-mode ultrasonography has been the most commonly described imaging modality to examine the equine ocular fundus, especially when there is opaque ocular media or changes in the anterior segment that block the direct imaging of the ocular fundus. The technique to image the ocular posterior segment by b-mode ultrasound imaging is the same as described previously in this article; however, a lower probe megahertz of 7.5 to 12 MHz may be needed to get adequate image of the deeper ocular structures. Common abnormalities that are seen include vitreal inflammation in posterior uveitis, vitreal degeneration, and retinal detachment (**Fig. 12**).[23,28] Additional findings may include endophthalmitis, axial length abnormalities (microphthalmos or buphthalmos [hydrophthalmos]), choroiditis, posterior segment masses, and phthisis bulbi.[25–27]

High resolution of normal equine ocular fundus structures, including the retina and optic nerve, have been evaluated by OCT (**Fig. 13**). The need for a clear ocular media to use this imaging modality limits is use in the horse and, to date, no description of the

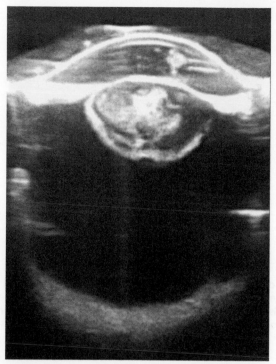

Fig. 10. Ultrasound image of a horse eye with a hypermature cataract. In this horse, the anterior chamber of the eye has hyperechoic debris, suggestive of uveitis, and there is a hypermature cataract, as determined by the hyperechoic lens and irregular lens capsule.

use of OCT in abnormal equine retinal disease has been reported, although there have been case reports of ocular trauma associated with retinal degeneration assessed by OCT (**Fig. 14**). Much more work is needed with this instrumentation, including assessment of glaucoma, chronic uveitis, and various unexplained retinopathies common in the equine retina.

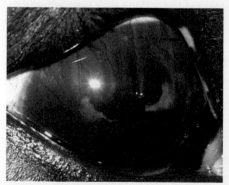
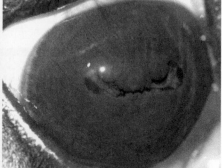

Fig. 11. Infrared photography (IR) of a horse with chronic uveitis. Because of corneal opacities, the detail of the anterior uveal tract is partially obstructed on standard color photography (*left*). However, with IR photography, the detail of the iris is visible because the long wavelengths of IR light penetrate the opaque cornea.

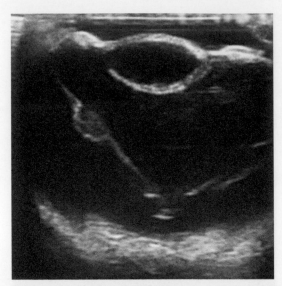

Fig. 12. Ultrasound image of a horse's eye indicating a complete retinal detachment. This horse was evaluated for a mature cataract and, on ultrasound imaging, a complete retinal detachment was visualized. The classic V-shaped retinal detachment is seen with the apex of the V extending to the optic nerve.

Fluorescein angiography (FA) has been used for many years in human and small animal ophthalmology to assess the blood–retinal barrier, but only in the past decade or so has there been descriptions of it use in the horse (**Box 4**).[29–31] The technique is accomplished by injecting intravenous fluorescein (10 mg/kg) followed by immediate imaging of the ocular fundus using a camera system with appropriate excitation and other filters, including use of handheld fundus cameras[30] or scanning digital ophthalmoscopes.[29] Fluoroangiographic phases described in the horse include the choriopapillary and retinal vascular phase, with the latter divided into the filling, maximum fluorescence, and fading phases (**Fig. 15**).[30] Hussey and colleagues[31] described the FA assessment of retinal lesions with the characteristic appearance of multifocal donut-shaped depigmented lesions with pigmented centers (focal or multifocal bullet hole lesions) induced experimentally by equine herpes

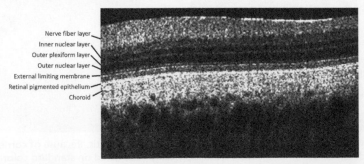

Nerve fiber layer
Inner nuclear layer
Outer plexiform layer
Outer nuclear layer
External limiting membrane
Retinal pigmented epithelium
Choroid

Fig. 13. Optical coherence tomography image of the equine central retina. The layers of the retina can be identified.

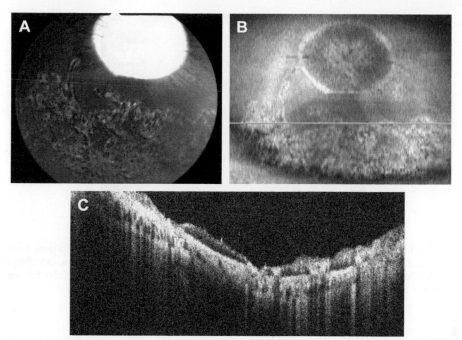

Fig. 14. Imaging of a young horse with blindness after a head injury. (*A*) Color ocular fundus photograph demonstrating depigmentation inferior to the optic nerve. (*B*) En face image of the ocular fundus as obtained by optical coherence tomography (OCT). (*C*) B-scan OCT image at the level of the green line in (*B*) demonstrating multifocal areas of retinal degeneration.

type 1 and on FA they demonstrated no leakage of fluorescein from choroidal or retinal vessels, but the underlying choroid was visible suggesting that the observed lesion was limited to retinal pigmented epithelium depigmentation (**Fig. 16**). Pachten and colleagues[29] described the use of FA in the diagnosis of optic nerve atrophy and recurrent uveitis.[29,32]

IMAGING OF THE ORBIT
Indications for Imaging

Imaging of the orbit is most commonly done after injury to determine if orbital fractures exist, but also for determining causes and extent of lesions associated with exophthalmos or other periocular swelling.

Advanced Imaging Modalities Described

There have been many descriptions of advanced techniques to image the orbit and periorbital tissues. The location of the suspected lesion determines which

---

Box 4
Technique for performing fluorescein angiography

After normal color photography of the ocular fundus of the horse, an ocular fundus camera with the appropriate blue excitation and yellow filters is used to image the ocular fundus after intravenous injection of fluorescein (10 mg/kg). Imaging of the equine fundus is typically continued for 10 minutes after injection.

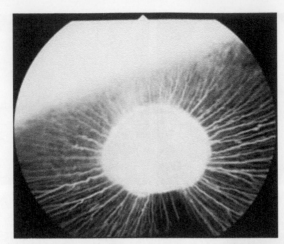

Fig. 15. Fluorescein angiography in the horse. Several fluorescein angiograph phases have been described in the horse, including maximum fluorescence as visualized here. (*Modified from* Molleda JM, Cervantes I, Galán A, et al. Fluorangiographic study of the ocular fundus in normal horses. Vet Ophthalmol 2008;11:2–7; with permission.)

modality is used. Ocular ultrasound imaging is the least invasive technique because it can be done routinely in a standing horse; however, it only images the retrobulbar space immediately adjacent to the eye, does not commonly provide imaging of the entire extent of the lesion, and does not provide information on changes to the boney structures of the orbit.[23,33,34] Therefore, it is recommended that CT and/or MRI be used for orbital disease.[8,35–40] Although there are systems that allow a standing horse to be imaged (ie, standing CT), most modalities require general anesthesia for detailed, well-focused studies with minimal motion artifact.

There have been several reports describing the imaging of retrobulbar disease with CT, including evaluation of a large sinonasal cyst,[36] a retrobulbar hematoma,[41] and several orbital neoplasms, including an optic nerve meningioma[40] and adenocarcinoma (**Fig. 17**).[42,43] The authors of 1 study of a case of ocular angiosarcoma concluded that the extent and exact definition of equine retrobulbar changes could only be made with MRI, with diagnostic yet incomplete descriptions of disease when using radiographic or ultrasonographic examinations.[39] CT scans are particularly helpful for identifying the location and extent of periorbital fractures (**Fig. 18**).[37]

MRI or CT scanning may also be needed to determine the cause and extent of central nervous system disease in horses with transient blindness, optic nerve atrophy, and upper respiratory tract disease (ie, sinusitis). In a small series of these equine cases, Barnett and colleagues[44] demonstrated the value of these imaging modalities for disease diagnosis and suggested in these cases that routine ophthalmic examination had relatively little diagnostic value. MRI was able to image an infection of the sphenopalatine sinuses with subsequent distension and compression of adjacent optic nerve(s) and optic chiasm (**Fig. 19**).[44] Equine head MRI has the advantage to provide localization of the lesions, their size, and relation of the lesion to surrounding structures. There was also good correlation between MRI findings and intraoperative or postmortem results.[38]

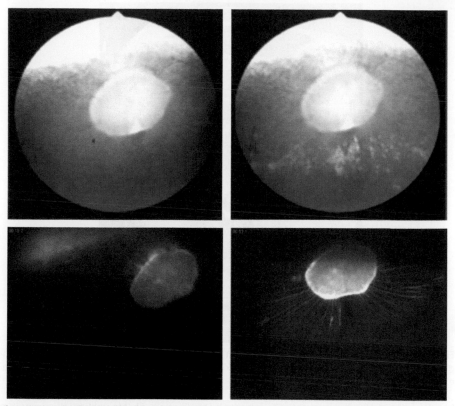

Fig. 16. Ocular lesions after experimental equine herpes virus-1 (EHV-1) infection in normal horses. (*Left*) A normal horse fundus image (*top*) and normal fluorescein angiography (FA) (*bottom*) before infection. (*Right*) Lesions suspected to be associated with EHV-1 at 3 months after infection. Because the vasculature is not disrupted, the classic bullet hole lesions on FA suggest that these lesions were likely caused by focal loss of retinal pigmented epithelium with exposure of the underlying choroid. (*Modified from* Hussey GS, Goehring LS, Lunn DP, et al. Experimental infection with equine herpesvirus type 1 (EHV-1) induces chorioretinal lesions. Vet Res 2013;44:118.

MISCELLANEOUS USE OF IMAGING: PROCEDURES
Indications for Imaging

Imaging can also be used to guide a needle behind the globe or in the eyelid to obtain samples, or to deliver therapeutics or anesthetics. It can also be used to guide aspiration, but not biopsy of intraocular structures, especially when the media or lesion is opaque and thus not allowing direct visualization of the needle placement.

Advanced Imaging Modalities Described

Few studies of this technique using ultrasound imaging to guide an aspiration or placement of a needle for retrobulbar nerve blocks have been reported. Ultrasound imaging has been used to visualize the intraorbital anatomic structures and to guide and accurately place a needle into the retrobulbar space to perform a retrobulbar nerve block.[45] Although this technique is possible, we have performed thousands of retrobulbar

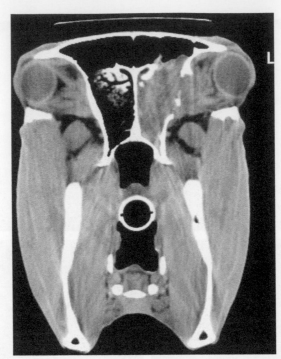

Fig. 17. Transverse computed tomography (CT) in a horse with exophthalmos. The CT scan demonstrates extension of a nasal mass (adenocarcinoma) through the orbital wall to cause exophthalmos in the left eye (L).

blocks without ultrasound guidance without complication, so it is unlikely this imaging is needed.[3] However, ultrasound-guided fine needle placement may be very useful for aspiration of retrobulbar lesions, as demonstrated in a report of an orbital hematoma where ultrasound-guided aspiration led to a definitive diagnosis.[41]

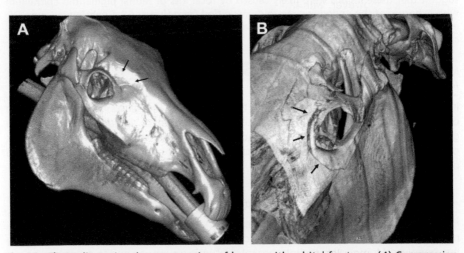

Fig. 18. Three-dimensional reconstruction of horses with orbital fractures. (*A*) Compression fracture of the superior orbital rim and frontal bones (*arrows*). (*B*) Comminuted and slightly displaced fracture of the superior and nasal orbital rim (*arrows*).

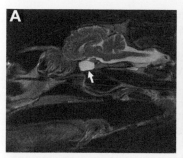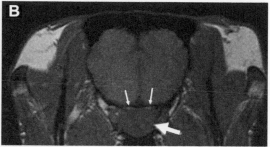

Fig. 19. MRI of a horse with sinusitis and blindness. (A) Sagittal T2-weighted MRI of the sphenopalatine sinus (*arrow*). (B) Transverse T1-weighted MARI of the sphenopalatine sinus (*large arrow*) with a moderate signal intensity material and a poorly defined dorsal wall and dorsoventral compression of the optic nerves (*small arrows*). (*Modified from* Barnett KC, Blunden AS, Dyson SJ, et al. Blindness, optic atrophy and sinusitis in the horse. Vet Ophthalmol 2008;11:20–6; with permission.)

SUMMARY

When considering advanced imaging of the eye, this review has shown that ultrasound imaging currently has the most uses and value for diagnosis of equine ocular disease, especially when the ocular media is opaque or damaged. Routinely, the ocular posterior segment is examined with ultrasound imaging to determine the extent of disease and prognosis in horse cases where the cornea is opaque, a cataract is present, or when there has been anterior segment trauma with the anterior chamber filled with blood and/or having an extremely miotic pupil. The main limitations of ultrasound imaging are the comparatively poor resolution (when compared with OCT or confocal microscopy) as well as the inability to thoroughly image the orbit and surrounding tissues. CT and MRI images are being used more routinely for evaluation of the equine head, but their widespread use is limited by the fact that general anesthesia is usually required and the high instrument costs and facility infrastructure needed to support the machines. However, with the advance of technology and further development of standing CT scans, the accessibility of these imaging techniques will no doubt increase. Finally, the extremely promising high-resolution and magnified imaging modalities, such as OCT and confocal microscopy, will provide much information of the pathogenesis of disease in vivo. As these technologies improve and the instruments become more practical for routine use in horses, more reports on their use to assess ocular disease in the horse will emerge. With the rapid development of clinical imaging technologies in humans, one would expect the rapid translation of the modalities to the equine eye.

ACKNOWLEDGMENTS

Thanks to Erin Barr for her expert photography and assistance with the figures.

REFERENCES

1. Srinivasan VJ, Wojtkowski M, Witkin AJ, et al. High-definition and 3-dimensional imaging of macular pathologies with high-speed ultrahigh-resolution optical coherence tomography. Ophthalmology 2006;113(11). http://dx.doi.org/10.1016/j.ophtha.2006.05.046.

2. de Sisternes L, Simon N, Tibshirani R, et al. Quantitative SD-OCT imaging bio-markers as indicators of age-related macular degeneration progression. Investig Ophthalmol Vis Sci 2014;55(11):7093–103.
3. Stoppini R, Gilger BC. Examination of the equine eye. In: Gilger BC, editor. Equine ophthalmology. 3rd edition. Ames (IA): Wiley-Blackwell; 2017. p. 1–56.
4. Greenberg SM, Plummer CE, Brooks DE, et al. Unilateral orbital lacrimal gland abscess in a horse. Vet Ophthalmol 2011;14(1):55–60.
5. Reimer JM, Latimer CS. Ultrasound findings in horses with severe eyelid swelling, and recognition of acute dacryoadenitis: 10 cases (2004-2010). Vet Ophthalmol 2011;14(2):86–92.
6. Nykamp SG, Scrivani PV, Pease AP. Computed tomography dacryocystography evaluation of the nasolacrimal apparatus. Vet Radiol Ultrasound 2004;45(1):23–8.
7. Spadari A, Spinella G, Grandis A, et al. Endoscopic examination of the nasolacri-mal duct in ten horses. Equine Vet J 2011;43(2):159–62.
8. Dawson C, Dixon J, Lam R, et al. Differential diagnoses, investigation, and man-agement of a periocular swelling close to the nasolacrimal duct in a horse - a case report of dacryops. Vet Ophthalmol 2016;19(5):427–31.
9. Gilger BC, Histed J, Pate DO, et al. Anomalous nasolacrimal openings in a 2-year-old Morgan filly. Vet Ophthalmol 2010;13(5):339–42.
10. Gibbs C, Lane JG. Radiographic examination of the facial, nasal and para-nasal sinus regions of the horse .2. Radiological findings. Equine Vet J 1987;19(5):474–82.
11. Elce YA, Wilkie DA, Santschi EM, et al. Metastasis or delayed local extension of ocular squamous cell carcinoma in four horses. Equine Vet Educ 2011;23(10):496–9.
12. Bentley E, Miller PE, Diehl KA. Diagnostic tool in veterinary ophthalmology. J Am Vet Med Assoc 2003;223(11):1617–22.
13. Pinto NI, Gilger BC. Spectral-domain optical coherence tomography evaluation of the cornea, retina, and optic nerve in normal horses. Vet Ophthalmol 2014;17(Suppl 1):140–8.
14. Pirie CG, Alario AF, Barysauskas CM, et al. Manual corneal thickness measure-ments of healthy equine eyes using a portable spectral-domain optical coher-ence tomography device. Equine Vet J 2014;46(5):631–4.
15. Pinto NI, Mcmullen RJ, Linder KE, et al. Clinical, histopathological and immuno-histochemical characterization of a novel equine ocular disorder: heterochromic iridocyclitis with secondary keratitis in adult horses. Vet Ophthalmol 2015;18(6):443–56.
16. Ledbetter EC, Scarlett JM. In vivo confocal microscopy of the normal equine cornea and limbus. Vet Ophthalmol 2009;12(Suppl 1):57–64.
17. Ledbetter EC, Irby NL, Schaefer DMW. In vivo confocal microscopy of corneal microscopic foreign bodies in horses. Vet Ophthalmol 2014;17(Suppl 1):69–75.
18. Ledbetter EC, Irby NL, Kim SG. In vivo confocal microscopy of equine fungal keratitis. Vet Ophthalmol 2011;14(1):1–9.
19. Pirie CG, Alario A. Anterior segment angiography of the normal canine eye: a comparison between indocyanine green and sodium fluorescein. Vet J 2014;199(3):360–4.
20. Pirie CG, Alario A. Use of indocyanine green and sodium fluorescein for anterior segment angiography in ophthalmologically normal cats. Am J Vet Res 2015;76(10):897–903.
21. Jancevski M, Foster CS. Anterior segment optical coherence tomography. Semin Ophthalmol 2010;25(5–6):317–23.

22. McMullen RJ, Clode AB, Gilger BC. Infrared digital imaging of the equine anterior segment. Vet Ophthalmol 2009;12(2):125–31.
23. Hughes K. Ultrasonographic examination of the painful equine eye. In Pract 2009; 31(2):70–6.
24. Hallowell GD, Bowen IM. Practical ultrasonography of the equine eye. Equine Vet Educ 2007;19(11):600–5.
25. Scotty NC. Ocular ultrasonography in horses. Clin Tech Equine Pract 2005;4(1): 106–13.
26. Scotty NC, Cutler TJ, Brooks DE, et al. Diagnostic ultrasonography of equine lens and posterior segment abnormalities. Vet Ophthalmol 2004;7(2):127–39.
27. Valentini S, Tamburro R, Spadari A, et al. Ultrasonographic evaluation of equine ocular diseases: a retrospective study of 38 eyes. J Equine Vet Sci 2010;30(3): 150–4.
28. Strobel BW, Wilkie DA, Gilger BC, et al. Retinal detachment in horses: 40 cases (1998 – 2005). Vet Ophthalmol 2007;10:380–5.
29. Pachten A, Wollanke B, Gerhards H, et al. Fluorescein angiography in the diseased ocular fundus of two horses. Equine Vet Educ 2008;20(1):11–5.
30. Molleda JM, Cervantes I, Galán A, et al. Fluorangiographic study of the ocular fundus in normal horses. Vet Ophthalmol 2008;11(Suppl 1):2–7.
31. Hussey GS, Goehring LS, Lunn DP, et al. Experimental infection with equine herpesvirus type 1 (EHV-1) induces chorioretinal lesions. Vet Res 2013;44(1): 1–15.
32. Pachten A, Niedermaier D, Wollanke B, et al. Fluorescein angiography in a horse with optic nerve atrophy. Pferdeheilkunde 2009;25(6):554–8.
33. Freesone JF, Glaze MB, Pechman R, et al. Ultrasonic identification of an orbital tumour in a horse. Equine Vet J 1989;21(2):135–6.
34. van den Top JGB, Schaafsma IA, Boswinkel M. A retrobulbar abscess as an uncommon cause of exophthalmos in a horse. Equine Vet Educ 2007;19(11): 579–83.
35. Dixon J, Lam R, Weller R, et al. Clinical application of multidetector computed tomography and magnetic resonance imaging for evaluation of cranial nerves in horses in comparison with high resolution imaging standards. Equine Vet Educ 2016;1–9. http://dx.doi.org/10.1111/eve.12629.
36. Annear MJ, Gemensky-Metzler AJ, Elce YA, et al. Exophthalmos secondary to a sinonasal cyst in a horse. J Am Vet Med Assoc 2008;233(2):285–8.
37. Gerding JC, Clode A, Gilger BC, et al. Equine orbital fractures: a review of 18 cases (2006-2013). Vet Ophthalmol 2014;17(Suppl 1):97–106.
38. Manso-Díaz G, Dyson SJ, Dennis R, et al. Magnetic resonance imaging characteristics of equine head disorders: 84 cases (2000-2013). Vet Radiol Ultrasound 2015;56(2):176–87.
39. Bischofberger AS, Konar M, Posthaus H, et al. Ocular angiosarcoma in a pony - MRI and histopathological appearance. Equine Vet Educ 2008;20(7):340–7.
40. Naylor RJ, Dunkel B, Dyson S, et al. A retrobulbar meningioma as a cause of unilateral exophthalmos and blindness in a horse. Equine Vet Educ 2010;22:503–10.
41. Boroffka S, Belt A. CT/Ultrasound diagnosis—retrobular hematoma in a horse. Vet Radiol Ultrasound 1996;37:441–3.
42. Davis JL, Gilger BC, Spaulding K, et al. Nasal adenocarcinoma with diffuse metastases involving the orbit, cerebrum, and multiple cranial nerves in a horse. J Am Vet Med Assoc 2002;221(10):1460–3, 1420.
43. Baptiste KE, Grahn BH. Equine orbital neoplasia: a review of 10 cases (1983-1998). Can Vet J 2000;41(4):291–5.

44. Barnett KC, Blunden AS, Dyson SJ, et al. Blindness, optic atrophy and sinusitis in the horse. Vet Ophthalmol 2008;11(Suppl 1):20–6.

45. Morath U, Luyet C, Spadavecchia C, et al. Ultrasound-guided retrobulbar nerve block in horses: a cadaveric study. Vet Anaesth Analg 2013;40(2): 205–11.

Genetic Testing as a Tool to Identify Horses with or at Risk for Ocular Disorders

Rebecca R. Bellone, PhD

KEYWORDS

- Genetics • Ocular disorders • Night blindness • Recurrent uveitis
- Squamous cell carcinoma • Multiple congenital ocular anomalies • Horses

KEY POINTS

- Genetic testing can help identify horses with ocular disorders and tests are available for congenital stationary night blindness and multiple congenital ocular anomalies.
- Genetic testing can also help identify horses at risk for developing ocular disorders, including equine recurrent uveitis and squamous cell carcinoma.
- Screening horses for genetic mutations can help inform management decisions for an earlier diagnosis and better prognosis.

INTRODUCTION

Sequencing the genome (the totality of an organisms DNA) of a gray thoroughbred mare named Twilight has allowed the rapid development of tools and resources to aid in the understanding of the genetics of economically and medically important traits in the horse.[1] Twilight's genome has served as a reference with which to compare sequence information from other horses and has enabled finding the causative mutations for several disorders, including those that can affect ocular function. These findings allow the creation of genetic tests offered by several commercial laboratories around the globe. Use of these tests can influence clinical management and breeding decisions.

Most inherited ocular disorders or those disorders with ocular manifestations are breed specific or affect breeds that are closely related. The genetics of 8 different ocular disorders have been investigated (**Table 1**). Approximately half of the disorders studied have an associated or causative variant identified. These disorders include congenital stationary night blindness (CSNB) and equine recurrent uveitis (ERU) in

Disclosure: R.R. Bellone is affiliated with the Veterinary Genetics Laboratory, a genetic testing laboratory offering diagnostic tests in horses and other species.
Department of Population Health and Reproduction, Veterinary Genetics Laboratory, UC Davis School of Veterinary Medicine, One Shields Avenue, Davis, CA 95616, USA
E-mail address: rbellone@ucdavis.edu

Vet Clin Equine 33 (2017) 627–645
http://dx.doi.org/10.1016/j.cveq.2017.08.005

Table 1
Inherited ocular disorders

Ocular Disorder	Alias Names	Breeds	DNA Test Available and Name	Important Clinical Considerations
Congenital stationary night blindness	CSNB	Appaloosa, American miniature horse, Knabstrupper, Noriker, Pony of the Americas	Yes: LP	All *LP/LP* horses are night blind
Equine recurrent uveitis	Moon blindness/ ERU	Appaloosa	Yes: LP	In the Appaloosa breed risk for ERU is defined as *LP/LP > LP > N > N/N*
		Warmblood breeds	No	
MCOA	Anterior segment dysgenesis/ MCOA	Rocky Mountain horse, Kentucky mountain saddle horse, Kentucky mountain pleasure horse, Icelandic horse, Shetland pony, American miniature horse, Comtois, and other breeds with silver, including American quarter horse and Morgan	Yes: silver	*Z/Z* horses typically have a more severe phenotype than *Z/N*
Limbal SCC	Ocular SCC	Haflinger	Yes: ocular SCC	*R/R* 5.5 times more likely to develop ocular SCC than *R/N* or *N/N*
Cataracts		Exmoor pony, American quarter horse, Arabian, thoroughbred, and Morgan	No	Females seem to be more frequently affected in the Morgan and Exmoor breeds
Corneal dystrophy		Friesian	No	May be related to other collagen disorders in the breed
Distichiasis		Friesian	No	Unknown mode of inheritance
Aniridia		Belgian and American quarter horse	No	Thought to be inherited as a dominant mutation so offspring of affected horses should be carefully monitored

Abbreviations: CSNB, congenital stationary night blindness; MCOA, multiple congenital ocular anomalies.

the Appaloosa and other breeds with the appaloosa spotting patterns, multiple congenital ocular anomalies in horse breeds with the silver mutation, and limbal squamous cell carcinoma (SCC) in the Haflinger breed.[2–5] Ocular manifestations have also been reported for 5 additional disorders, with genetic tests available for all but 1 (**Table 2**). Genetic testing has the potential to help clinicians identify causes of ocular anomalies and can greatly aid in the identification of those horses at highest risk of developing diseases such as ERU and SCC. Careful screening of horses at highest risk may allow early detection and better prognosis. The inheritance of many of these disorders is recessive, meaning those horses that are affected or at highest risk for disease must inherit 2 copies of the mutant form of the gene. For these disorders, identifying horses that are carriers (1 copy of the mutant version) is essential to inform breeding decisions. The focus of this article is to provide clinicians with a comprehensive description of known inherited ocular disorders and manifestations and to discuss when genetic testing is useful in clinical practice.

CONGENITAL STATIONARY NIGHT BLINDNESS

CSNB is characterized by impaired vision in dark conditions. This condition is present at birth and is nonprogressive. Definitive clinical diagnosis is determined by a so-called negative dark electroretinography (ERG), in which the b-wave (ON bipolar cell activation) is absent and the a-wave (photoreceptor cell activation) has an increased amplitude.[6] This condition has been reported most frequently in the Appaloosa breed but has also been reported in the American Miniature Horse, Knabstrupper, as well as 1 reported case in each of the Paso Fino and Thoroughbred breeds.[2,7–14] The reported incidence of Appaloosas in the literature and anecdotal evidence from breeders, suggesting Appaloosa horses with 2 copies of the mutation responsible for their unique coat patterning were the ones with night blindness, led to extensive investigation of the genetics for this trait.[2,11,15,16]

Appaloosa horses are best known for their white patterning in the coat, termed leopard complex spotting. The white patterning is typically symmetric and centered over the hips (**Fig. 1**). It can occur with and without pigmented spots in the white area. Additional characteristics include visible sclera; stripes of pigment on an otherwise unpigmented hoof; mottled skin around the muzzle, anus, and genitalia; and progressive roaning (progressive occurrence of white hairs in the coat as the animal ages). Although most horses with a leopard complex spotting pattern have these characteristics and some white patterning, there is considerable variability in phenotype. The extent of the white pattern can range from a few white flecks on the rump to nearly completely white from birth. The extent of roaning can also vary because some horses roan a great deal, whereas others show little roaning in their coat even by the late teens (**Fig. 2**). In addition, variability can occur with regard to the size and number of pigmented spots in the white pattern area. Leopard complex spotting is thought to be a polygenic trait with the presence of the coat pattern and associated characteristics inherited by an incompletely dominant form of a gene known as *LP*, for leopard complex spotting. The extent of the white patterning is thought to be caused by additional genes (the exact number is still under investigation). Horses that are heterozygous for *LP* (*LP/N*; 1 copy of the allele controlling for the presence of the spotting pattern and 1 copy of the wild-type allele) tend to have more oval spots of pigment in the white patterned area compared with homozygotes (those with 2 copies of *LP*). However, it is not always easy to predict genotype and thus affection status for CSNB based on the horses' variable coat pattern (see **Fig. 1**). This spotting pattern also occurs in other breeds of horses, specifically the American Miniature Horse and the

Table 2
Ocular manifestations of other equine disorders and genetic testing

Disorder	Ocular Manifestations	Breeds	Mode of Inheritance	DNA Test Available
Hyperkalemic periodic paralysis	Third eyelid prolapse	Quarter horse and related breeds	Dominant with variable expression	Yes
Hereditary equine regional dermal asthenia	Thin corneas and increased incidence of corneal ulcers	Quarter horse and related breeds	Recessive	Yes
Junctional epidermolysis bullosa	Corneal ulcers	Draft breeds	Recessive	Yes
		American Saddlebreds	Recessive	Yes
Incontinentia pigmenti	Developmental ocular anomalies	Quarter horse (?)	X-linked dominant	Yes
Neuroaxonal dystrophy/equine degenerative myeloencephalopathy	Pigment retinopathy	Warmbloods	Unknown	No

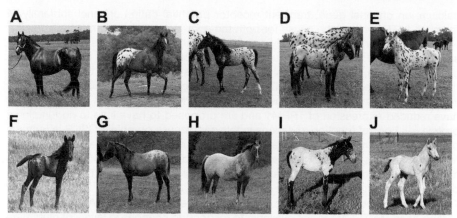

Fig. 1. Leopard complex spotting patterns and ocular disorders. Leopard complex spotting patterns in horses have been linked to both CSNB and ERU. This coat pattern is best characterized as a group of white spotting patterns that can range on a continuum from a few white flecks on the rump (A and F) to a horse that is almost completely white, known as a fewspot (J). Horses that are homozygous for *LP* (F–J) have few to no spots of pigment in the white patterned area, have CSNB, and are also at highest risk of developing ERU. Those horses that are heterozygous (*LP/N*) have pigmented spots in the white patterned area, are not night blind, but have an increased risk for ERU compared with solid non–leopard complex spotted horses (A–E). It is not always evident based on appearance what the genotype of the horse is with respect to *LP* (A, F, G, J), thus genotyping for the *LP* mutation is recommended to determine whether the horse has, or is a carrier for, CSNB and to determine level of risk for ERU. (*Photographs Courtesy of* Sheila Archer, Cheryl Woods, Petra Davidson, and Lisa Estridge.)

Knabstrupper, two breeds with documented cases of CSNB.[12,14] In addition pony of the Americas, British Spotted Ponies, Norikers, and Mustangs can have a leopard complex spotting pattern.

Several molecular genetic studies and the availability of the horse reference genome led to the identification of an insertion of 1378 base pairs (bp) in the first intron of the

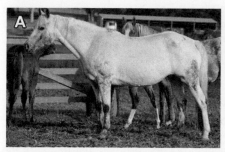
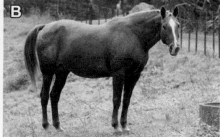

Fig. 2. Extensive loss of pigment in leopard complex spotting and connection to ocular disorders. Some horses with leopard complex spotting can roan extensively (A), whereas others show little evidence of roaning (B). Both mares are 17 years old at the time of photography and have the same base color. By appearance alone their genotype with respect to LP may be misleading because both are heterozygous for *LP* (*LP/N*) and hence are only carriers for CSNB. It has been speculated that horses like the one in (A), with extensive roaning, have a higher chance of developing ERU, although this remains to be investigated. (*Courtesy of* Petra Davidson.)

calcium ion channel gene, transient receptor potential cation channel subfamily M member 1 (TRPM1) as the cause for both the spotting pattern and night blindness.[2] Homozygosity for LP was perfectly concordant with CSNB and was documented in several studies.[2,11,12] Thus, although the coat spotting phenotype is inherited in a dominant fashion, CSNB is recessive. The LP allele is thought to be an old mutation, having been detected in ancient DNA that dates back at least 17,000 years.[2] This insertion disrupts the normal transcription of TRPM1. Horses with 2 copies of LP have reduced expression of TRPM1 and are proposed to have little to no functional protein.[2,15] Loss of function mutations in this gene cause complete CSNB in humans but with no known pigmentation defects.[17] Work in humans and mice has shown that reduction in levels of glutamate released by retinal rod cells when light is detected signals the opening of the TRPM1 channels. Calcium signaling through TRPM1 results in depolarization of the ON bipolar cells (the b-wave on the ERG).[18,19] Absence of TRPM1 in LP homozygous horses explains the negative ERG of Appaloosas with CSNB, because TRPM1 is not available to respond to changes in levels of glutamate release by the retinal rod cells.

CLINICAL PERSPECTIVE ON GENETIC TESTING FOR CONGENITAL STATIONARY NIGHT BLINDNESS IN BREEDS WITH LEOPARD COMPLEX SPOTTING

Horses homozygous for the leopard complex spotting mutation are night blind.[2] A horse's coat pattern does not always indicate genotype. Therefore, one way to diagnose horses with CSNB is by DNA testing for the LP mutation. For horses with obvious coat patterns, genetic testing is not necessary. For example, a horse with many pigmented spots in the white pattern area will be heterozygous (LP/N) and thus will not have the LP-associated form of CSNB (see **Fig. 1**F). However, in horses with spotting patterns on either end of the white patterning continuum it is not easy to discern the LP genotype with certainty based on appearance alone. Therefore, these animals should be tested for LP to determine whether they are night blind or are carriers for the night blind allele. Care should be taken when handling or examining potential homozygous animals in low light conditions because some are more apprehensive than others. A complete ophthalmic examination should be performed, including an ERG to confirm genetic diagnosis. Management strategies and breeding considerations should be discussed with clients who own horses that test homozygous for the LP mutation (LP/LP). Although breeding away from CSNB is not possible, because homozygous horses give the highest chances of passing this desirable coat color pattern on to the next generation, care should be taken and owners advised on breeding, handling, training, and riding these animals in low light or dark conditions.

EQUINE RECURRENT UVEITIS

ERU, also known as moon blindness, is characterized by repeated episodes of inflammation of the iris, ciliary body, and choroid. The cumulative effects of the immune-mediated process can lead to glaucoma, cataracts, and complete loss of vision. ERU is the most common cause of blindness in horses, blinding 1% to 2% of the American horse population.[20] The breeds with the highest occurrence reported in the United States include the Appaloosa, Quarter horse, Thoroughbred, Warmblood, Hanoverian, and the American Paint Horse.[21] Of these, Appaloosas have been reported to be 8 times more likely to develop ERU and significantly more likely to go blind in 1 or both eyes, as a result of the inflammatory process, than any other breed (**Fig. 3**).[20] In the most recent retrospective study, 62.5% of the horses diagnosed with ERU were Appaloosas.[22]

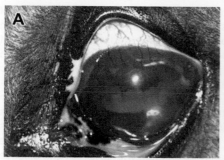
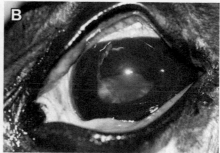

Fig. 3. ERU in the Appaloosa horse. (*A*) Insidious uveitis in an Appaloosa horse shown by conjunctival hyperemia, corneal vascularization, diffuse corneal edema, aqueous flare, and miosis. The pupil is irregular because of posterior synechia. Corneal mineralization is evident in the ventrolateral cornea. (*B*) Active uveitis shown by conjunctival hyperemia, epiphora, and miotic pupil. Cataract is present and the vitreous appears yellow. (*Courtesy of* Dr Lynne Sandmeyer.)

Clinically, ERU has been subclassified into 3 syndromes: classic, insidious, and posterior ERU. Classic ERU is the most common and is explained by periods of active, apparently painful inflammation followed by a quiescent phase. The repeated attacks are what often lead to vision loss. Insidious ERU is distinguished by a persistent low-grade intraocular inflammation with gradual and cumulative destruction that does not typically manifest in outward painful episodes.[23] Appaloosa horses frequently have this form of ERU. The continual gradual destruction of the eye can lead to vision loss. The third classification is posterior ERU, which is characterized by inflammation primarily present in the vitreous, retina, and choroid. Commonly, retinal degeneration is observed with this form of ERU and is most often observed in warmbloods and draft breeds.[24] Although the pathogenesis of ERU is not entirely elucidated, all 3 subclassifications of ERU are thought to have a complex autoimmune component with environmental factors and genetics contributing to risk and severity of disease. It is unclear whether the inciting cause of inflammation and breakdown of the blood-ocular barrier is triggered by a cross-reactive microbial antigen or an autoantigen derived from the ocular tissue, or some combination of both.[25] It is also unclear whether immune mechanisms are different for the 3 subclassifications of ERU. However, the involvement of leptospirosis in ERU risk and progression has been documented at least in some cases.[26–29] Specifically, intraocular antibodies to *Leptospira* were identified in horses with ERU.[26–28,30] Further, horses testing positive for *Leptospira* antibodies were more likely to go blind from ERU than those testing negative.[21] The precise mechanism causing the recurring nature is not known but cross-reactive immunity between *Leptospira* and equine ocular antigens has been identified. One hypothesis is that infection with *Leptospira* leads to autoimmunity because autoantigens are presented by class II molecules to the CD4+ T cells in the uveal tract.[20,31] Several different autoantigens have been identified, only some of which help to explain the role of *Leptospira* in ERU risk.[32] Further, many studies support the involvement of *Leptospira* in ERU risk but not all cases can be explained by the presence of *Leptospira* antibodies,[21,24,33] thus identifying other risk factors is essential to elucidating the cause of this disease.

Genetic background likely plays a vital role in antigen production and may help to explain why Appaloosas are more likely to present with the insidious form and why warmbloods present more frequently with posterior ERU. Genetic contributors likely also explain why not all horses with ERU test positive for *Leptospira* and why Appaloosas are more likely to go blind than other breeds.[20,21,24] Studying the Appaloosa and the

German warmblood breeds showed associations with different markers in the region of the major histocompatibility complex in horses known as the equine leukocyte antigen (ELA).[3,34] The homologous region in humans has been associated with several different types of uveitis and these have become important tests for inherited risk for ocular and other inflammatory diseases.[35,36] However, genetic typing for ELA to ascertain genetic risk for ERU in the horse is not available. Nonetheless, German warmblood horses carrying the ELA-A9 haplotype had the highest risk of ERU. This haplotype was present in 41% of the cases but absent in the controls.[37] Genome-wide association studies (GWAS) are often used to investigate thousands to millions of markers spread across the genome to identify loci of association with disease. A GWAS performed in the German warmblood identified 2 loci significantly associated with ERU risk and disease severity.[34] A single nucleotide polymorphism (SNP) located on horse chromosome 20 (ECA20) was significantly associated with disease status, and this SNP is near 2 interleukin (IL) 17 genes (*IL-17A* and *IL-17F*) and these loci may play a role in ERU risk. An SNP on horse chromosome 18 (ECA18) was associated with disease severity; this SNP is near crystalline genes (*CRYGA-CRYGF*) and the investigators proposed that mutations in 1 or more of these genes may contribute to the cataract formation that is typical of disease progression. Causal variants for the associated loci on ECA18 or ECA20 have not been reported and no genetic tests are currently being offered for warmbloods. In the Appaloosa, a candidate gene approach was used to investigate the *LP* spotting locus (described earlier) as well as the major histocompatibility complex (MHC) locus.[3] Specifically, 7 microsatellites and 2 SNPs encompassing the *LP* locus and 13 microsatellites encompassing the ELA on ECA20 were used. Significant associations with the maker linked with *LP* (denoted as TRPM1 RFLP) as well as 2 microsatellites on ECA20 (microsatellite 472-260 located in the MHC class I region and microsatellite EqMHC1 located in intron 1 of the class II *DRA* gene) were detected. The *LP*-associated allele, the 224-bp allele at microsatellite 472-260, and the 207-bp allele at microsatellite EqMHC1 are thought to increase risk for ERU in an additive fashion. Genotypes from these loci could predict ERU risk with approximately 80% accuracy in a second population; however, DNA testing for the microsatellites are not commercially performed. Further, this study investigated an *LP*-associated SNP and not the causal mutation, and, given the high level of linkage disequilibrium between this associated SNP and the LP causal variant,[16] the *LP* test is the most effective and only DNA test currently commercially available to ascertain risk for ERU. Identification of causal variants for robust genetic predictions in the Appaloosa and warmblood breeds is needed and the genetics of ERU risk is an active area of research in several laboratories.

CLINICAL PERSPECTIVE ON GENETIC TESTING FOR EQUINE RECURRENT UVEITIS

A genetic risk for both insidious and posterior ERU has been documented in the Appaloosa and German warmblood, respectively.[3,34] Only 1 commercial genetic test, the *LP* test, is available for the Appaloosa breed. Risk for ERU based on this genetic test can be evaluated as *LP*/*LP* > *LP*/*N* > *N*/*N*. Horses homozygous for *LP* are at the highest risk of developing ERU. Horses heterozygous for the *LP* mutation are at a higher risk of developing ERU than those without the breed-identifying white spotting pattern. Thus genotype with respect to *LP* can be used to identify which horses to frequently evaluate and treat for signs of ocular inflammation. Furthermore, the *LP* test can be used to identify horses with CSNB (as described earlier and in **Figs. 1** and **2**) in multiple horse breeds but to date the only breed with *LP* that has been investigated for its role in ERU risk is the Appaloosa.[3] More work is needed to determine the validity of this test in other *LP* breeds. Further, it is not yet known whether the *LP* mutation is the causal risk factor or whether it is simply being inherited with *LP* (ie, whether the causative mutation is located close by on the DNA). Careful management of at-risk horses should be considered and include any practices that decrease the risk of injury or inflammatory stimuli. One study showed that Appaloosas that were seropositive for *Leptospira interrogans* serovar Pomana had the worst visual prognosis, with 50% of the cases becoming completely blind.[38] Although genotype with respect to *LP* was not known for the horses in that study, consideration for vaccination with the Lepto Eq Innovator (Zoetis Inc, Florham Park, NJ) may be advisable for the at-risk groups that show no clinical signs or past history of disease. However, there are no published studies to indicate the efficacy of this vaccine on different *LP* genotypes.

MULTIPLE CONGENITAL OCULAR ANOMALIES

Multiple congenital ocular anomalies (MCOA) is a syndrome of ocular disorders. This disorder was first characterized in the Rocky Mountain horse and was previously termed anterior segment dysgenesis.[39,40] Subsequent studies have identified the same phenotypes in other breeds, including the Kentucky mountain saddle and pleasure horses, the Icelandic horse, the Shetland pony, the American miniature horse, and the Comtois.[41–46] Clinically, this syndrome is divided into 2 phenotypic categories, termed cystic phenotype and MCOA. The cysts phenotype is characterized by temporal cysts that originate from the ciliary body or the peripheral retina; these cysts are translucent and range up to a centimeter in size. The MCOA phenotype is considered to be more severe and is characterized by ciliary or peripheral retina cysts with additional abnormalities, including iris hypoplasia, corneal globosa, megaloblepharon, retinal dysplasia, immature nuclear cataracts, and iridocorneal hypoplasia[40,41,47] (Fig. 4).

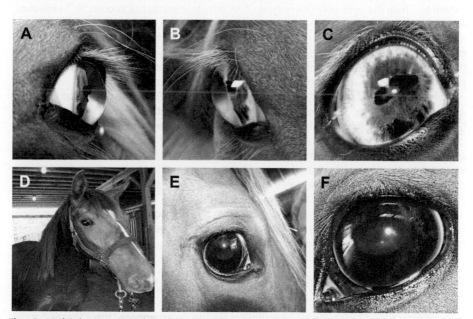

Fig. 4. Multiple congenital ocular anomalies. Silver dapple miniature horse showing the MCOA phenotype, including cornea globosa and iridal hypoplasia of the (*A*) left eye and (*B*) right eye, and (*C*) close-up view of iridal hypoplasia and dyscoric pupil. (*D*) Chestnut Rocky Mountain horse mare with MCOA phenotype, including (*E*) bilateral dyscoria, iridocorneal angle abnormality, and (*F*) cataract changes OS (oculus sinister). (*Courtesy of* Dr Ann Dwyer.)

The genetics of MCOA were first investigated by Ewart and colleagues[39] in 2000, who reported a codominant mode of inheritance with the more severe MCOA pheno-type thought to be explained by homozygosity for the mutant form of the gene. Another study also reported a dominant mode of inheritance but suggested incom-plete penetrance, meaning horses could carry the mutation but not express the phenotype.[41] Several molecular studies have since shown, similar to leopard complex spotting and CSNB, that MCOA results from a pleiotropic effect of a gene involved in pigmentation.[4,48,49] Specifically, the silver coat color has been associated with MCOA. Silver dilutes black pigment (eumelanin) but leaves red pigment (pheomelanin) unaf-fected. The mane and the tail are typically more dilute than the body but there is a great deal of variation (**Fig. 5**). Dappling often appears in the coat of silver horses. A missense mutation, or single base change in the DNA, results in an amino acid change from arginine to cysteine (Arg625Cys) in premelanosome protein (PMEL) causing both silver coat color and MCOA.[4,49] Horses heterozygous for the silver mutation most often have the cyst-only phenotype, whereas homozygotes have multiple ocular de-fects. PMEL forms amyloid fibrils within the melanosome and this protein is essential for proper formation of this organelle and intracellular transfer of eumelanin.[50,51] A PMEL knockout mouse cell line shows reduced pigment in skin, choroid, and retinal pigment epithelium, but an electroretinogram did not show any impaired function of the retina.[52] However, mutations in PMEL also regulate hypopigmentation with con-current ocular anomalies in dogs and zebrafish.[53,54] The precise role of this variant in ocular defects in horses remains to be determined. Several commercial laboratories offer a DNA test for silver in horses and breeds with the silver allele (*Z*) and all have reported cases of MCOA.

Horses homozygous for the silver mutation (*Z/Z*) have impaired vision or are blind. The extent to which the cyst-only phenotype (*Z/N*) affects vision is not known.[46,49] However, a study in Comtois and Rocky Mountain horses reported deeper anterior chambers in horses with the silver mutation (*Z/Z* and *Z/N*) compared with wild type (*N/N*), suggesting that perhaps vision is affected in the heterozygotes. However, the same study reported that homozygotes (*Z/Z*) had deeper chambers than heterozygotes (*Z/N*),[55] again sup-porting the notion that homozygotes have the most severe phenotype.

Horses heterozygous for the *PMEL* mutation are most often reported to have the cyst-only phenotype; however, a recent study noted that 8 out of 71 heterozygotes (*Z/N*) had mild cornea globosa in 1 or both eyes and 1 older horse had bilateral mitotic pupils and abnormal pupillary reflexes in both eyes.[55] This study also reported that only 32% of the heterozygotes (*Z/N*) had detectable cysts. It is possible that the incomplete penetrance may explain some of the cases of heterozygotes without cysts or that detection methods used in this report were not sensitive enough to identify all cysts. In this same study heterozygotes (*Z/N*) older than 16 years of age were more likely to be myopic than nonsilver horses (*N/N*), suggesting for the first time that there may be a progressive change in vision related to this disorder. More work is needed to better understand vision deficits in heterozygotes.

CLINICAL PERSPECTIVE ON GENETIC TESTING FOR MULTIPLE CONGENITAL OCULAR ANOMALIES

Horses from breeds with the silver mutation should be considered candidates for ge-netic testing for silver and screening for clinical symptoms of disease. The reported cases of incomplete penetrance make genetic screening important to determine which animals should be evaluated more closely. In addition, cysts vary in size and some may go undetected, thus horses with the silver mutation warrant additional

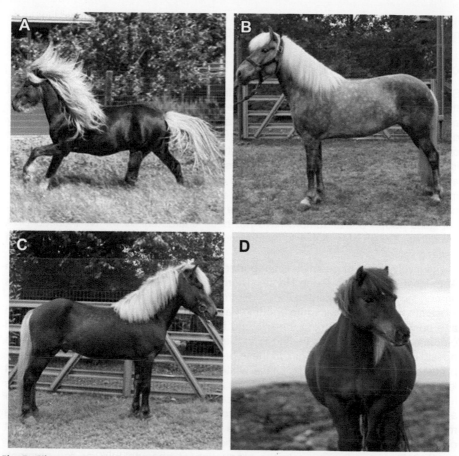

Fig. 5. Silver coat color is associated with multiple congenital ocular anomalies. Black horses with the silver mutation can range in phenotype from dark body with light mane and tail (*A*) to a light body known as light chocolate silver (*B*). Also note the dappling (*B*) that is present in some horses with the silver mutation. (*C*) Bay horses with the silver mutation, known as red silver, retain a red shade of the body but the mane and tail are dilute. (*D*) Chestnut horses with the silver allele only appear chestnut because silver does not dilute red pigment. Therefore, chestnut horses with or without the silver allele coat are phenotypically indistinguishable. Chestnut horses with the silver allele have MCOA (see **Fig.** 4D–F). Horses *A*, *C*, and *D* are heterozygous for the silver mutation and thus most likely have the cyst phenotype, whereas the horse in *B* is homozygous for the silver mutation and thus is likely more severely affected. (*Courtesy of* Lucinda Nold, Dawn Shaw, and þórhildur Gunnarsdottir.)

ocular screenings. Further, because recent evidence suggests that there may be a progressive nature to this syndrome,[55] knowing the genotype with respect to silver can help to determine which horses should be examined more carefully as they age. Chestnut horses with the silver mutation do not show the silver phenotype and thus should be screened for the silver allele to help inform breeding decisions. For example, breeding 2 chestnut horses that are heterozygous for the PMEL mutation has a 25% chance of producing an offspring with the most severe phenotype and vision deficits (*Z/Z*). Because the silver mutation causes both the popular coat color and ocular anomalies, breeding away from the disorder is not possible. However, heterozygotes are thought to have a milder form of disease and thus matings that do not produce the homozygous phenotype (Z/Z) are advised.

OCULAR SQUAMOUS CELL CARCINOMA

SCC is the second most common tumor of the horse and the most common cancer of the equine eye.[56] Ocular SCC can originate at the limbus, the nictitans, or the upper and lower eyelids. Tumors at the limbus are particularly concerning because they can spread axially into the cornea and can lead to visual impairment and destruction of the eye.[43] The cause of SCC is not entirely understood but ultraviolet (UV) radiation is among the most documented risk factors. In horses, increased longitude, altitude, and mean annual solar radiation have been correlated with ocular SCC prevalence.[57] Increased UV exposure has been linked to accumulating mutations that lead to cancer, although, with the exception of a single mutation identified in the tumor suppressor gene p53,[58] ocular tumors have not been characterized for UV-induced DNA mutations. Other potential risk factors include viruses, hormonal regulation, and genetics.[5,57,59]

The involvement of genetics is supported again by breed predisposition, with the Appaloosa, American Paint Horse, Thoroughbred, Haflinger, and draft breeds among those overrepresented.[57,60–62] Both the American paint horse and the Appaloosa are known for their white spotting patterns that often lack pigment in the skin and conjunctiva surrounding the eye and this is attributed to mutations in several pigmentation genes. DNA testing is available for approximately 13 of these. It is possible that the increased risk in these breeds can be attributed to lack of photoprotective pigment caused by these white spotting mutations, although it is not known which of these are specifically associated with SCC risk. Several studies have also implicated an increased risk of ocular SCC with chestnut coat color and gray coat depigmentation pattern across breeds, suggesting that these genes may explain increased incidence in some horse breeds.[60,63,64] The chestnut coat color results from a recessive loss of function mutation in the melanocortin 1 receptor (MC1R) gene allowing only the production of pheomelanin, or red pigment, which may be less photoprotective than eumelanin.[65] People with MC1R mutations tend to have red hair and fair skin and are generally photosensitive, prone to sunburn when exposed to UV light, and have an increased risk of melanomas tied to UV associated somatic C > T transitions.[66] UV mutations have not been examined in chestnut horses. The gray coat color is a gradual loss of pigment caused by a 4.6-kb duplication in the syntaxin-17 gene (STX17), which has been associated with increased risk for melanomas in horses.[67] Genetic testing for both the chestnut and the gray mutations is available and may help to explain the risk in some cases of ocular SCC.

To investigate other genetic contributors aside from pigmentation or lack thereof, recently the Haflinger breed, which is fixed for the chestnut allele, was investigated (**Fig. 6**). Two retrospective studies indicate that Haflingers are overrepresented for limbal SCC, with prevalence estimated to be 35% in this breed.[61,62] An autosomal recessive mode of inheritance best explains the genetic risk for limbal SCC in the breed. Using a GWAS approach, a strongly associated locus on horse chromosome 12 (ECA12) was detected.[5] Sequencing a candidate gene from this locus, damage-specific DNA binding protein 2 (DDB2), identified a missense mutation (c.1013 C > T p.Thr338Met) that was strongly but not perfectly associated with limbal SCC status. Because the identified allele was not perfectly associated (ie, homozygosity for the T allele explained 77% and

A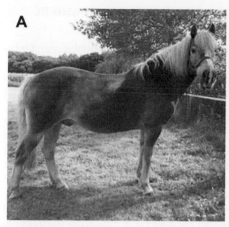

B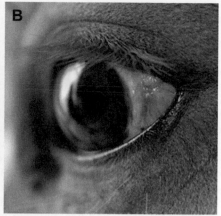

Fig. 6. Ocular SCC. (*A*) Haflinger horse showing chestnut coloration with flaxen main and tail typical of the breed. (*B*) Left eye of horse with limbal SCC. (*Courtesy of* Anouk Schurink and Dr Mary Lassaline.)

not 100% of the SCC cases), it is likely that additional loci may also contribute to risk for SCC in this breed. However, Haflingers homozygous for the T allele had 5.89 times greater risk of developing limbal SCC than horses with *T/C* or *C/C* genotypes. This risk allele is predicted to impair the ability of DDB2 to recognize and bind UV-damaged DNA, thus linking genetic and environmental risk. The SCC genetic risk variant was also detected in 2 other closely related breeds with reported cases of ocular SCC, the Belgian and the Percheron, suggesting that it may also be an SCC risk factor in these breeds. A DNA test for ocular SCC risk is commercially available at the Veterinary Genetics Laboratory University of California–Davis and this laboratory reports alleles as R for risk, and N for normal.

CLINICAL PERSPECTIVE ON GENETIC TESTING FOR SQUAMOUS CELL CARCINOMA

Genetic testing can help to identify horses at risk for ocular SCC and can be used to inform clinical and breeding decisions. Lack of photoprotective pigment and absence of eumelanin explains some of the risk for ocular SCC in horse breeds and more than 15 genetic tests could help to determine which allele may be tied to increased risk caused by pigmentation. However, the precise contribution of each pigmentation allele to genetic risk is not currently known.

A mutation identified in the Haflinger breed can be used to screen horses in this breed for the highest risk of developing ocular SCC (https://www.vgl.ucdavis.edu/services/HaflingerSCC.php). Horses with the *R/R* genotype are more likely to develop SCC than *R/N* or *N/N*. These (*R/R*) horses should be examined more frequently for earlier detection, and excision of any suspicious lesions should be carefully considered. Horses with ocular lesions who test *R/R* likely have a higher risk for recurrence and thus these horses should be examined more frequently. To reduce the incidence in the breed, breeding decisions should be advised so as to avoid mating *R/R* or *R/N* to one another. Many of the risks for ocular SCC are tied to UV radiation exposure, and it is therefore recommended that at-risk horses should have minimized UV light exposure, especially during peak hours. UV-protective fly masks should also be advised for these animals.

OCULAR MANIFESTATIONS OF EQUINE DISEASES CAUSED BY KNOWN GENETIC MUTATIONS

Inherited equine disorders affecting other systems can also result in ocular manifestations. Performing genetic testing can assist with clinical diagnosis. Hyperkalemic periodic paralysis is an autosomal disorder that is found in Quarter Horses and breeds that allow outcrossing to quarter horses. Typically, as its name suggests, this disorder is characterized by episodes of muscle fasciculations that can lead to weakness, although some horses remain asymptomatic throughout their lives. A missense mutation in a sodium ion channel (SCN4A) leads to the persistent depolarization of skeletal muscle cells and causes weakness.[68] Ocular manifestations can result from muscle weakness and include third eyelid prolapse secondary to globe retraction.[69] Another condition affecting quarter horses and related breeds is hereditary equine regional dermal asthenia (HERDA), which is an autosomal recessive disorder and thus carrier identification is extremely important. HERDA is characterized by hyperextensible skin that tears easily and has impaired healing caused by a missense mutation in the cyclophilin B gene (PPIB). PPIB is thought to play a role in collagen fibrillogenesis.[70] Horses with HERDA have thinner corneas and thus have an increased risk for corneal ulcers.[71] A second condition that can also cause corneal ulcers is junctional epidermolysis bullosa (JEB), which is characterized by mechanical stress–induced lesion of the skin and mucosal membranes.[72] This condition is also a recessive disorder and carrier-to-carrier matings should be avoided. Mutations in laminin genes cause separation of the dermis and epidermis. A mutation in LAMC2 causes JEB in draft breeds, whereas in American saddlebreds a large deletion in LAMA3 causes this disorder.[73,74] Incontinentia pigmenti in horses has been characterized by a brindle pigmentation pattern and skin lesions that evolve over time; it has a dominant X-linked mode of inheritance in which males are thought to die in utero. A single nucleotide change in the X-chromosomal IKBKG gene is predicted to produce a truncated protein, resulting in this disorder in a single family of horses. This family is also reported to have teeth, hoof, and ocular developmental abnormalities but the specifics of those abnormalities were not reported.[75] Neuroaxonal dystrophy (NAD), also referred to as equine degenerative myeloencephalopathy, is characterized by general proprioceptive ataxia with both genetics and vitamin E deficiencies during the first year of life and is thought to contribute to disease risk.[76] Recently a pigment retinopathy characterized by granular dark pigment was observed in 4 NAD warmblood horses but was not identified previously in quarter horses with NAD, indicating that genetic differences between breeds may contribute to differences in ocular manifestations.[77,78] Genetic mutations have not been reported for this disorder.

INHERITED OCULAR DISORDERS WITH UNKNOWN GENETIC CAUSES

Several additional ocular disorders are thought to be inherited but the investigations have been limited to studying the modes of inheritance and therefor causal mutations have not been determined. Friesian horses have several reported inherited collagen disorders, including megaesophagus, aortic rupture, dwarfism, and hydrocephalus, and these may be related to 2 corneal disorders in the breed.[79–81] Corneal dystrophy in Friesian horses is characterized by stromal loss that is bilateral and has a higher occurrence in males, making an inherited X-linked recessive hypothesis likely.[80] Distichiasis is a condition in which cilia aberrantly emerge from the meibomian gland openings, and, when pointing toward the cornea, these can cause corneal irritation or ulceration.[81] The breed predisposition implies a genetic cause, and a dominant mode of inheritance has been proposed for a similar disorder in humans,[82] but mode of inheritance is unknown for horses. Developmental and congenital cataracts have been reported in several breeds (American Quarter horse, Arabian, Thoroughbred, Morgan, and Exmoor), and the breed predisposition and bilateral nature together again support a genetic basis but no mutations have been reported. A pedigree analysis of congenital nuclear cataracts in Morgan horses suggested a dominant mode of inheritance that may be sex influenced (females more often and more severely affected), whereas in Exmoor ponies a sex-linked mode of inheritance has been proposed.[83,84] Aniridia and iridial hypoplasia have been documented as dominantly inherited in Belgians and American quarter horses.[85,86] Given the proposed dominant mode of inheritance proposed for congenital cataracts and aniridia, offspring of affected horses should be evaluated carefully. Although at this time it is not possible to genetically test for these disorders, knowing the breeds that are most likely to be affected by these ocular disorders can help to identify additional cases, which inevitably will make genetic discoveries possible.

SUMMARY

Genetic testing can complement ocular examinations and assist with clinical diagnoses. At present, genetic testing to identify horses with ocular disorders is available for CSNB and MCOA. Genetic testing is also useful to identify horses at risk for developing ocular disorders, including ERU and SCC. Screening horses for genetic mutations can help inform management decisions for an earlier diagnosis and better prognosis. Genetic testing can also identify horses that have a higher chance of producing offspring with ocular anomalies. With continued advances in knowledge of the equine genome, a better understanding of the biochemical pathways that lead to ocular disorders should be achieved. In some cases, this could lead to more effective treatments. With the help of clinicians identifying and contributing affected cases for genetic investigations, genetic testing for additional ocular disorders should be available in the future.

REFERENCES

1. Wade CM, Giulotto E, Sigurdsson S, et al. Genome sequence, comparative analysis, and population genetics of the domestic horse. Science 2009;326(5954): 865–7.
2. Bellone RR, Holl H, Setaluri V, et al. Evidence for a retroviral insertion in TRPM1 as the cause of congenital stationary night blindness and leopard complex spotting in the horse. PLoS One 2013;8:e78280.
3. Fritz KL, Kaese HJ, Valberg SJ, et al. Genetic risk factors for insidious equine recurrent uveitis in Appaloosa horses. Anim Genet 2014;45:392–9.
4. Brunberg E, Andersson L, Cothran G, et al. A missense mutation in PMEL17 is associated with the silver coat color in the horse. BMC Genet 2006;7:46.
5. Bellone RR, Liu J, Petersen JL, et al. A missense mutation in damage-specific DNA binding protein 2 is a genetic risk factor for limbal squamous cell carcinoma in horses. Int J Cancer 2017;141:342–53.
6. Sandmeyer LS, Grahn BH, Breaux CB. Diagnostic ophthalmology. Congenital stationary night blindness (CSNB). Can Vet J 2006;47:1131–3.
7. Witzel DA, Joyce JR, Smith EL. Electroretinography of congenital night blindness in an Appaloosa filly. J Equine Med Surg 1977;1:226–9.
8. Witzel DA, Riis RC, Rebhun WC, et al. Night blindness in Appaloosa - sibling occurrence. J Equine Med Surg 1977;1:383–6.

9. Witzel DA, Smith EL, Wilson RD, et al. Congenital stationary night blindness: an animal model. Invest Ophthalmol Vis Sci 1978;17:788–95.
10. Rebhun WC, Loew ER, Riis RC, et al. Clinical manifestations of night blindness in the Appaloosa horse. Compend Contin Educ Pract Vet 1984;6:S103–6.
11. Sandmeyer LS, Breaux CB, Archer S, et al. Clinical and electroretinographic characteristics of congenital stationary night blindness in the Appaloosa and the association with the leopard complex. Vet Ophthalmol 2007;10:368–75.
12. Sandmeyer LS, Bellone RR, Archer S, et al. Congenital stationary night blindness is associated with the leopard complex in the miniature horse. Vet Ophthalmol 2012;15:18–22.
13. Nunnery C, Pickett JP, Zimmerman KL. Congenital stationary night blindness in a thoroughbred and a Paso Fino. Vet Ophthalmol 2005;8:415–9.
14. de Linde Henriksen M, Blaabjerg K, Baptiste KE, et al. Congenital stationary night blindness (CSNB) in the Danish Knabstrupper horse. Vet Ophthalmol 2007;10:326.
15. Bellone RR, Brooks SA, Sandmeyer L, et al. Differential gene expression of TRPM1, the potential cause of congenital stationary night blindness and coat spotting patterns (LP) in the Appaloosa horse (*Equus caballus*). Genetics 2008;179:1861–70.
16. Bellone RR, Forsyth G, Leeb T, et al. Fine-mapping and mutation analysis of TRPM1: a candidate gene for leopard complex (LP) spotting and congenital stationary night blindness in horses. Brief Funct Genomics 2010;9:193–207.
17. Zeitz C, Robson AG, Audo I. Congenital stationary night blindness: an analysis and update of genotype-phenotype correlations and pathogenic mechanisms. Prog Retin Eye Res 2015;45:58–110.
18. Morgans CW, Brown RL, Duvoisin RM. TRPM1: the endpoint of the mGluR6 signal transduction cascade in retinal ON-bipolar cells. Bioessays 2010;32:609–14.
19. Morgans CW, Zhang J, Jeffrey BG, et al. TRPM1 is required for the depolarizing light response in retinal ON-bipolar cells. Proc Natl Acad Sci U S A 2009;106:19174–8.
20. Dwyer AE, Crockett RS, Kalsow CM. Association of leptospiral seroreactivity and breed with uveitis and blindness in horses: 372 cases (1986-1993). J Am Vet Med Assoc 1995;207:1327–31.
21. Gerding JC, Gilger BC. Prognosis and impact of equine recurrent uveitis. Equine Vet J 2016;48:290–8.
22. Sandmeyer LS, Bauer BS, Feng CX, et al. Equine recurrent uveitis in western Canadian prairie provinces: a retrospective study (2002-2015). Can Vet J 2017;58:717–22.
23. Gilger BC. Equine recurrent uveitis: the viewpoint from the USA. Equine Vet J Suppl 2010;(37):57–61.
24. Kulbrock M, von Borstel M, Rohn K, et al. Occurrence and severity of equine recurrent uveitis in warmblood horses–a comparative study. Pferdeheilkunde 2013;29:27–36.
25. Deeg CA, Kaspers B, Gerhards H, et al. Immune responses to retinal autoantigens and peptides in equine recurrent uveitis. Invest Ophthalmol Vis Sci 2001;42:393–8.
26. Davidson MG, Nasisse MP, Roberts SM. Immunodiagnosis of leptospiral uveitis in two horses. Equine Vet J 1987;19:155–7.
27. Brem S, Gerhards H, Wollanke B, et al. Demonstration of intraocular leptospira in 4 horses suffering from equine recurrent uveitis (ERU). Berl Munch Tierarztl Wochenschr 1998;111:415–7 [in German].

28. Brem S, Gerhards H, Wollanke B, et al. 35 leptospira isolated from the vitreous body of 32 horses with recurrent uveitis (ERU). Berl Munch Tierarztl Wochenschr 1999;112:390–3 [in German].
29. Wollanke B, Rohrbach BW, Gerhards H. Serum and vitreous humor antibody titers in and isolation of *Leptospira interrogans* from horses with recurrent uveitis. J Am Vet Med Assoc 2001;219:795–800.
30. Brandes K, Wollanke B, Niedermaier G, et al. Recurrent uveitis in horses: vitreal examinations with ultrastructural detection of leptospires. J Vet Med A Physiol Pathol Clin Med 2007;54:270–5.
31. Pearce JW, Galle LE, Kleiboeker SB, et al. Detection of *Leptospira interrogans* DNA and antigen in fixed equine eyes affected with end-stage equine recurrent uveitis. J Vet Diagn Invest 2007;19:686–90.
32. Witkowski L, Cywinska A, Paschalis-Trela K, et al. Multiple etiologies of equine recurrent uveitis–a natural model for human autoimmune uveitis: a brief review. Comp Immunol Microbiol Infect Dis 2016;44:14–20.
33. Gilger BC, Salmon JH, Yi NY, et al. Role of bacteria in the pathogenesis of recurrent uveitis in horses from the southeastern United States. Am J Vet Res 2008;69: 1329–35.
34. Kulbrock M, Lehner S, Metzger J, et al. A genome-wide association study identifies risk loci to equine recurrent uveitis in German warmblood horses. PLoS One 2013;8:e71619.
35. Feltkamp TE. HLA and uveitis. Int Ophthalmol 1990;14:327–33.
36. Zamecki KJ, Jabs DA. HLA typing in uveitis: use and misuse. Am J Ophthalmol 2010;149:189–93.e2.
37. Deeg CA, Marti E, Gaillard C, et al. Equine recurrent uveitis is strongly associated with the MHC class I haplotype ELA-A9. Equine Vet J 2004;36:73–5.
38. Dwyer AE, Kalsow CM. Visual prognosis in horses with uveitis. Proceedings of the American Society of Veterinary Ophthalmology Annual Meeting. Chicago (IL), March 14, 1998.
39. Ewart SL, Ramsey DT, Xu J, et al. The horse homolog of congenital aniridia conforms to codominant inheritance. J Hered 2000;91:93–8.
40. Ramsey DT, Ewart SL, Render JA, et al. Congenital ocular abnormalities of Rocky Mountain horses. Vet Ophthalmol 1999;2:47–59.
41. Grahn BH, Pinard C, Archer S, et al. Congenital ocular anomalies in purebred and crossbred Rocky and Kentucky Mountain horses in Canada. Can Vet J 2008;49: 675–81.
42. Andersson LS, Axelsson J, Dubielzig RR, et al. Multiple congenital ocular anomalies in Icelandic horses. BMC Vet Res 2011;7:21.
43. Kaps S, Richter M, Philipp M, et al. Primary invasive ocular squamous cell carcinoma in a horse. Vet Ophthalmol 2005;8:193–7.
44. Komaromy AM, Rowlan JS, La Croix NC, et al. Equine multiple congenital ocular anomalies (MCOA) syndrome in PMEL17 (silver) mutant ponies: five cases. Vet Ophthalmol 2011;14:313–20.
45. Plummer CE, Ramsey DT. A survey of ocular abnormalities in miniature horses. Vet Ophthalmol 2011;14:239–43.
46. Segard EM, Depecker MC, Lang J, et al. Ultrasonographic features of PMEL17 (Silver) mutant gene-associated multiple congenital ocular anomalies (MCOA) in Comtois and Rocky Mountain horses. Vet Ophthalmol 2013;16:429–35.
47. Ramsey DT, Hauptman JG, Petersen-Jones SM. Corneal thickness, intraocular pressure, and optical corneal diameter in Rocky Mountain horses with cornea globosa or clinically normal corneas. Am J Vet Res 1999;60:1317–21.

48. Andersson LS, Lyberg K, Cothran G, et al. Targeted analysis of four breeds narrows equine multiple congenital ocular anomalies locus to 208 kilobases. Mamm Genome 2011;22:353–60.

49. Andersson LS, Wilbe M, Viluma A, et al. Equine multiple congenital ocular anomalies and silver coat colour result from the pleiotropic effects of mutant PMEL. PLoS One 2013;8:e75639.

50. Berson JF, Harper DC, Tenza D, et al. Pmel17 initiates premelanosome morphogenesis within multivesicular bodies. Mol Biol Cell 2001;12:3451–64.

51. Theos AC, Berson JF, Theos SC, et al. Dual loss of ER export and endocytic signals with altered melanosome morphology in the silver mutation of Pmel17. Mol Biol Cell 2006;17:3598–612.

52. Hellstrom AR, Watt B, Fard SS, et al. Inactivation of Pmel alters melanosome shape but has only a subtle effect on visible pigmentation. PLoS Genet 2011;7: e1002285.

53. Gelatt KN, Powell NG, Huston K. Inheritance of microphthalmia with coloboma in the Australian shepherd dog. Am J Vet Res 1981;42:1686–90.

54. Schonthaler HB, Lampert JM, von Lintig J, et al. A mutation in the silver gene leads to defects in melanosome biogenesis and alterations in the visual system in the zebrafish mutant fading vision. Dev Biol 2005;284:421–36.

55. Johansson MK, Jaderkvist Fegraeus K, Lindgren G, et al. The refractive state of the eye in Icelandic horses with the Silver mutation. BMC Vet Res 2017;13:153.

56. Strafuss AC. Squamous cell carcinoma in horses. J Am Vet Med Assoc 1976;168: 61–2.

57. Dugan S, Curtis C, Roberts S, et al. Epidemiologic study of ocular/adnexal squamous cell carcinoma in horses. J Am Vet Med Assoc 1991;198:251–6.

58. Pazzi KA, Kraegel SA, Griffey SM, et al. Analysis of the equine tumor suppressor gene p53 in the normal horse and in eight cutaneous squamous cell carcinomas. Cancer Lett 1996;107:125–30.

59. Newkirk KM, Hendrix DV, Anis EA, et al. Detection of papillomavirus in equine periocular and penile squamous cell carcinoma. J Vet Diagn Invest 2014;26:131–5.

60. Plummer CE, Smith S, Andrew SE, et al. Combined keratectomy, strontium-90 irradiation and permanent bulbar conjunctival grafts for corneolimbal squamous cell carcinomas in horses (1990–2002): 38 horses. Vet Ophthalmol 2007;10:37–42.

61. Bosch G, Klein WR. Superficial keratectomy and cryosurgery as therapy for limbal neoplasms in 13 horses. Vet Ophthalmol 2005;8:241–6.

62. Lassaline M, Cranford TL, Latimer CA, et al. Limbal squamous cell carcinoma in Haflinger horses. Vet Ophthalmol 2015;18:404–8.

63. Mosunic CB, Moore PA, Carmicheal KP, et al. Effects of treatment with and without adjuvant radiation therapy on recurrence of ocular and adnexal squamous cell carcinoma in horses: 157 cases (1985-2002). J Am Vet Med Assoc 2004;225:1733–8.

64. Michau TM, Davidson MG, Gilger BC. Carbon dioxide laser photoablation adjunctive therapy following superficial lamellar keratectomy and bulbar conjunctivectomy for the treatment of corneolimbal squamous cell carcinoma in horses: a review of 24 cases. Vet Ophthalmol 2012;15:245–53.

65. Marklund L, Moller MJ, Sandberg K, et al. A missense mutation in the gene for melanocyte-stimulating hormone receptor (MC1R) is associated with the chestnut coat color in horses. Mamm Genome 1996;7:895–9.

66. Robles-Espinoza CD, Roberts ND, Chen S, et al. Germline MC1R status influences somatic mutation burden in melanoma. Nat Commun 2016;7:12064.

67. Rosengren Pielberg G, Golovko A, Sundström E, et al. A cis-acting regulatory mutation causes premature hair graying and susceptibility to melanoma in the horse. Nat Genet 2008;40:1004–9.
68. Rudolph JA, Spier SJ, Byrns G, et al. Periodic paralysis in quarter horses: a sodium channel mutation disseminated by selective breeding. Nat Genet 1992;2:144–7.
69. Cullen CL, Webb AA. Ocular manifestations of systemic disease. Part 3: the horse. In: Gelatt KN, Gilger BC, Kern TJ, editors. Veterinary ophthalmology. 5th edition. Ames (IA): John Wiley & Sons, Inc; 2013. p. 2037–70.
70. Tryon RC, White SD, Bannasch DL. Homozygosity mapping approach identifies a missense mutation in equine cyclophilin B (PPIB) associated with HERDA in the American quarter horse. Genomics 2007;90:93–102.
71. Mochal CA, Miller WW, Cooley AJ, et al. Ocular findings in quarter horses with hereditary equine regional dermal asthenia. J Am Vet Med Assoc 2010;237:304–10.
72. Kohn CW, Johnson GC, Garry F, et al. Mechanobullous disease in two Belgian foals. Equine Vet J 1989;21:297–301.
73. Milenkovic D, Chaffaux S, Taourit S, et al. A mutation in the LAMC2 gene causes the Herlitz junctional epidermolysis bullosa (H-JEB) in two French draft horse breeds. Genet Sel Evol 2003;35:249–56.
74. Graves KT, Henney PJ, Ennis RB. Partial deletion of the LAMA3 gene is responsible for hereditary junctional epidermolysis bullosa in the American saddlebred horse. Anim Genet 2009;40:35–41.
75. Towers RE, Murgiano L, Millar DS, et al. A nonsense mutation in the IKBKG gene in mares with incontinentia pigmenti. PLoS One 2013;8:e81625.
76. Finno CJ, Estell KE, Katzman S, et al. Blood and cerebrospinal fluid alpha-tocopherol and selenium concentrations in neonatal foals with neuroaxonal dystrophy. J Vet Intern Med 2015;29:1667–75.
77. Finno CJ, Aleman M, Ofri R, et al. Electrophysiological studies in American quarter horses with neuroaxonal dystrophy. Vet Ophthalmol 2012;15(Suppl 2):3–7.
78. Finno CJ, Kaese HJ, Miller AD, et al. Pigment retinopathy in warmblood horses with equine degenerative myeloencephalopathy and equine motor neuron disease. Vet Ophthalmol 2017;20:304–9.
79. Boerma S, Back W, Sloet van Oldruitenborgh-Oossterbaan MM. The Friesian horse breed: a clinical challenge to the equine veterinarian? Equine Vet Educ 2012;24: 66–71.
80. Lassaline-Utter M, Gemensky-Metzler AJ, Scherrer NM, et al. Corneal dystrophy in Friesian horses may represent a variant of pellucid marginal degeneration. Vet Ophthalmol 2014;17:186–94.
81. Hermans H, Ensink JM. Treatment and long-term follow-up of distichiasis, with special reference to the Friesian horse: a case series. Equine Vet J 2014;46: 458–62.
82. Samlaska CP. Congenital lymphedema and distichiasis. Pediatr Dermatol 2002; 19:139–41.
83. Beech J, Irby N. Inherited nuclear cataracts in the Morgan horse. J Hered 1985; 76:371–2.
84. Pinard CL, Basrur PK. Ocular anomalies in a herd of Exmoor ponies in Canada. Vet Ophthalmol 2011;14:100–8.
85. Eriksson K. Hereditary aniridia with secondary cataract in horses. Nord Vet Med 1955;7:773–93.
86. Joyce JR, Martin JE, Storts RW, et al. Iridial hypoplasia (aniridia) accompanied by limbic dermoids and cataracts in a group of related quarterhorses. Equine Vet J Suppl 1990;(10):26–8.

Moving?

Make sure your subscription moves with you!

To notify us of your new address, find your **Clinics Account Number** (located on your mailing label above your name), and contact customer service at:

Email: journalscustomerservice-usa@elsevier.com

800-654-2452 (subscribers in the U.S. & Canada)
314-447-8871 (subscribers outside of the U.S. & Canada)

Fax number: 314-447-8029

**Elsevier Health Sciences Division
Subscription Customer Service
3251 Riverport Lane
Maryland Heights, MO 63043**

*To ensure uninterrupted delivery of your subscription, please notify us at least 4 weeks in advance of move.

Printed and bound by CPI Group (UK) Ltd, Croydon, CR0 4YY

03/10/2024

01040395-0002